Ankylosing Spondylitis

Diagnosis
and
Management

Ankylosing Spondylitis

Diagnosis
and
Management

Edited by

Barend J. van Royen
Ben A. C. Dijkmans

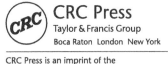

CRC Press
Taylor & Francis Group
Boca Raton London New York

CRC Press is an imprint of the
Taylor & Francis Group, an **informa** business

A TAYLOR & FRANCIS BOOK

First published in 2006 by Taylor & Francis Group

Published 2019 by CRC Press
Taylor & Francis Group
6000 Broken Sound Parkway NW, Suite 300
Boca Raton, FL 33487-2742

© 2006 by Taylor & Francis Group, LLC
CRC Press is an imprint of Taylor & Francis Group, an Informa business

First issued in paperback 2019

No claim to original U.S. Government works

ISBN 13: 978-0-367-45387-9 (pbk)
ISBN 13: 978-0-8247-2751-2 (hbk)

Library of Congress Cataloging-in-Publication Data

Catalog record is available from the Library of Congress

Visit the Taylor & Francis Web site at
http://www.taylorandfrancis.com

and the CRC Press Web site at
http://www.crcpress.com

Preface

Ankylosing spondylitis is a chronic inflammatory disease that primarily affects the spine and sacroiliac joints, causing pain, stiffness, and a progressive thoracolumbar kyphotic deformity. In about one-third of the patients, peripheral joints are also affected. The aim of treatment is reduction of pain and stiffness, and to prevent a thoracolumbar kyphotic deformity or at least to minimize progression. Current conservative therapy consists of exercise programs and medical treatment, including nonsteroidal anti-inflammatory drugs and disease modifying anti-rheumatic drugs. Recently, biologicals (anti-tumor necrosis factor-α drugs) proved to be very effective in the treatment of ankylosing spondylitis. Most patients can be treated successfully with these conservative treatment modalities. A small group of patients, however, do develop a severe thoracolumbar or cervical kyphotic deformity. In these patients, corrective osteotomy of the spine may be considered. These osteotomies proved to be advantageous for numerous patients. However, occasional poor results and complications have diminished their acceptance by rheumatologists and orthopedic surgeons. This is not surprising, because there are still many unsolved questions concerning pre- and postoperative assessment of the deformity, and surgical procedures.

This book is designed to carry basic, biomechanical, and clinical essentials of ankylosing spondylitis and related rheumatological and orthopedic issues on applied research, medical, and surgical treatment. Emphasis is laid on difficulties with making a diagnosis (still mean eight years) and therapeutic advances. Potential readers include rheumatologists, orthopedic surgeons, orthopedic and rheumatological residents, orthopedic and rheumatological researchers, fellows, and graduate students. This is the first inclusive and interdisciplinary organized reference book on basic science and relevance to medical and surgical treatment of ankylosing spondylitis, a topic that has not been covered in any existing books.

Barend J. van Royen, M.D.
Ben A. C. Dijkmans, M.D.
Amsterdam, The Netherlands

Contents

PART V: ACUTE SPINAL INJURIES IN ANKYLOSING SPONDYLITIS

Contributors

Francisco J. Aceves-Avila Department of Rheumatology, Centro Médico Nacional de Occidente, IMSS, Guadalajara, Mexico

Antonio Barrera-Cruz Department of Rheumatology, Centro Médico Nacional de Occidente, IMSS, Guadalajara, Mexico

Sigurd H. Berven Department of Orthopaedic Surgery, University of California, San Francisco, California, U.S.A.

Heinrich Boehm Department of Orthopaedics, Spinal Surgery and Paraplegiology, Zentralklinik Bad Berka, Bad Berka, Germany

Sandra D. M. Bot Institute for Research in Extramural Medicine, VU University Medical Center, Amsterdam, The Netherlands

David S. Bradford Department of Orthopaedic Surgery, University of California, San Francisco, California, U.S.A.

Juergen Braun Rheumazentrum Ruhrgebiet, Herne and Ruhr-University, Bochum, Germany

Matthew A. Brown The Botnar Research Centre, Nuffield Orthopaedic Centre, Headington, Oxford, U.K.

Margo Caspers BGZ Wegvervoer, Gouda, The Netherlands

Arthur de Gast Department of Orthopaedic Surgery, VU University Medical Center, Amsterdam, The Netherlands

Marinus de Kleuver Institute for Spine Surgery and Applied Research, Sint Maartenskliniek, Nijmegen, The Netherlands

Jaap J. de Lange Department of Anesthesiology, VU University Medical Center, Amsterdam, The Netherlands

Kurt de Vlam   Department of Rheumatology, University Hospital K.U.Leuven, Leuven, Belgium

Jan Dequeker   Department of Rheumatology, University Hospital K.U.Leuven, Leuven, Belgium

Maxime Dougados   Department of Rheumatology, Cochin Hospital, AP-HP, René Descartes University, Paris, Cedex, France

Hesham El Saghir   Department of Orthopaedics, Spinal Surgery and Paraplegiology, Zentralklinik Bad Berka, Bad Berka, Germany

Paul Emery   Academic Unit of Musculoskeletal Disease, Chapel Allerton Hospital, Leeds, U.K.

Aaron M. From   Department of Neurosurgery, University Hospitals, Iowa City, Iowa, U.S.A.

Sohrab Gollogly   Department of Orthopaedic Surgery, Centre Des Massues, Lyon, France

Jürgen Harms   Department of Spinal Surgery, Klinikum Karlsbad-Langensteinbach, Karlsbad, Germany

David M. Hasan   Department of Neurosurgery, University Hospitals, Iowa City, Iowa, U.S.A.

Patrick W. Hitchon   Department of Neurosurgery, University Hospitals, Iowa City, Iowa, U.S.A.

Muhammad Asim Khan   Division of Rheumatology, Department of Medicine, MetroHealth Medical Center, Case Western Reserve University, Cleveland, Ohio, U.S.A.

Idsart Kingma   Department of Human Movement Sciences, VU University Amsterdam, Amsterdam, The Netherlands

Miguel A. Macias-Islas   Department of Neurology, Centro Médico Nacional de Occidente, IMSS, Guadalajara, Mexico

Jean Francis Maillefert   University of Burgundy and Department of Rheumatology, Dijon University Hospital, Hôpital Général, Dijon, France

Dennis McGonagle   Academic Unit of Musculoskeletal Disease, Chapel Allerton Hospital, Leeds, U.K.

Corinne Miceli-Richard   Department of Rheumatology, Cochin Hospital, AP-HP, René Descartes University, Paris, Cedex, France

John Minnich   Department of Orthopaedics, Rothman Institute, Philadelphia, Pennsylvania, U.S.A.

Viktor Moser   Department of Spinal Surgery, Klinikum Karlsbad-Langensteinbach, Karlsbad, Germany

Javad Parvizi   Department of Orthopaedics, Rothman Institute, Philadelphia, Pennsylvania, U.S.A.

Cesar Ramos-Remus   Department of Rheumatology, Centro Médico Nacional de Occidente, IMSS, Guadalajara, Mexico

Pierre Roussouly   Department of Orthopaedic Surgery, Centre Des Massues, Lyon, France

Christian Roux   Department of Rheumatology, René Descartes University and Institut de Rhumatologie, Cochin Hospital, Paris, France

Michael Ruf   Department of Spinal Surgery, Klinikum Karlsbad-Langensteinbach, Karlsbad, Germany

Frederic Sailhan   Department of Orthopaedic Surgery, Centre Des Massues, Lyon, France

Joachim Sieper   Department of Medicine and Rheumatology, University Medicine Charité, Freie Universität Berlin, Universitatsklinikum Benjamin Franklin, Berlin, Germany

Theo H. Smit   Department of Physics and Medical Technology, VU University Medical Center, Amsterdam, The Netherlands

David H. Sochart   The Manchester Arthroplasty Unit, North Manchester General Hospital, Crumpsall, Manchester, U.K.

Ai Lyn Tan   Academic Unit of Musculoskeletal Disease, Chapel Allerton Hospital, Leeds, U.K.

Andrew E. Timms   The Botnar Research Centre, Nuffield Orthopaedic Centre, Headington, Oxford, U.K.

Vincent C. Traynelis   Department of Neurosurgery, University Hospitals, Iowa City, Iowa, U.S.A.

Désirée van der Heijde   Division of Rheumatology, Department of Internal Medicine, University Maastricht, Maastricht, The Netherlands

Irene E. van der Horst-Bruinsma   Department of Rheumatology, VU University Medical Center, Amsterdam, The Netherlands

Sjef van der Linden   Division of Rheumatology, Department of Internal Medicine, University Maastricht, Maastricht, The Netherlands

Astrid van Tubergen   Division of Rheumatology, Department of Medicine, University Maastricht, Maastricht, The Netherlands

Debby Vosse   Division of Rheumatology, Department of Internal Medicine, University Maastricht, Maastricht, The Netherlands

Richard Wakefield   Academic Unit of Musculoskeletal Disease, Chapel Allerton Hospital, Leeds, U.K.

B. Paul Wordsworth   The Botnar Research Centre, Nuffield Orthopaedic Centre, Headington, Oxford, U.K.

Wouter W. A. Zuurmond   Department of Anesthesiology, VU University Medical Center, Amsterdam, The Netherlands

1

The History of Ankylosing Spondylitis

Jan Dequeker and Kurt de Vlam
Department of Rheumatology, University Hospital K.U.Leuven, Leuven, Belgium

INTRODUCTION

The antiquity of ankylosing spondylitis (AS) is controversial because early descriptions of ancient remains did not clearly differentiate between ankylosing skeletal diseases affecting the axial and peripheral joints (1).

It is now well recognized that on the one hand there are a number of chronic inflammatory rheumatic diseases, which may result in ankylosis of multiple spine and peripheral joints, but clinically they can be differentiated in separate entities. They are usually grouped under the name seronegative spondylarthropathies. Most of these entities affect young adults and are strongly associated with a genetic predisposition identifiable by the antigen HLA-B27. In this group sacroiliac joints and spinal joints are affected.

On the other hand, ankylosis of the spine can also be the result of noninflammatory chronic skeletal disorders as primary and secondary hyperostosis vertebralis. Primary hyperostosis is seen mainly in elderly cases and is considered to be a degenerative-metabolic disorder. In this group the sacroiliac joints are not fused. Secondary hyperostosis can be due to fluor- or vitamin A intoxication or to chronic use of retinoids. Ankylosis of a joint can be the result of direct local infection (e.g., toe), trauma, or immobilization. The characteristic of ankylosis due to infection, trauma, or immobilization is that in the majority of these cases only one joint will be involved.

The study of the history of AS has some limitations, which should be recognized. In paleopathology (study of fossil remains), the only evidence of AS consists of alterations in skeletal remains, as fusion of joints, ligamentous calcifications, and erosions. The latter erosions, compared to complete fusion, can be biased and must be differentiated from other inflammatory diseases such as calcium pyrophosphate dihydrate (CPPD) deposition disease or rheumatoid arthritis (RA). Moreover, after a hundred or even a thousand million years, corrosion and chemical interactions with soil may create artifacts, which have to be interpreted carefully in order to eliminate any bias.

In historical images (paintings, drawings, and etches), general clinical appearance can give additional information for the historian. In longstanding AS, the entire spine is stiff, the lumbar lordosis is flattened, and there is a smoothly curved thoracic kyphosis. In Pott's disease (tuberculosis of the spine), there is an angular curve.

SKELETAL PALEOPATHOLOGY

The commonly observed osseous alterations of spondylosis deformans and AS have been described in both humans and animals, dating back to prehistoric times. Rogers et al. (1) reviewed the available literature and concluded that many paleopathological specimens, previously reported as AS, are examples of diffuse idiopathic skeletal hyperostosis (DISH) or other seronegative spondylarthropathies. So the antiquity and paleopathology of AS need reappraisal.

The differential diagnosis of ankylosis of the axial skeleton, spine and pelvis in skeletal remains should include AS, DISH, fluorosis, hypervitamin A, and inflammatory spondylarthropathies associated with related rheumatic disorders as juvenile onset chronic arthritis, reactive arthritis, and psoriatic arthritis.

Paleopathology in Animals

Rotschild et al. (2) identified erosive arthritis of the spondylarthropathy variety in the Paleocene of North America 40 million years ago. In 7 out of 37 fossils of the Eocene examined (19%), sacroiliac fusion was noted.

Rotschild and Wood (3) assessed for evidence of spondylarthropathy in 1699 nonhuman Old World primates from 10 different collections. Syndesmophytes and sacroiliac erosions or fusion was present in 2.1% of Old World primates, in 3.2% of lesser apes, and in 6.7% of the great apes (but none of the orangutans was affected).

A detailed description of the pathologic findings of a case of spontaneous AS in an 18.5-year-old Rhesus monkey, compared with another monkey, diagnosed postmortem as hyperostotic spondylosis, is given by Sokoloff et al. (4).

In a radiological study of 48 saber-toothed cat vertebral specimens, Bjorkengren et al. (5) found changes typical of AS in 11 specimens and changes resembling those of DISH in nine specimens. The saber-toothed cat species existed during most of the Pleistocene epoch and became extinct approximately 12,000 years ago. This carnivore was of comparable size but of much heavier build compared to the modern day African lion.

The existence of disease of the spine has been described in two crocodiles, one from Egypt and one from Cuba, dating from the Miocene and Pliocene periods, respectively (6–8). Whether these lesions are developmental or pathological, or whether they have any relation to human AS is impossible to judge.

It is well known that in many domestic animals, including dogs, cats, sheep, bulls, cows, pigs, and horses, the incidence of osteophytic outgrowths increases with the age of the animal and is thought to be secondary to degenerative changes in the annulus fibrosus of the intervertebral disc. Thus it is not surprising that similar lesions were present in the mummies of the sacred animals in ancient Egypt (6).

Paleopathology in Humans

Short (9), reviewing the paleopathological literature on RA, concluded that AS, with or without peripheral joint involvement, existed with some frequency in the ancient world but not what we see today as RA. A description of a Stone Age skeleton with complete ankylosis of the lumbosacral and sacroiliac joints is indisputable evidence for the existence of AS in ancient remains (10). Findings on Egyptian mummies concerning arthritis and in particular AS have been criticized (1). Most of the cases found in mummies represent more likely hyperostosis vertebralis, also called DISH, which can cause fusion of the upper third of the sacroiliac joints.

Many Egyptian skeletons, ranging from 3000 B.C. to the beginning of the Christian era, were examined by Ruffer and Rietti and others (7,8,11,12). They described "AS" or "spondylitis deformans" in many cases, but the terms are not clearly defined. Sacroiliac changes were often ignored or absent, and the spinal changes described included asymmetrical fusion with "roughness of bones" elsewhere. Nubian skeletons examined by Smith and Wood Jones (13) were also said to show frequent spinal fusion. Salib describes frequent "spondylitis" and spinal "arthritis deformans" in Egyptian material and Shore states that spinal fusion was seen in 7 of 274 vertebral columns from Ancient Egypt, although he concluded that infection was the most likely cause (12,14). Bourke (15) also looked at Egyptian and Nubian material and reported some possible cases of AS. However, only one case, an individual from Hou, is convincing (Fig. 1), and in others the asymmetrical changes with large paravertebral osteophytosis suggest possible DISH or psoriatic arthritis. Zorab (16) was unable to find convincing evidence of AS in Egyptian material and thought that the previous authors had misdiagnosed osteophytosis.

Two examples of peripheral joint disease and cervical spine ankylosis were found in the tomb of the third Dynasty (2700 B.C.). The first bony specimens involved the distal joint of one finger, with bony ankylosis in a flexed position. An accompanying fragment demonstrates two cervical vertebrae firmly joined by anterior and posterior paravertebral calcification (11). The other is an ankylosed knee, with patella fused to the femur. In this subject, definite cervical spondylitis is pictured, with bony bridging (9). Ruffer (12) describes a possible case of AS: a third dynasty (2980–2900 B.C.) Egyptian named Nefermaat. This unfortunate patient has bony ankylosis of his apophyseal joints, along with bone formation in his long ligaments. His spine is a solid block from the fourth cervical vertebra to the coccyx. According to a recent publication by Feldtkeller et al. (17) reviewing the published material about the remains of the pharaohs of ancient Egypt's 18th and 19th dynasty, at least three had AS: Amenhotep (Amenophis) II, Ramses II ("The Great") and his son Mezenptah.

Rogers et al. (1) concluded that there are surprisingly few convincing descriptions of human AS in other paleopathological literature. A possible French case from the Neolithic period was described by Snorrason (18). Morse (19) and Kidd (20) have both examined suspected cases from ancient midwestern skeletons; Zivanovic (21) records a case of medieval Anglo-Saxon origin with probable AS (although he diagnosed RA); and Kramar (22) gave a detailed description of a very convincing case from medieval Geneva. Calvin Wells (23,24) describes many examples of spinal fusion from Anglo-Saxon skeletons; in many of these cases DISH seems the likely diagnosis. It is apparent from examining this literature that most authors, with the notable exception of Kramar (22) and Feldtkeller (17), were not aware of DISH or of other possible causes of spinal fusion such as fluorosis or psoriatic spondylitis. Evaluation of the zygapophyseal joints can be useful for the diagnosis of AS, since ankylosis of the zygapophyseal joints occurs very often prior to ankylosis of the vertebral body in AS (25).

The skeletal remains of a man of the post-classic period (900–1521) of Mesoamerica suggest AS (26). It showed fusion of the vertebral column T8 to L5 due to ankylosis of the apophyseal joints and of the spinal processes. The pelvis was not preserved. Radiographs demonstrated ossification of both supraspinous and interspinous ligaments. This finding suggests that AS was present in Mesoamerica before the arrival of Europeans.

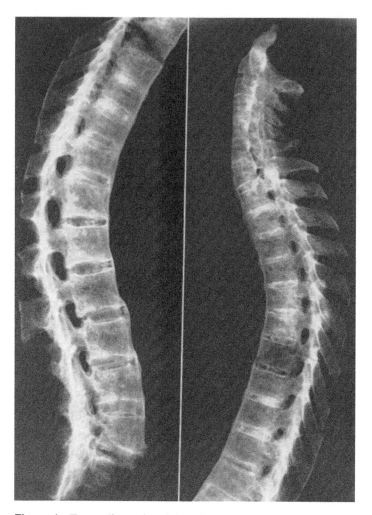

Figure 1   Two radiographs of the spine of an individual from Hou, 12th Dynasty, Museum Cambridge. They show an increased thoracic kyphosis and a decreased lumbar lordosis, and squaring of the vertebral bodies with calcification of the spinal ligaments and apophyseal joints.

Zorab (16), who made an M.D. thesis (London) on AS in 1959, mentions several excellent accounts of AS occurrence in ancient men. It has been found in Swedish skeletons of Neolithic times, in a middle-aged male Jute of the Bronze Age, in Germans of pre-Roman days, and in skeletons from a Viking ship of the 10th century A.D. (27,28).

In 2 cases out of 83 skeletons from a 17th century Hungarian necropolis, advanced radiological features of AS of the spine were observed. The radiological alterations were convincingly differentiated from hyperostosis (29).

An example of bamboo spine was found in a 3500-year-old Neolithic tumulus (Fontenay-le-Marmion near Caen in France) (Fig. 2) (30).

Rothschild and Wood (3), analyzing an extensive search for spondylarthropathy in North American skeletal remains of 16 populations dated from 4700-years ago up to less than 500-years ago, found 35 cases with spondylarthropathies. Spondyloarthropathy was defined as zygapophyseal or sacroiliac joint erosion or fusion, asymmetrical pattern of arthritis, reactive new bone formation, enthesopathy, or peripheral joint fusion. Considering that erosion can be an artifact in skeletal remains, in 6 individuals

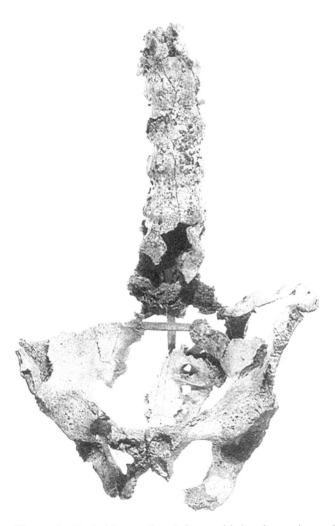

Figure 2 Neolythic tumulus skeleton with bamboo spine and sacroiliac fusion 3500 years ago. Fontenay-le-Marmion.

out of 31, fusion of sacroiliac bones was present. One hundred sixty-five individual skeletons were examined. Six of them had definite sacroiliac fusion (0.3%), and 2.1% had skeletal signs of peripheral or axial arthritis. These prevalence of sacroiliac fusion (0.3%) and 2.1% for peripheral arthritis are in line with what one would expect in modern times.

HISTORY OF AS IN THE LITERATURE

Many physicians in the past have written on AS. Evidence that AS existed thousands of years before Christ has been found in Egyptian and Nubian skeletons. Hippocrates mentioned a disease in which "the vertebrae of the spine, and neck may be affected with pain, and it extends to the os sacrum." Caelius Aurelianus in the fifth century referred to a patient who was afflicted with pain in the nates, moved slowly, and could only bend or stand erect with difficulty (31). The celebrated English physician, Thomas Sydenham, described what he termed "rheumatic lumbago" (32). It is likely from this description that the disease was AS.

The earliest attempts at a pathological account is by Connor (33), who in 1694 to 1695 described a skeleton found in a French churchyard or charnel house in which the vertebrae and ribs "were so straightly and intimately joined, their ligaments perfectly bony, and their articulations so effaced, that they really made but one uniform continuous bone; so that it was as easy to break one of the vertebrae into two, as to disjoint or separate it from the other vertebrae, or the ribs" (Fig. 3). Connor surmised that this individual had been unable to bend and had problems with breathing.

It was not, however, until the latter part of the last century that the disease came to be regarded as a separate entity, and more accurate attempts to understand its pathology were made. In a textbook from 1850, the English surgeon Sir Benjamin

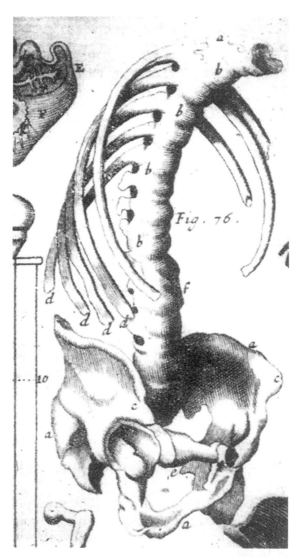

Figure 3   Skeletal findings described by O'Connor in 1694.

Brodie (34) described a 31-year-old man with pronounced stiffness of the spine, recurrent gonitis, and inflammation of the eyes. Fagge (35) described the disease in patients attending Guy's Hospital. It was a few years later that Bechterew in Russia, Strümpell in Germany, and Marie in France reported cases (Fig. 4A–C). Bechterew (36) described an upper dorsal type of case, but one that was complicated by meningeal involvement with degeneration of the spinal cord and in which there was degeneration of the intervertebral discs. Strümpell (37) briefly referred to two cases, which he had seen "of a remarkable and unique disorder leading very gradually and painlessly to a complete ankylosis of the entire spinal column and hip joints." But it was not by any means so detailed an account as that which followed in 1898 by Pierre Marie (38). The latter stressed the involvement of shoulder and hip joint by suggesting the name "spondylose rhizomélique," derived from the Greek words spondylos = vertebra, rhiza = root and melos = extremity. Pierre Marie's paper entitled "La Spondylose Rhizomélique" contains a remarkably accurate description of AS, including such characteristic features as the typical gait, the flattened lumbar spine, the forward craning of the neck, the flexing of the hips and knees, and the Z-shaped posture. From postmortem examinations he was aware of the fusion of the spine, chest, and hips, and commented on the difficulty in breathing and walking that must have resulted from such extensive joint ankylosis. Later on his pupil André Leri (39) perfected the clinical description and added details based on pathologic-anatomical observations.

Until this time no very clear differentiation had been made between this and other forms of spinal arthritis. Indeed, Pierre Marie in his memoirs remarks that the first of the three original cases, which he described while working in Charcot's clinic, suggested the possibility of Paget's disease of bone. In these cases there was complete fixity of the chest, the spine being "fait rigide comme un baton." Marie obtained an autopsy on two cases and then showed that the lesions present in the spine consisted essentially "en une ossification tout particulièrement localisée aux ligament; aux bourrelets et aux menisques articulaires." Connor's (33) account 200 years earlier is perhaps even more descriptive: "a layer of new bone may be seen covering the whole length of dorsal and lumbar spine as if some soft liquid osseous material had been poured over them and this had subsequently hardened."

Leden (40) reviewed at the occasion of the centennial of Bechterew's original report the controversial story, who described first AS, between Bechterew (Russian), Pierre Marie (French), and Strümpell (German). For all those interested in the medical history of AS, a copy of the review in detail of Leden's analysis, "Did Bechterew describe the disease which is named after him?," is added.

In 1892, prior to the works of Marie and Strümpell, Bechterew (36) published a report in the Russian journal Wratch about five cases with remarkable stiffness of the spine accompanied by slight neurological signs. The next year a revised version was published in Germany with the title: "Steifigkeit der Wirbelsäule und ihre Werkrümmerung als besondere Erkrankungsform" (Stiffness and deformity of the spine as a special disease) (36). In this article Bechterew chose to omit two incomplete case histories. Instead he gave an extended description of the remaining three cases. They are regarding two women, 52 and 56 years old, and a 39-year-old male. Of the three, the disease of the 39-year-old male was the most severe. It started 15 years earlier when a heavy bale struck his left shoulder. Since then he suffered from pain, muscular weakness, and a pronounced flexion of the upper spine. When breathing he only used the abdominal muscles. He died a few years later but unfortunately no autopsy was performed.

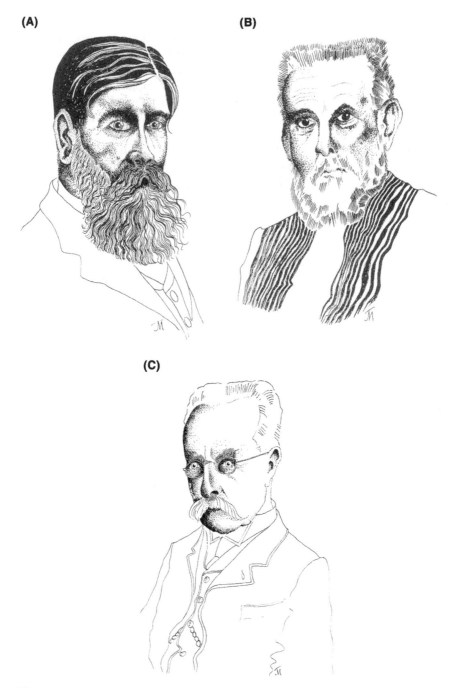

Figure 4 Historical authorities in relation to the description of AS: (**A**) V.M. Bechterew (Russia), (**B**) P. Marie (France), (**C**) A. Strümpell (Germany), reproduced from V. Wright and J. Moll in Seronegative polyarthritis. North Holland Publishing Company, 1976. *Abbreviation*: AS, ankylosing spondylitis.

The two women also had stiffness and flexion deformity of their spines. The younger woman's symptoms also started after a trauma, when she slipped and fell on her back. The older had a hereditary predisposition as several relatives had a similar flexion deformity of the spine. Bechterew was well aware that the diseases of his patients were far from uniform but still he saw several common manifestations. Besides the flexion deformity and immobility of the spine, all had pronounced pain, paresthesia, hyperesthesia, slight pareses, and muscular atrophy. He ended the article with a pathogenetic discussion, and hypothesized that the symptoms may be explained by a diffuse chronic inflammation of the spinal dura and adjacent tissues. In 1897 he gave a detailed description of a new case and two years later he reported a further case (41,42). This patient succumbed from pneumonia and thus an autopsy was possible (42). By microscopy, degenerative lesions were seen in cross-sections of the spinal cord at the thoracic level and dura mater spinalis was chronically inflamed—findings that could explain the pains and the other neurological symptoms and signs in the upper extremities and trunk.

Some years late, when Pierre Marie and Strümpell had published their observations, a discussion was started on priorities and whether the reported disorders were identical. Throughout his life Bechterew claimed that the disorder he had described was different from that of Marie and Strümpell. Bechterew stressed that his disorder was characterized by:

- Greater or slighter stiffness in the whole or parts of the spine,
- Kyphosis of the thoracic spine accompanied by forward movement of the head,
- Signs of paresis and atrophy of the muscles in the neck, trunk, and shoulders, and
- Sensory disturbances of the skin over the back, loins, and upper extremities.

According to Bechterew, the most important differences between his disorder and that of Marie and Strümpell were the following:

- There were no signs of disease of the peripheral joints,
- The prominent changes of the spine were located in the thoracic part,
- Neurological signs were obligatory, and
- Probable pathogenetic factors were heredity, trauma, and ongoing syphilis.

In polemic articles published in 1899 against Marie and Strümpell, Bechterew stressed the earlier facts (42,43). It is also clear that he has seen and treated cases similar to those described by Marie and Strümpell.

As a modern reader of Bechterew's original report (36), it is easy to agree with Bechterew's opinion. His report from 1893 does not concern patients with the disease we today call pelvispondylitis and which was described by Strümpell in 1897 (44), Marie in 1898 (38), and Leri in 1899 (39). In the case, which was autopsied, there is no bony bridging (42). The spine was taken out in extenso and Bechterew stresses that the mobility between the lumbar vertebrae was normal and that the decreased motion in the thoracic part was due to severe disk degeneration. The spinal nerves in the thoracic region had a gray color, which was interpreted as a sign of degeneration.

However, in one of his articles from 1889, Bechterew (43) clearly describes two cases with a disease similar to the cases of Strümpell and Marie. Bechterew disliked the nosological designations by Strümpell (37) and Marie (38) and therefore suggested a new one—"chronische ankylosirende Entzündung der grossen

Gelenke und der Wirbelsäule" (a chronic ankylosing inflammation of the large joints and the spine). The immobility of the spine in this disorder is primary and has a "so-called rheumatic cause," in contrast to the cases he described in 1893, where the immobility is secondary and due to factors like heredity, trauma, and syphilis. Bechterew also seems to have a more open mind for the new nosology, which appeared during the 19th century, while Marie and Leri are more rigid and more influenced by the "old" nosology system, which had its roots in the antique classification partially based on anatomical regions. They tried to treat back disorders as a disease entity and to solve dissimilarities by extended subclassification. Some decades later at least Leri seems to have changed his mind and accepted that Bechterew in his original report described a special disease different from that of Strümpell and Marie. At that time Leri in a monograph refers to Bechterew when describing a special disorder classified as "Cyphose hérédo-traumatique" (45).

The initial question can be answered both yes and no. Yes: Bechterew clearly recognized cases seen in his practice similar to those of Marie and Strümpell—that is, pelvispondylitis, the disorder which now bears his name. No: his primary reports from 1892 and 1893 concern a disorder clearly separated from that reported by Marie and Strümpell. Bechterew himself was well aware of the differences but his contemporaries had difficulty in seeing the distinction. Studies of Bechterew's original reports show that he was in fact correct (46,47). This conclusion merely reveals the extraordinary acuity of Bechterew's powers of clinical observation. Bechterew's report is an early description of patients with a deformity of the spine associated with cervical cord affection. Such cases are uncommon even today.

At present, the evaluation of the zygapophyseal joints, as well as the determination of human leukocyte antigen B27 (HLA-B27), can be helpful in the differentiation of AS and other rheumatic diseases (25).

PALEOPATHOLOGY OF AS IN VISUAL ARTS

Visual arts, especially in combination with historical data, can be an important tool for paleopathological research (48). Works of art of different kinds may serve as a source of evidence of disease and contribute to a better understanding of the natural history of the disease. Diagnostic acumen, however, applied to paintings can be misleading if not tempered with the knowledge of artistic conventions and historical context.

When searching for the paleopathology of AS in pictures, we have encountered five pictures related to this disease.

Figure 5 shows the full-length portraits of a young and an old man in the famous church of de Decani Monastery in Kosovo. The pictures are details of a large fresco "Christ healing the Innocent," made by unknown masters in 1335. The sorrows and vicissitudes of human existence are all to be found on the walls of Decani: the crippled and the sick, the martyrs and the tormentors, the robbers and the sinners, peasants, men working in the fields and in the vineyards, fishermen, stonemasons, and preachers are included in an unending procession.

In the case of Figure 5A, a young man is visible, showing a marked high dorsal kyphosis, forward protrusion of the neck, limited cervical mobility, flexion contracture of the hips and compensatory flexion of the knees, and some muscle wasting of the left lower limb, awkwardly using two axilla crutches, and his visual field seems restricted.

The association of this typical posture, and the sex and age of the case, strongly suggests the possible diagnosis of ankylosing spondylarthropathy with associated coxitis on the left side.

Figure 5B shows an older man with similar spine deformities, in a more accentuated stage (Z-shaped posture). Note the craned neck, high dorsal kyphosis, rounded shoulders, obliterated lumbar lordosis, and wasted buttocks. Because of his clothes, a flattened chest and ballooned abdomen are not visible. His right foot is possibly also involved with ankylosis of the midtarsal joints.

The observation of advanced stage spinal deformities suggests the clinical diagnosis of AS. Furthermore, the fact that the two cases—the younger and the older—are represented in the same fresco, raises the suggestion that the older man may be the father or the uncle of the younger crippled man described, indicating the first illustration of the at present well documented hereditary familial factor linked to the presence of HLA-B27 in typical cases of AS.

As mentioned in the introduction, in elderly cases the differential diagnosis of a spinal stenosis with diffuse idiopathic hyperostosis has to be considered.

(A)   **(B)**

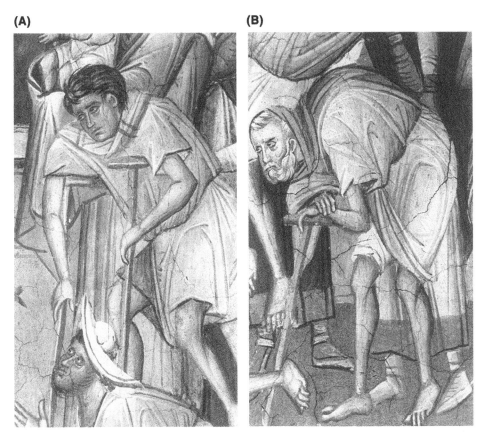

Figure 5 Decani Monastery Frescos, Kosovo (1335), Christ healing the Innocent. (**A**) Young crippled male with advanced spinal deformities, high dorsal kyphosis, forward protrusion of the neck, flexion contracture of the hip and compensatory flexion of the knees. (**B**) Old crippled male with advanced spinal deformities and hip flexion (*Z-shaped posture*), craned neck and rounded shoulders.

Figure 6 shows a copper engraving of Albrecht Dürer (Kupferstichkabinett Basel, 1526) showing Erasmus writing on his desk in a standing position. From Erasmus' letters we know his medical history of fever, pustulotic skin eruptions, backache, renal stones, oligo-polyarthritis, and dysentery. Because of his backache he was writing his books in a standing position. In paintings by Quinten Metsys (1517) and Hans Holbein the Younger (1523), signs of arthritis in the hands have been noted (49). From the information in paintings of two famous artists, letters of Erasmus himself, and the engraving of Dürer, a clinical diagnosis of AS can be considered in association with pustulotic arthro-osteitis synovitis, acne, pustulosis, hyperostosis, and osteitis (SAPHO-syndrome).

Figure 7 shows the title page of Stefaan Blankaart's book "Verhandelingen van het Podagra en Vliegende Jigt" (1684) (Dissertation on Podagra and "flying" Gout). In the middle of the drawing—showing a treatment place—a young male sits with a stiff back, a high dorsal kyphosis, a left knee in extension (ankylosed?), and semi-flexed hips, in a specially designed wheelchair. His unusual position and his age and sex, suggest a possible clinical diagnosis of AS or psoriatic arthropathy, despite the

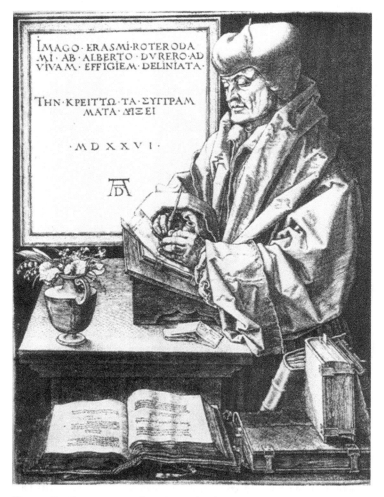

Figure 6 Copper engraving, Portrait of Erasmus of Rotterdam by Albrecht Dürer (1526), Kupferstichkabinett Basel.

title of the dissertation: podagra and gout. Psoriatic arthritis is often misdiagnosed as gout (50). In the past centuries, most rheumatic complaints were classified as gout, without any subdivision. Even the first description of RA by A.J. Landré-Beauvais in Paris (1800) was called "Doit-on admettre une nouvelle espèce de goutte sous la dénomination de goutte asthénique primitive?"

Figure 8 shows Cosimo de Medici by Pontormo Jacopo ca 1520, Galleria degli Uffizi, Florence. The picture shows a rigid position of Cosimo de Medici who, according to his profiled head, is cachectic with muscle atrophy of the face, a dorsal kyphosis, and a strange position of the right index finger. This painting is a posthumous representation based on previous portraits. The Medici family in Florence is of

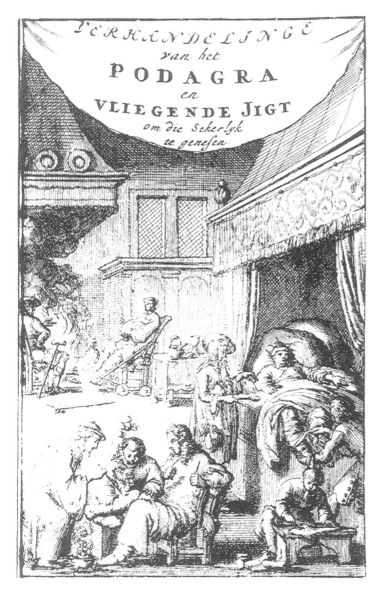

Figure 7　Title page of Stefaan Blankaart's dissertation on podagra and gout (1684). The young man sitting in a wheelchair has an ankylosed back and knee joint.

particular interest for the history of AS. From four members of four generations of de Medici, rulers of Florence, it is known that they had a medical history, clinical and postmortem, of interest for rheumatologists. When the bodies of four generations of Medici's were removed from the family chapel in 1945, Costa and Weber (51) and Pizon (52) studied the skeletons of Cosimo il Vecchio, his son Piero il Gottoso, his grandson Lorenzo il Magnifico, and his great-grandson Giulano. They were known to be sufferers of so-called "gout" characterized by fever, skin alterations, and arthritis of the lower and upper limb joints, starting at a young age and giving trouble for years.

Table 1 and Figures 9–14 summarize the medical history of these four cases in the same family. The fact that in skeletal remains of two of them sacroiliac ankylosis was seen and in all of them ankylosis of the peripheral joints (ankles, fingers), there can be no doubt that this family had a genetic predisposition for spondylarthropathy. The description of a "chronic skin disorder" severe enough to be remembered in

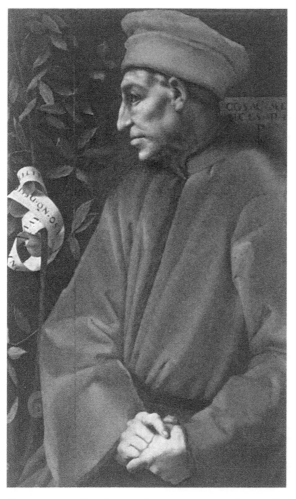

Figure 8 Cosimo il Vecchio, painted ca 1518–1519 by Jacopo di Pontorno, Galleria degli Uffizi, Florence.

Table 1 Summary Medical History of Four Generations of Male Members of the Famous Florentine Medici Family

	Cosimo il Vecchio °1389 †1464 father	Piero il Gottoso °1416 †1469 son	Lorenzo il Magnifico °1449 †1492 grandson	Giuliano, Duca di Nemours °1478 †1516 great-grandson
Age				
Onset	43-arthritis, fever	26-fever 40-joints	18-dermatosis 33-joints, spa therapy	9-fever 33-joints++
Death	75	53	43	38
Joints affected	Feet: ankylosis tarsus Hands: wrist ankylosis, index ankylosis Ankle ankylosis tibia, fibula	Wrist: ankylosis Knee: flexion deformity Ankle: synostosis tibia-fibula-talus, cuneiform	Humerus: enthesitis Feet	Hands: distal phalanx left index missing First phalanx fused IV metacarpal
Spine X-ray findings	Syndesmophytes ++ Apophyseal ankylosis	Loss lumbar lordosis Coxitis, syndesmophytes dorsal		
Sacroiliac joints	?	Fusion sacroiliac joints		
Systemic features	Fever Renal failure	Fever Chronic skin disease Renal stones	Fever Chronic skin disease Renal colics	Skin disease Weight loss

° born.
† died.

historical reports indicates that this spondylarthropathy could be related to psoriatic spondylarthropathy.

MODERN HISTORY OF AS

The modern history of AS has recently been summarized by Sieper et al. (53).

By the mid-1900s, radiographic, epidemiological, and clinical reports disclosed relationships between AS and several other forms of arthritis, including reactive arthritis (Reiter's disease), psoriatic arthritis, and arthropathies associated with inflammatory bowel disease (54–56). As a result, the concept of the spondyloarthropathies was introduced by Moll et al. (56) as a family of interrelated disorders sharing clinical and genetic characteristics distinct from RA. The original group of disorders known as spondyloarthropathies included AS, reactive arthritis (Reiter's syndrome), psoriatic arthritis, juvenile onset spondyloarthropathy (a subgroup

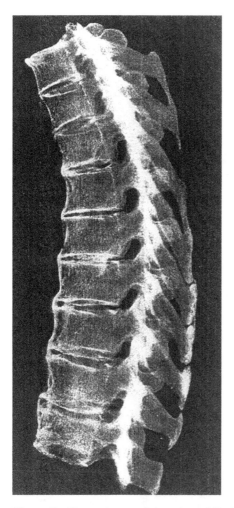

Figure 9   X-ray picture of the spine of Cosimo il Vecchio. Syndesmophytes and calcificated discs. *Source*: From Ref. 51.

(A)   **(B)**

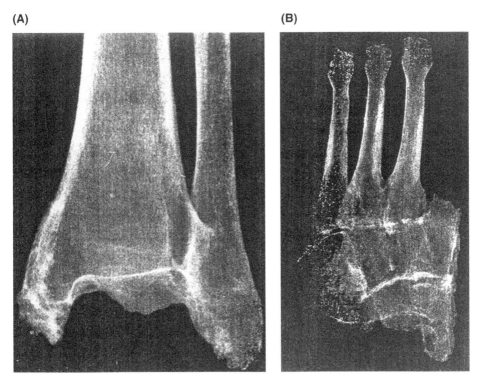

Figure 10   X-ray picture ankle (**A**) and forefeet (**B**) Cosimo il Vecchio. Ankylosis tibia, fibula and tarsus bones. *Source*: From Ref. 51.

of juvenile chronic arthritis), and arthritis associated with inflammatory bowel disease (56–58). In 1991, the European Spondyloarthropathy Study Group (ESSG) modified this disease grouping to accommodate undifferentiated forms of spondyloarthropathy (59).

Among the many landmarks in the history of AS and its relationship to the other spondyloarthropathies, perhaps the most important were the revelations of an infectious etiology and a genetic predisposition to AS. With respect to the latter, medical historians consider the discovery of the human leukocyte antigens in the 1940s to 1950s and the subsequent characterization of the human major histocompatibility complex as the most important contribution to the understanding of spondyloarthropathies. An infectious etiology was originally proposed based on the correlation between AS and reactive arthritis, perhaps the best understood of the spondyloarthropathies. In 1916, Reiter's syndrome was described by Hans Reiter as non-gonococcal urethritis, peripheral arthritis, and conjunctivitis following dysentery (60). Subsequent documentation of the syndrome following dysentery, *Shigella flexneri* infection, and venereally acquired genito-urinary infections established the relationship between Reiter's syndrome and preceding gastrointestinal or genito-urinary infection (61,62). The term "reactive arthritis" was introduced in 1969 (63). The presence of some of the clinical signs of AS (for example, spondylitis and uveitis) in patients with reactive arthritis suggested a correlation between the two diseases. This hypothesis was confirmed in 1973 by the discovery of a high frequency of HLA-B27 in both AS and Reiter's syndrome (64,65). Based upon its clinical and genetic association with reactive arthritis, it suggested a correlation

(A)   (B)

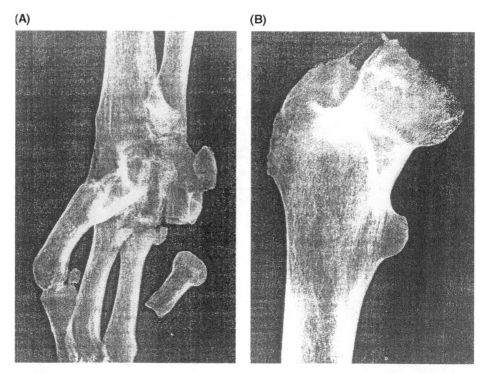

Figure 11 (**A**) X-ray picture wrist of Piero il Gottoso showing carpal bone fusion. (**B**) Proximal femur of Piero il Gottoso showing loss of bone tissue femoral head and enthesopathy greater trochanter. *Source*: From Ref. 51.

(A)   (B)

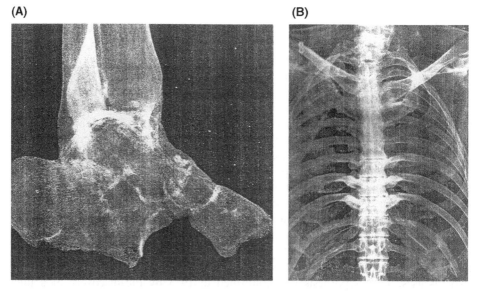

Figure 12 (**A**) X-ray tarsus ankylosis of Piero il Gottoso. (**B**) X-ray dorsolumbar spine with syndesmophytes of Piero il Gottoso. *Source*: From Ref. 51.

(A) (B)

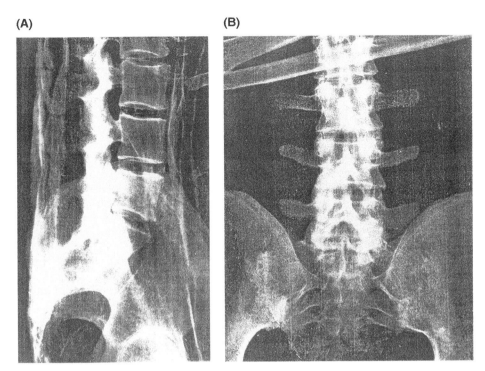

Figure 13 (**A, B**) X-ray lumbar spine and pelvis of Piero il Gottoso showing flattening lumbar lordosis, joint space narrowing hip, and ankylosis sacroiliac joints. *Source*: From Ref. 51.

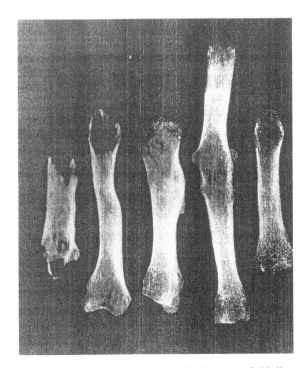

Figure 14 Metacarpal bones of left hand of Giuliano dei Medici, and Duca di Nemour. Note fusion of first phalanx fourth metacarpal. *Source*: From Ref. 51.

between the two diseases. Indeed, enteric infections with *Klebsiella pneumoniae* and *Escherichia coli* have been implicated in the pathogenesis of AS in genetically susceptible hosts (66,67). Furthermore, observation of a close link between inflammatory bowel disease and AS suggested that normal gut bacteria might stimulate the immune system once the mucosal barrier was broken (68).

REFERENCES

1. Rogers J, Watt I, Dieppe P. Palaeopathology of spinal osteophytosis, vertebral ankylosis, ankylosing spondylitis, and vertebral hyperostosis. Ann Rheum Dis 1985; 44:113–130.
2. Rotschild BM, Sebes JI, Rotschild C. Antiquity of arthritis: Spondyloarthropathy identified in Paleocene of North America. Clin Exp Rheumatol 1998; 16:573–575.
3. Rotschild BM, Woods RJ. Character of pre-Columbian North American spondyloarthropathy. J Rheumatol 1992; 19:1229–1235.
4. Sokoloff L, Snell KC, Steward H. Spinal ankylosis in old Rhesus Monkeys. Clin Orthop 1968; 61:285–293.
5. Bjorkengren AG, Sartoris D, Shermis S, Resnick D. Patterns of paravertebral ossification in the prehistoric Saber-Toothed Cat. Am J Roentgenol 1987; 148:779–782.
6. Spencer DG, Sturrock RD, Watson Buchanan W. Ankylosing spondylitis: yesterday and today. Med Hist 1980; 24:60–64.
7. Ruffer MA. In: Moodie RL, ed. Studies in the paleopathology of Egypt. Chicago: University of Chicago Press, 1921:187–201.
8. Moodie RL. Paleopathology: an introduction to the study of ancient evidence of disease. Urbana: University of Illinois Press, 1923.
9. Short Ch L. The antiquity of rheumatoid arthritis. Arthritis Rheum 1974; 17:193–205.
10. Raymond P. Les maladies de nos ancêtres à l'âge de la pierre. Aesculape 1912; 2:121–123.
11. Ruffer MA, Rietti A. On osseous lesions in ancient Egyptians. J Pathol Bacteriol 1912; 16:439–447.
12. Ruffer MA. Arthritis deformans and spondylitis in ancient Egypt. J Pathol Bacteriol 1918; 22:152–159.
13. Smith GE, Wood Jones F. Archaeological survey of Nubia. Report for 1907–1908. Cairo: National Print Department, 1910; 2:273.
14. Shore LR. Some examples of disease of the vertebral column found in skeletons of ancient Egypt. A contribution to paleopathology. Br J Surg 1936; 24:256–271.
15. Bourke JB. A review of paleopathology of arthritic disease. In: Brothwell D, Sandison AT, eds. Diseases in antiquity. Springfield: Thomas, 1967:352–370.
16. Zorab PA. The historical and prehistorical background to ankylosing spondylitis. Proc R Soc Med 1961; 54:23–28.
17. Feldtkeller E, Lemmel E-M, Russell AS. Ankylosing spondylitis in the pharaohs of ancient Egypt. Rheumatol Int 2003; 23:1–5.
18. Snorrason ES. Rheumatism past and present. Can Med Assoc J 1942; 46:589–594.
19. Morse D. Ancient disease in the Midwest. Illinois State Mus Rep Invest 1969; 15.
20. Kidd KE. A note on the paleopathology of Ontario. Am J Phys Anthropol 1954; 12:610–615.
21. Zivanovic S. Ancient diseases: the elements of paleopathology. London: Methuen, 1982.
22. Kramar C. A case of ankylosing spondylitis in mediaeval Geneva. OSSA 1982; 8:115–129.
23. Wells C. Romano-British cemeteries at Cirencester. Cirencester Excavation Committee, 1982.
24. Wells C. Joint pathology in ancient Anglo-Saxons. J Bone Jt Surg 1962; 44B:948–949.
25. de Vlam K, Mielants H, Verstraete KL, Veys EM. The zygapophyseal joint determines morphology of the enthesophyte. J Rheumatol 2000; 27:1732–1739.

26. Martinez-Lavin M, Mansilla J, Pineda C, Pijoan C. Ankylosing spondylitis is indigenous to Mesoamerica. J Rheumatol 1995; 22:2327–2330.
27. von Hölder H. Untersuchungen über die Skelettefunde in den vorrömischen Hügelbräbern Württembergs und Hohenzollerns. Fundberichte aus Schwaben. Stuttgart, 1895; 2.
28. Nicoloysen N. The Viking Ship discovered at Gothstadt in Norway. Christiania, 1882.
29. Palfi GY, Panuel M, Gyetvay A, Molnar E, Bende L, Dutour O. Advanced-stage ankylosing spondylitis in a subject in the 8th century. J Radiol 1996; 77:283–285.
30. Dastugue J. Les maladies de nos ancêtres. La Recherche 1982; 13:980–988.
31. Mettler CC. History of medicine. Philadelphia: Blakiston, 1947.
32. O'Connell D. Ankylosing spondylitis. The literature up to the close of the nineteenth century. Ann Rheum Dis 1956; 15:119–123.
33. Connor B. An abstract from a letter to Sir Charles Walgrave, published in French at Paris: Giving an account of an extraordinary human skeleton, whose vertebrae of the back, the ribs and several bones down to the os sacrum, were firmly united into one solid bone, without jointing or cartilage. Philos Trans 1695; 19:21–27.
34. Brodie BC. Pathological and surgical observations on diseases of the joints. London: Longman, Hurst, Rees, Orne and Brown, 1818:55.
35. Fagge CH. A case of simple synostosis of the ribs to the vertebrae, and of the arches and articular processes of the vertebrae themselves, and also of one hip-joint. Trans Pathol Soc Lond 1877; 28:201–209.
36. Bechterew W. Steifigkeit der Wirbelsaule und ihre Verkrummung als besondere Erkrankungsform. Neurol Centralbl 1893; 12:426–434.
37. Strümpell E. Lehrbuch der speciellen Pathologie und Therapie der inneren Krankheiten, Leipzig, 1884; Bd.2.
38. Marie P. Sur la spondylose rhizomélique. Rev Méd 1898; 18:285–315.
39. Leri A. La spondylose rhizomélique. Rev Méd 1899; 19:597–624, 691–733 and 801–833.
40. Leden I. Did Bechterew describe the disease which is named after him? A question raised due to the centennial of his primary report. Scand J Rheumatol 1994; 23:42–45.
41. Bechterew W. Von der Verwachsung oder Steifigkeit der Wirbelsäule. Deutsche Zeitschrift für Nervenheilkunde 1897; 11:327–337.
42. Bechterew W. Neue Beobachtungen mit patologisch-anatomische Undersuchungen über Steifigkeit der Wirbelsäule. Deutsche Zeitschrift für Nervenheilkunde 1899; 15:45–57.
43. Bechterew W. Über ankylosirende Entzündung der Wirbelsäule und der grossen Erxtremitätengelenke. Deutsche Zeitschrift für Nervenheilkunde 1899; 15:37–45.
44. Strümpell A. Bemerkungen über chronisch-ankylosierende Entzündung der Wirbelsaule und der Huftergelenks. Deutsche Zeitschrift für Nervenheilkunde 1897; 11:338–342.
45. Leri A. Etudes sur les affections de la colonne vertébrale. Paris: Masson et Cie, 1926:309.
46. Leden I. Wladimir Bechterew. Ryssen som "Sowed confusion and reaped glory." Läkartidningen 1987; 84:2960–2962.
47. Ljungren B. Vladimir Bekhterev—The professor who diagnosed the state of Stalin. In: Ljungren B, ed. Great men with sick brains & other essays. Parkeridge Il: American Association of Neurological Surgeons, 1990:49–68.
48. Dequeker J. Paleopathology of rheumatism in painting. In: Ortner DJ, Aufderheide AC, eds. Human paleopathology: current synthesis and future options. Washington: Smithsonian Institution Press, 1991:216–221.
49. Dequeker J. Art, history and rheumatism: the case of Erasmus of Rotterdam (1466–1536) suffering from pustulotic arthro-osteitis. Ann Rheum Dis 1991; 50:517–521.
50. Wolfe F, Cathey MA. The misdiagnosis of gout and hyperuricemia. J Rheumatol 1991; 18:1232–1234.
51. Costa A, Weber G. Le Alterazioni morbose del sistema sclerotico in Cosimo dei Medici il Vecchio. In: Piero il Gottoso, in Lorenzo il Magnifico, in Guiliano duca di Nemours. Arch De Vecchi Anat Patol 1955; 23:1–69.

52. Pizon P. La pathologie ostéoarticulaire de quatre Médicis. Presse Médicale 1956; 64:1483–1484.

53. Sieper J, Braun J, Rudwaleit M, Boonen A, Zink A. Ankylosing spondylitis: an overview. Ann Rheum Dis 2002; 61(suppl III):iii8–iii18.

54. Forestier J. Gilbert Scott memorial oration. Ankylosing spondylitis at the beginning of the century. Rheumatism (J Charterhouse Rheumatism Clinic) 1964; 20:28–53.

55. Forestier J, Jacqueline F, Rolesquerol J, eds. Ankylosing spondylitis: clinical considereations, roentgenology, pathologic anatomy, treatment. Springfield IL, Charles C. Thosmas, 1956. (Translated by AU Desjardins).

56. Moll JM, Haslock I, Macrae IF, Wright V. Associations between ankylosing spondylitis, psoriatic arthritis, Reiter's disease, the intestinal arthropathies, and Behçet's syndrome. Medicine (Baltimore) 1974; 53:343–364.

57. Wright V, Moll JMH, eds. Seronegative polyarthritis. Amsterdam: North Holland Publishing, 1976.

58. Arnett FC. Seronegative spondylarthropathies. Bull Rheum Dis 1987; 37:1–12.

59. Dougados M, van der Linden S, Juhling R, et al. The European spondylarthropathy study group preliminary criteria for the classification of spondylarthropathy. Arthritis Rheum 1991; 34:1218–1230.

60. Benedek TG. The first reports of Dr. Hans Reiter on Reiter's disease. J Albert Einstein Med Center 1969; 17:100–105.

61. Bauer W, Engleman EP. A syndrome of unknown etiology characterized by urethritis, conjunctivitis and arthritis (so-called Reiter's disease). Trans Assoc Am Physicians 1942; 57:307–313.

62. Paronen I. Reiter's disease. A study of 344 cases observed in Finland. Acta Med Scand 1948; 131(suppl):1–114.

63. Alvonen P, Sievers K, Aha K. Arthritis associated with Yersinia enterocolitica infection. Acta Rheumatol Scand 1969; 15:232–253.

64. Schlosstein L, Terasaki PI, Bluestone R, Pearson CM. High association of and HL-A antigen, W27, with ankylosing spondylitis. N Engl J Med 1973; 288:704–706.

65. Brewerton DA, Caffrey M, Nicholls A, Walters D, Oates JK, James DC. Reiter's disease and HL-A 27. Lancet 1973; ii:996–998.

66. Ebringer RW, Cawdell DR, Cowling P, Ebringer A. Sequential studies in ankylosing spondylitis. Association of Klebsiella pneumoniae with active disease. Ann Rheum Dis 1978; 37:146–151.

67. Maki-Ikola O, Lehtinen K, Granfors K, Vainionpaa R, Toivanen P. Bacterial antibodies in ankylosing spondylitis. Clin Exp Immunol 1991; 84:872–875.

68. Mielants H, Veys EM, Joos R, Noens I, Cuvelier C, De Vos M. HLA antigens in seronegative spondylarthropathies. Reactive arthritis and arthritis in ankylosing spondylitis: relation to gut inflammation. J Rheumatol 1987; 14:466–467.

2

Epidemiology, Pathogenesis, and Genetics of Ankylosing Spondylitis

Andrew E. Timms, B. Paul Wordsworth, and Matthew A. Brown
The Botnar Research Centre, Nuffield Orthopaedic Centre, Headington, Oxford, U.K.

EPIDEMIOLOGY

Ankylosing spondylitis (AS) is one of the most common inflammatory rheumatic diseases, but estimates of its prevalence vary considerably, even in similar ethnic groups. The prevalence of AS generally varies with the prevalence of histocompatibility leukocyte antigen (HLA)-B27 (referred to as B27 hereafter), but determination of the precise prevalence in populations is affected by the sensitivity of the screening modality employed. Populations with a high prevalence of B27, such as Scandinavians and among the Inuit, Haida, and Bella Coola North American Indians, have correspondingly high levels of AS (1–3). In contrast, ethnic groups with a low prevalence of B27 such as Africans and Australian Aboriginals have a low prevalence of AS (4–7). Rare exceptions to this rule occur, as will be discussed subsequently. Estimates of the proportion of B27-carriers that develop AS also vary significantly, most likely related to the screening procedures that were used to identify cases. Where plain radiography was the screening modality, the prevalence of AS in B27-carriers has been estimated at 1.3–1.9%, whereas where magnetic resonance imaging (MRI) scanning was employed, the reported rate was 6.8% (8–12). Estimates of the overall prevalence of AS are similarly quite varied, ranging from 0.1% to 0.86% in Caucasian populations (9,12).

Early estimates of the magnitude of the increased risk of the disease in males are now recognized to be inflated. This appears to have been due to under-reporting of the disease in women, and possibly also ascertainment bias due to men having more severe disease. In studies designed to minimize this bias, the gender ratio has been estimated at 2.4:1 (13). In spondyloarthritis complicating psoriasis, the gender ratio is 3.5:1, and complicating inflammatory bowel disease (IBD), it is 1:1 (13). With increasing age, the gender ratio in AS declines, such that in patients with disease onset <20 years old the gender ratio is 3:1, compared to 1.8:1 for those with an onset at >40 years (14).

Men do have more severe disease than women in terms of measured loss of mobility and radiographic spinal disease, although women may have more severe acute symptoms (13,15). Young age of onset correlates with increased disease severity, and increased frequency of hip disease (16,17). Other determinants of disease severity include cigarette smoking, educational levels, and employment and socioeconomic status (18–20).

A large genetic component in susceptibility to AS has been inferred from twin studies, which have demonstrated a monozygotic (MZ) twin concordance rate of 63% as compared to a dizygotic (DZ) twin concordance rate of 12% (21). The heritability of susceptibility has been estimated at 97% [95% confidence interval (CI) 92–99%]. The remainder of the variance is due to environmental factors, which are likely to be widespread. Evidence for the environmental trigger of AS being ubiquitous include: (i) the lack of significant difference between DZ and sibling concordance rates (21), (ii) the observation that B27-transgenic rats do not develop inflammatory, intestinal, or peripheral joint disease in germ-free environments, but do when exposed to normal enteric conditions (22), and (iii) that the disease and therefore the environmental trigger occur in such varied conditions as equatorial and Arctic regions. Although a clustered "outbreak" of AS has been reported, this condition is pandemic (23).

The role of B27 (or a very closely linked gene) has been well established by population genetic studies in many ethnic groups. As discussed above, only a small fraction of B27-positive individuals develop spondyloarthritis, but for B27-positive individuals with an affected first-degree relative, the risk of AS is 6 to 16 times greater than for B27-positive individuals with no family history (9,10). The presence of non-B27 susceptibility factors has also been highlighted in twin studies in which the concordance rate for B27-positive DZ twin pairs (23%) is considerably below that of MZ pairs (63%) (Table 1) (21).

The number of genes involved in susceptibility to AS is unknown, but family recurrence risk modeling has suggested that a limited number are involved. It has been demonstrated, in diseases with a significant genetic component, that the pattern of reduction of disease concordance in increasingly distant relatives of patients is determined by the number of genes involved and their interactions (24). Recurrence risk modeling suggests the model operating in AS is an oligogenic model with predominantly multiplicative interaction between loci (25).

Table 1 Pairwise Twin Concordance Rates in Ankylosing Spondylitis

Category	Brown (21)	All previous studies	Total
MZ			
Affected	6	11	17
Total	8	19	27
% (95% CI)	75	58	63 (42–81)
DZ			
Affected	4	3	7
Total	32	24	56
% (95% CI)	12.5	15	12.5 (5–24)
B27-positive DZ			
Affected	4	3	7
Total	15	15	30
% (95% CI)	27	20	23 (10–42)

Abbreviations: MZ, monozygotic; DZ, dizygotic; CI, confidence interval.

Recurrence risk in families has been shown to differ according to the gender of the proband, with an increased risk associated with younger, female patients (26). There is also a reduction in the prevalence of disease in daughters and sisters of male probands, compared to sons and brothers (26). This cannot be explained by greater exposure to environmental risks, since this would suggest that children of affected men would be at higher risk than children of affected women. If women actually have a higher genetic threshold for developing disease, then affected women may have more susceptibility genes than men, which could explain the increased risk in relatives. This is consistent with a polygenic contribution to susceptibility to AS. A role for the X chromosome in influencing this gender bias has been discounted by the exclusion of a significant susceptibility locus on the X chromosome (27).

The role of genetics in determining disease severity for AS has also been examined in twins. Although the numbers of twin pairs were small, measures of disease activity and functional impairment were more similar in MZ twin pairs than DZ pairs (21). A major genetic contribution to disease severity, as assessed by the Bath AS Disease Activity Index (BASDAI) and functional impairment as assessed by the Bath AS Functional Index (BASFI), has been demonstrated by a complex segregation study (28). A high degree of familiality was observed for both BASDAI and BASFI, with heritability estimated at 51% and 68%, respectively. Segregation studies reject polygenic and environmental models, with a monogenic model fitting the data most closely. We have identified the loci involved in controlling measures of clinical manifestations as assessed by the BASDAI, BASFI, and age of disease onset; heritability estimates for these traits were estimated at 49%, 76%, and 33%, respectively (29).

PATHOGENESIS

The Role of B27

The association of B27 with AS is among the strongest of any disease. Evidence of the role of B27 in AS comes from association and linkage studies in humans and from transgenic animal studies. Association between B27 and AS was first noted by two groups in 1973, and has been confirmed in most populations worldwide (30–32). This worldwide association strongly suggests that B27 is involved directly in the etiology of AS; if B27 were merely a marker for a further susceptibility gene, recombination would be expected to reduce the degree of association in some ethnic groups. Although various populations including West Africa, Sardinia, and some Southeast Asian populations show either weak or no association between B27 and AS, this may be due to the differences in strength of association of the B27-subtypes present (B*2706 in Asia, B*2709 in Sardinia) (33–38). However, in West Africa the disease does not occur even in B*2705 carriers, suggesting that other environmental or genetic protective factors must be operating (39).

Strong linkage of the HLA with AS has been reported in several studies (40,41). A study of multicase Newfoundland pedigrees demonstrated a likely autosomal dominant pattern of inheritance, with penetrance of approximately 20%. A maximum logarithm of odds (LOD) score of 15.6 at the HLA region has also been reported in whole genome screens of British families (42).

A direct role for B27 in the etiology of AS is supported by animal studies. A study of AS-like disease in cattle demonstrated linkage and association of a bovine major histocompatibility complex (MHC) class I antigen bovine lymphocyte antigen A8 (BoLA-A8) with disease (43). Although BoLA-A8 does not cross-react with anti-HLA-B27 antibodies, this still supports direct involvement of the MHC class I antigen in disease. B27-transgenic rats develop psoriasis, colitis, orchitis, and spondyloarthritis, but only if large copy numbers of the transgenes are present (44,45). B7-transgenic rats do not develop any of these features (46). The development of a transgenic rat expressing a nondisease-associated B27 subtype (B*2706 or B*2709), with a large copy number is required as a true control. Concerns about this model include the disease characteristics which are not shared with human AS (especially severe colitis and orchitis), and the large copy number of transgenes which is required for development of disease.

B27-transgenic mice spontaneously develop an inflammatory arthritis, but only when lacking mouse beta-2 microglobulin (β_2m). Mice expressing human β_2m also develop disease, whereas B27-transgenic mice which express mouse β_2m normally (B27$^+$ mβ_2m$^+$) do not (47). This appears to be associated with the expression of free B27 heavy chains (HC) which would normally be associated with β_2m. These findings are further complicated by the finding that β_2m deficiency alone can cause spondyloarthritis in mice, independent of B27 (48).

A further mouse model of spondyloarthritis, ankylosing enthesopathy (ANKENT), is a naturally occurring joint disease characterized by progressive ankylosis of the ankle and tarsal joints of the hind paw, but not by axial arthritis. ANKENT has a reported male predominance, and generally occurs in relatively young males (between four and eight months of age) (49). A role for environmental factors has been suggested by the finding that B10.BR male mice in a germ-free environment did not develop ANKENT, compared with 20% of their litter mates brought up in a conventional environment (50). A similar finding has been reported in B27-transgenic rats (22,50,51). In contrast to the mouse models described above, in this model insertion of HLA-B*2702 increases the frequency of disease in the presence of mouse β_2m. In the absence of β_2m, ANKENT occurs much less frequently; B*2702 is not expressed on the cell surface, and does not increase the risk of ANKENT (52).

In BALB/c mice immunised with the proteoglycan component versican or peptides derived from it, spondylitis and sacroiliitis develop (53). Nine percent of these mice also develop uveitis, a common complication of human AS. Following the onset of inflammation, chondrocyte proliferation occurs, leading to ossification. The influence of B27 on this model has not yet been tested.

Structure and Function of B27

The MHC comprises three regions (class I, II, and III), containing over 200 genes within a 4-Mb region. The principal function of class I molecules is the presentation of endogenous peptides to CD8$^+$ T lymphocytes to induce protective immune responses. Class I molecules conventionally consist of polymorphic HLA heavy chains which form a heterodimer with β_2m (54). The membrane distal domains of the HC form a peptide-binding groove, which consists of several strands of β-pleated sheets topped by two antiparallel walls of α helices. MHC class I molecules can bind many different peptides with restrictions with regard to the length and sequence of the peptide (55). The peptide-binding groove is closed at both ends, so class I molecules are generally only able to bind peptides that are between 8 and 10 residues in length. Certain anchor residues in the peptide are required to bind specific pockets in the floor of the antigen-binding site of the class I molecule. The charge and shape of these antigen-binding pockets are major determinants of the specificity of binding seen in different class I molecules. For B27, presented peptides are characterized by the presence of arginine at position 2, and a high proportion carrying basic residues such as arginine or lysine at position 9.

Antigenic peptides bind to HLA class I molecules in the endoplasmic reticulum (ER). Typically such peptides are derived from the degradation of complex antigens in the cytosol by large molecular weight proteosomes. These peptides are then actively transported into the ER by transporters associated with antigen processing (TAP). Newly synthesized class I HC bind a membrane-bound chaperone known as calnexin. The binding of β_2m to the HC dissociates calnexin and the HC-β_2m heterodimer binds to a complex of proteins including the TAP-associated protein, tapasin. Tapasin then binds to the TAP1 unit of the TAP complex, and the heterodimer associates with a suitable peptide. Binding of an appropriate 8 to 12 residue peptide by the HC-β_2m heterodimer is crucial to the correct folding and stability of the class I molecule and its release from the ER. The peptide–HC-β_2m trimeric complex then trafficks to the cell surface, where it interacts with specific CD8[+] T cells.

Given the function of MHC class I antigens in peptide presentation to CD8[+] T cells, there has been much work on identification of B27-restricted CD8[+] T cells in spondyloarthritis patients. Autoreactive CD8[+] T cells have been identified, which show restriction to B27, B27-restricted responses to intracellular bacteria, and B27-restricted responses to cross-reactive self- and bacteria-derived peptides (56–59). These findings are all consistent with the "arthritogenic peptide" theory of the AS-pathogenesis (see following sections). However, some of these responses occur in both spondyloarthritis patients and healthy controls, and therefore their relevance to the pathogenesis of AS is uncertain.

As described earlier, the requirement for the presence of β_2m is inconsistent between mouse models. Nonetheless, the development of spondyloarthritis in the absence of B27 has led to the hypothesis that B27 may not be causing spondyloarthritis by a mechanism involving traditional peptide presentation to cytotoxic T-lymphocytes. B27 has been demonstrated to have many unusual properties in comparison with other class I antigens which may explain these findings. An unusual structural feature of B27 is the presence of an unpaired cysteine residue at position 67 (Cys67) in the B pocket of the peptide-binding groove. Although the Cys67 is seen in other HLA molecules not associated with AS (HLA-B38, -B39, -B14, -B15, and -B73), the presence of Cys67 with other unusual residues in the B pocket, such as the lysine at position 70, may result in some of the unique properties of B27 (60). Misfolding of B27 occurs to a greater extent than with other class I antigens, and appears to be related to the composition of its B pocket (61). B27 molecules can form homodimers, through the formation of disulfide bonds involving the unpaired B-pocket Cys67 residue, and possibly other residues. Misfolded and homodimeric B27 tends to accumulate in the ER and be slowly degraded in the cytosol, and it has been hypothesized that this may cause disease, perhaps through the generation of "stress responses" in the ER (62,63). B27 homodimer formation and accumulation in the ER has recently been demonstrated to occur in B27-transgenic rats (64). Interestingly, this did not appear to be dependent on the presence of Cys67, contradicting earlier in vitro studies (65). Strains with serine substituted for Cys67-produced homodimers, although to a lesser extent than rats not carrying the substitution. They also developed disease, albeit milder than Cys67 B27-transgenic rats (63).

Whether these unusual properties of B27 have any relevance to human disease remains unproven. A further level of complexity is that there are different hypotheses as to how homodimers may cause disease. One hypothesis suggests that B27-homodimers induce disease as a consequence of intracellular accumulation. However, it has also been proposed that they may act by some extracellular mechanism such as aberrant presentation of peptides or recognition by immune cells [either natural killer (NK) cells or cytotoxic T-lymphocytes] (66). B27 can be expressed on the surface of cells in the absence of the TAP complex, tapasin, and peptide (67–70). This may explain the finding that mice B27$^+$ mβ_2m$^{-/-}$ hβ_2m$^+$ TAP1$^-$ mice develop arthritis as do mice with intact TAP (B27$^+$ mβ_2m$^{-/-}$ hβ_2m$^+$ TAP1$^+$), although with a lower frequency (54% vs. 69%) (71). B27 homodimers are expressed on the cell surface, but do not appear to be derived from intracellular sources; rather they are produced from B27 heterodimers either at the cell surface or in endocytic compartments (66). High affinity peptide-binding by B27 heterodimers appears to reduce the homodimer formation (66). Further, high affinity binding of a B27-specific peptide in B27-transgenic rats reduces the incidence of spondyloarthritis, perhaps by effects on homodimer formation (72). It has therefore been postulated that bacterial triggering infections may promote homodimer formation by interference with the peptide-loading complex, or by changing the intracellular oxidative conditions promoting disulfide bond formation (66). It has been demonstrated that a variety of B and T lymphocytes and synovial and peripheral blood monocytes express receptors for B27 homodimers (73). Whether these have any pathogenic significance remains unknown.

B27 Subtypes

There are 24 reported subtypes of B27 (Tables 2 and 3). Subtypes B*27052, -053, and -054 have also been reported but encode the same mature protein as B*2705. The subtype B*2722 is no longer regarded as a legitimate subtype, but is a variant of B*2706 having an additional noncoding single nuclear polymorphism (SNP) (74,75). B*2705 shows a worldwide distribution and is thought to be the ancestral allele (76,77). The other subtypes are related to B*2705 by one or more genetic events, either gene conversion or point mutation. Most variations are in exons 2 and 3, which encode the α1 and α2 domains, respectively. The subtypes can be divided into at least three groups (Table 3): (i) the first is seen in Caucasians and Africans and involve substitutions in the alpha 1 domain, (ii) the second is seen predominantly in Asians, involving one shared substitution in the α1 domain and a variable number in the α2 domain, and (iii) the third group which is seen predominantly in Caucasians involves substitutions only in the second domain. Subtypes which do not fit into these groups include B*2713, which differs from B*2705 outside of the α1 and α2 domains [an alanine (Alu) to glutamic acid (Glu) substitution 20 base pairs before the start of exon 1] and B*2718, which appears to have evolved separately.

There has been considerable interest in the level of disease association seen with different B27 subtypes as this may yield clues to the role of B27 in AS. Association with disease is clearly seen with B*2705, except in the Western African populations of Senegal and Gambia (78,79). Clear disease association is also observed with the following subtypes:

- B*2702, which is present in 4–10% of B27-positive individuals of Northern European descent, and up to 55% of Arab and Jewish populations (36,80,81),
- B*2704, the predominant allele among the Chinese and Japanese,
- B*2707, a rare Indian subtype (36,81),

Table 2 Amino Acid Changes of HLA-B27 Subtypes

Residue number

B27 subtype	AS association	L	α1												α2												α3
		-20	59	63	67	69	70	71	74	77	80	81	82	83	94	95	97	103	113	114	116	131	143	152	156	163	211
B*2705	Yes	A	Y	E	C	A	K	A	D	D	T	L	L	R	T	L	N	V	Y	H	D	S	T	V	L	E	A
B*2701	Yes	ND	–	–	–	–	–	–	Y	N	–	A	–	–	–	–	–	–	–	–	–	–	–	–	–	–	–
B*2702	Yes	–	–	–	–	–	–	–	–	N	I	A	–	–	–	–	–	–	–	–	–	–	–	–	–	–	–
B*2703	Yes	–	H	–	–	–	–	–	–	–	–	–	–	–	–	–	–	–	–	–	–	–	–	–	–	–	–
B*2704	Yes	–	–	–	–	–	–	–	–	S	–	–	–	–	–	–	–	–	H	D	Y	–	–	E	–	–	G
B*2706	No	–	–	–	–	–	–	–	–	S	–	–	–	–	–	–	–	–	–	N	Y	–	–	E	–	–	G
B*2707	Yes	ND	–	–	–	–	–	–	–	S	N	–	R	G	–	–	S	–	H	–	–	R	–	–	–	–	–
B*2708	Yes	–	–	–	–	–	–	–	–	–	–	–	–	–	–	–	–	–	–	–	H	–	–	–	–	–	–
B*2709	No	ND	–	–	–	–	–	–	–	–	–	–	–	–	–	–	–	–	–	–	–	–	–	–	–	–	–
B*2710	Yes	ND	–	–	–	–	–	–	–	–	N	–	R	G	–	–	S	–	H	N	Y	R	–	E	–	–	ND
B*2711	Not known	–	–	–	–	–	–	–	–	S	–	–	–	–	–	–	–	–	–	–	–	–	–	–	–	–	–
B*2712	Not known	–	–	–	–	T	N	T	–	S	–	–	–	–	–	–	–	–	–	–	–	–	–	–	–	–	–
B*2713	Not known	E	–	–	–	–	–	–	–	–	–	–	–	–	–	–	–	–	–	–	–	–	–	–	–	–	–
B*2714	Yes	–	–	–	–	–	–	–	–	–	–	–	–	–	–	W	–	L	–	–	–	–	–	–	–	–	ND
B*2715	Yes	ND	–	–	–	–	–	–	–	S	–	–	–	–	–	–	–	–	–	–	–	–	–	E	–	T	ND
B*2716	Not known	ND	–	–	–	T	N	T	–	–	–	–	–	–	–	–	–	–	–	–	–	–	–	–	–	–	ND
B*2717	Not known	ND	F	–	–	–	–	–	–	–	–	–	–	–	–	–	–	–	–	D	Y	–	–	–	–	–	ND
B*2718	Not known	–	–	–	S	T	N	–	Y	S	N	–	R	G	–	–	–	–	–	–	Y	–	–	E	–	–	ND
B*2719	Yes	ND	–	–	–	–	–	–	–	–	–	–	–	–	I	–	R	–	H	N	Y	–	–	–	–	–	ND
B*2720	Not known	ND	–	–	–	–	–	–	–	S	–	–	–	–	–	–	–	–	H	N	Y	R	–	E	–	–	ND
B*2721	Not known	ND	–	–	F	T	N	T	–	S	–	–	–	–	–	–	R	–	–	–	Y	–	–	E	–	–	ND
B*2723	Not known	ND	–	N	–	–	–	–	Y	S	–	–	–	–	–	–	S	–	H	N	Y	R	S	E	–	–	ND
B*2724	Not known	ND	–	–	–	–	–	–	–	S	–	–	–	–	–	–	–	–	–	–	–	–	–	–	W	–	ND
B*2725	Not known	ND	–	–	–	–	–	–	–	S	–	–	–	–	–	–	–	–	–	–	L	–	–	E	–	L	ND

The amino acid sequence of each B27 subtype is defined using the standard single letter amino acid code, where identity with B*2705 is indicated by dashes (–), and any difference noted; ND, not determined. If an association with AS has been reported it is noted in the second column.

Table 3 Possible Origins of HLA-B27 Alleles

	α1	α2	Group
B*27052	0	0	Caucasian, other
B*27052	0	0	Unknown
B*27052	0	0	Unknown
B*2713	0	0	Unknown
B*2703	1	0	African
B*2717	1	0	Unknown
B*2701	3	0	Mestizo
B*2702	3	0	Unknown
B*2716	3	0	Caucasian
B*2708	4	0	Caucasian
B*2712	7	0	Caucasian
B*2723	7	0	Caucasian
B*2704	1	1	Asian
B*2715	1	2	Asian
B*2706	1	3	Asian
B*2725	1	3	Unknown
B*2721	1	4	Unknown
B*2711	1	5	Asian
B*2720	1	5	Asian
B*2724	1	7	Unknown
B*2709	0	1	Caucasian
B*2710	0	1	Caucasian
B*2714	0	3	American Indian
B*2719	0	3	Caucasian, Middle East
B*2707	0	5	Caucasian, Central America
B*2718	9	1	Unknown

Numbers under α1 and α2 respond to the number of amino acid substitutions within that region.

- B*2701, a very rare subtype observed in Caucasian, Asian, Mestizo, and African American populations, and spondyloarthritis has only been reported in one kindred (82), and
- B*2708, a rare European subtype, which has been associated with AS in a large family from the Azores (83).

The association of B*2703 with AS or spondyloarthritis is unclear; the subtype is restricted to West African and African American populations. In a study of the Fula group of Gambia' disease association was not observed with B*2703 or B*2705 and AS (78). Three B*2703-positive AS patients from Senegal have been identified, suggesting a role for B*2703 in disease susceptibility (84).

B*2706 and B*2709 have been reported to be either weakly or not associated with AS in populations where other B27 subtypes have been associated with AS. It is unlikely that individuals with different B27 subtypes would have different genetic or environmental factors influencing their susceptibility to AS. B*2706 differs from the disease-associated subtype B*2704 by two amino acid substitutions at residues 114 and 116 (Table 2). In a study in the Thai population, B*2704 was more frequent in AS patients (91%) as compared to healthy controls (47%), however,

B*2706 was seen in 47% of controls but not observed in AS patients (35). This lack of association was confirmed in a follow-up study, and independent studies in a Singapore Chinese population, and Chinese Indonesians from Java (37,75,85).

The B*2708 subtype is of particular interest because it carries a different "public epitope" to the other allelic forms of B27, carrying the sequence specifying the Bw6 epitope in contrast to most B27 alleles which carry a Bw4 sequence. These serological epitopes are known to be important in NK cell recognition, and therefore it was postulated that a lack of association of B*2708 with AS would point to involvement of NK cells in AS-pathogenesis. However B*2708 has now been reported in cases with AS (83). B*2709 differs from the disease-associated subtype B*2705 by an amino acid substitution at residue 116. B*2709 is primarily observed in Sardinians, and is seen in 25% of B27-positive healthy controls, but not among B27-positive AS patients (34). B*2709 is also seen in approximately 3% of B27-positive individuals from mainland Italy. Although no B*2709 positive AS patients have been identified in mainland Italy, three patients with an undifferentiated form of spondyloarthritis have been reported (86,87). These data suggest that B*2709 may play a role in some form of spondyloarthritis, but appears not to be involved in the pathogenesis of AS. These data suggest that in some populations it is not just the presence of B27 which is crucial in susceptibility to AS, but also the B27 subtype. However, this is not true in western Europeans, where the B27 subtype does not play a role in determining which B27-positive individuals develop AS (88).

The Role of B27 in the Causation of AS

Despite extensive research since the association with AS of B27 was first described in 1973, the role of B27 in disease pathology is still unknown. Numerous theories have been proposed, and are reviewed in the following sections.

Linked Gene

It is widely accepted that B27 plays a critical role in the pathogenesis of AS. However, it has been postulated that B27 is in linkage disequilibrium with the true disease-causing gene. The worldwide association of B27 with AS is strong evidence that B27 is the true disease-causing gene, as recombination would be expected to reduce the range of linkage disequilibrium (80). In the majority of ethnic groups the prevalence of AS also tends to reflect the underlying level of B27. Various studies in different ethnic groups have examined haplotype patterns in B27 and closely related genes, such as MHC class I chain-related gene (MICA) and tumor necrosis factor α (TNFα) (89–91). Different patterns of linkage disequilibrium are observed with the B27 subtypes, suggesting that B27 is the primary gene involved in susceptibility to AS. However, it is highly possible that other MHC genes on B27 haplotypes are involved in conferring susceptibility to disease. The linked-gene model of AS does not explain the occurrence of spondyloarthritis in B27-transgenic mice and rats (44,51). However, neither model is entirely representative of the human condition, as discussed earlier.

Arthritogenic Peptide Hypothesis

The arthritogenic peptide model is based on the natural function of HLA class I molecules to present endogenous peptides to T lymphocytes. Recognition of antigens as "foreign" by the T-cell receptor (TCR) can trigger an immune response, typically via CD8 positive cytotoxic T lymphocytes (CTLs). It is postulated that after infection with a pathogen, B27 may specifically bind and present an arthritogenic peptide, which elicits an inflammatory immune response. Evidence for the role for peptides and CTLs in AS is the finding of B27-restricted CD8$^+$ CTL in the synovial fluid of reactive arthritis patients and B27-restricted CTL directed against self-epitopes in reactive arthritis and AS patients (56,58,59). In addition, alteration of an endogenous B27-bound peptide in B27-transgenic rats (by the introduction of a minigene construct) resulted in a reduction in the prevalence of arthritis (72). As discussed before, this finding is also consistent with models involving immune reactions to B27 homodimers, as high affinity peptide binding by B27 heterodimers reduces the rate of B27 homodimer formation.

If the arthritogenic peptide hypothesis is correct, one would postulate that the B27 subtypes' which show weak or negative association with AS should not be able to bind the arthritogenic peptide. B*2704 and B*2706 peptide repertoires overlap by 88% and 90%, respectively, and B*2705 and B*2709 peptide repertoires overlap by 79% and 88%, respectively (92,93). This shows that the substitution of one or two amino acid residues within the B pocket can result in a significant change in peptide repertoires, consistent with the arthritogenic peptide hypothesis.

Molecular Mimicry

As originally described, this theory proposed pathological antibodies to bacteria such as the Klebsiella species which cross-reacted with B27 (94,95). A variant of these theories is the peptide homology theory: B27 bears homology to the antigenic peptides with which B27 is predicted to bind (96,97). This model suggests that the endogenous arthritogenic peptide is usually presented at levels too low to initiate an immune response. A stimulus, such as an infection' sensitizes the T cells to cross-react with the low level peptide and trigger an extended inflammatory immune response.

Studies have found a self-peptide, with homology to a B27-restricted virus-derived epitope, shows evidence of CTL cross-reaction (59,98). The self-peptide bound B*2709 better than B*2705, and elicited CTL from B*2705, but not B*2709 individuals. An additional B27-derived peptide with homology to protein sequences derived from Chlamydia has been reported to be presented by three disease-associated subtypes (B*2702, B*2704, and B*2705) but not by B*2706 and B*2709 (99). These findings are consistent with both the molecular mimicry and arthritogenic peptide models. However, strong direct evidence for the involvement of these peptides in spondyloarthritis, such as the triggering of disease by exposure to a single cross-reactive B27 peptide or bacterial antigen, is lacking.

GENETICS

MHC Genes Other than B27

Although B27 appears to be crucial in susceptibility to AS, there is considerable evidence that other genes are involved, including genes within the MHC (Fig. 1). The extensive linkage disequilibrium that occurs within the MHC region complicates any attempts to identify genes by population genetics. Studies to date have largely compared B27-positive cases with healthy controls, ignoring the fact that while the HLA-B locus is in Hardy–Weinberg equilibrium in controls, this is not the case in affected individuals. To what extent this will affect the findings of the studies of non-HLA-B MHC loci described later is unknown, and until B27-matched haplotypic studies have been reported, these studies must be interpreted with caution.

Chromosome 6

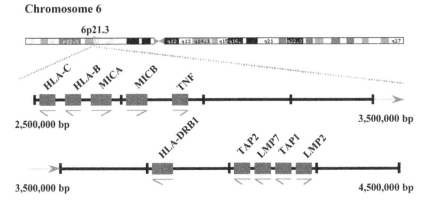

Figure 1 A graphical representation of the relative locations within the MHC of the genes. For each labeled gene the light gray arrow indicates the direction of transcription, and the base pair values are distances from the *p*-telomere.

HLA-B60

HLA-B60 (B60) has been shown to increase the risk for AS threefold in B27-positive individuals, and has been replicated in some but not all studies of Caucasian and Asian groups. Several small studies have also implicated B60, or a gene in linkage disequilibrium with B60, in B27-negative AS (21,88,92).

TNF α

Studies in some European populations have demonstrated association with the TNFα promoter polymorphism TNF-308 and AS (101–103). Although other small studies have produced negative results, this could be due to a lack of power to detect the small effects being investigated. However, in a large study no association was noted in British Caucasians, whereas a positive association was reported in a population from southern Germany (103). This suggests that TNF may be in linkage disequilibrium with a true disease-causing variant, rather then being involved in disease susceptibility itself. A possible role of the TNF-308 polymorphism has been suggested by the finding that the TNF-308.2 allele, when found on a B27-bearing haplotype, is associated with higher TNF production, possibly explaining its protective effect (104).

HLA-DRB1

Many reports have found association between HLA-DRB1 alleles and susceptibility to and the clinical manifestations of AS, although some may be due to linkage disequilibrium with B27. To overcome the problem of linkage disequilibrium, case–control and within-family studies of B27-DRB1 haplotypes have identified association of the B27-DR1 haplotype with AS in British and French groups (21,105, 106). The association with HLA-DR1 is of interest because of the association of the rare allele HLA-DRB1*0103 and IBD, increased severity of IBD, and arthritis complicated IBD (107,109). The strong association with DRB1*0103 is seen in patients with both AS and IBD, and is also found in B27-negative cases (109,110). Thus, it appears that B27-DRB1*0101 haplotypes are associated with primary AS, and B27-DRB1*0103 haplotypes with AS complicating IBD.

Association of HLA-DR4 with spondyloarthritis has recently been reported in a family study, but this study used multiple cases per family in the analysis, and therefore the validity of the conclusions are uncertain (111).

DR7 has been associated with a younger age of onset in British Caucasian patients with AS, and the presence of peripheral arthritis in AS (105,112,113). This is consistent with the associations seen between DR7 and psoriatic arthritis, and the association of the B27-DR7 haplotype and disease progression in psoriatic arthritis (114,115). DR8 is associated with iritis and age of onset in Norwegian AS patients, iritis in Japanese AS patients, and DR8 homozygosity is associated with AS, but not iritis in a group of British Caucasians (105,115,116). These findings indicate a role for a further MHC gene in susceptibility and the clinical manifestations of AS, and when complicated with disorders such as IBD and psoriasis.

Other MHC Genes

Various genes within the MHC class II region have been investigated due to their possible interaction with B27, including LMP2 and LMP7 (large multi-functional proteases), and TAP1 and TAP2, which are involved in antigen processing and peptide transport, respectively. LMP2 and LMP7 have been reported to be associated with acute anterior uveitis or extraspinal disease in AS patients in some studies, but not in others (117–122). TAP1 and TAP2 variants have been reported to have either marginal or no association with spondyloarthritis (122–124).

Studies of MICA in various populations have demonstrated no B27-independent association in AS, indicating any association of MICA alleles is due to linkage disequilibrium (100,125,126). Studies of heat shock protein 70 (HSP70), have observed no association with AS (127,128). One study did demonstrate association with disease but the control population were not B27-matched (therefore, did not control for linkage disequilibrium with B27), and genotypes were not in Hardy–Weinberg equilibrium (129).

These studies all suggest a role for additional MHC genes in various aspects of the AS phenotypes, although these studies are not able to pinpoint exact genes. Larger studies of different ethnic groups are required to take into account the extensive linkage disequilibrium within the MHC region. Studies with full matching for B27 are required to conclusively demonstrate the existence of further MHC loci independent of B27.

Non-MHC Genes

Two whole genome studies in British Caucasians have been published, involving a total of 188 families with 255 affected sibling pairs (130,131). These screens provide strong evidence as to the loci encoding the non-MHC genetic susceptibility to AS. Regions on chromosomes 1, 2, 6, 9, 10, 16, and 19 were identified with at least moderate linkage to the disease. The strongest linkage observed outside of the MHC is on chromosome 16q, where maximum linkage was observed at 101 cm from the p-telomere (LOD = 4.7), equivalent to a genome-wide significance level of <0.005 (132). Both screens showed significant support for this locus, with screen 1 achieving LOD = 4.1 at 106 cm and screen 2 LOD = 1.2 at 99 cm, making it quite unlikely that either represents a chance finding. Independent support of this finding has been reported in a preliminary report on a further genome-wide screen (133). The region of linkage is very broad, with the 3-LOD confidence interval extending from 84 to 114 cm, and contains numerous potential candidate genes. Further refinement of this interval by high density association/linkage disequilibrium mapping will be required to identify the actual genes involved. The magnitude of the genetic effect observed in affected sibling pair linkage screens is measured by the statistic λ, which is the ratio of the observed/expected number of pairs sharing zero alleles identical by descent. The magnitude of the chromosome 16q locus is $\lambda = 1.8$ (95% CI 1.3–2.4), equivalent to 13% or 2.2% of the recurrence risk ratio for polygenic multiplicative or additive models, respectively. This is roughly equivalent to the magnitude of the genetic effect of HLA-DRB1 in rheumatoid arthritis.

Two further screens in the North American (134) and French population (135) have subsequently been published which provide varying levels of support for these findings. To help synthesize the data from these different studies, the International Genetics of Ankylosing Spondylitis (GAS) Consortium performed a meta-analysis of the studies involving 3744 subject. Regions on chromosome 10q and 16q achieved 'suggestive' evidence of linkage, and regions on chromosomes 1q, 3q, 5q, 6q, 9q, 17q, and 19q showed at least nominal linkage in 2 or more scans and in the weighted meta-analysis. Regions previously associated with AS on chromosome 2q (the *IL-1* gene cluster) and 22q (*CYP2D6*) exhibited nominal linkage in the meta-analysis, providing further statistical support for their involvement in susceptibility to AS. These findings provide a useful guide for future studies aiming to identify the genes involved in this highly heritable condition.

Positional candidate gene studies have identified two non-MHC genes likely to be involved in AS susceptibility. The poor metabolizer phenotype or genotype of cytochrome P450 2D6 (*CYP2D6*) has been implicated in case–control studies in both German and British AS patients (129,136). Additional support comes from within-family association ($p = 0.01$) and linkage (LOD 1.0) analysis (130).

The interleukin 1 receptor antagonist (*IL-1RN*) gene has been implicated in susceptibility to AS. Significant over-representation of the *IL-1RN* variable number of tandem repeats (VNTR) allele 2 has been noted in two case–control association studies of AS patients; although a lack of association was noted in an additional study, this could be due to a lack of power, due to a small sample number (137–139). A case–control study examining SNPs within the *IL-1RN* gene also noted a significant association with AS in two SNPs in exon 6 of the gene (140). Allele 2 of *IL-1RN* VNTR is associated with an increase in IL-1RA production, which would be expected to inhibit the action of the pro-inflammatory cytokine IL-1, which is contrary to the expectations in AS. It is possible that the association with *IL-1RN* reflects linkage disequilibrium with a nearby gene, such as another gene encoded within the IL-1 complex on chromosome 2. This hypothesis is strongly suggested by the findings of an extensive study of the *IL-1* gene complex which demonstrated widespread association across the region in families and case-control analysis (141). This study suggested that AS-susceptibility was influenced by genes at both the *IL-1β* and *IL-1RN* ends of the *IL-1* gene complex, and further studies will be required to determine which are the primary genes involved.

Transforming growth factor beta-1 (TGF-β1) is a protein involved in inflammatory processes, tissue fibrosis, and bone remodeling. A study in Scottish AS patients reported an association between the SNP *TGFβ1* +915 and AS, and demonstrated association of that genotype with higher serum concentrations of TGF-β1 (142). However, in a large study of Finnish and British families with AS, the only positive finding was a weak association with *TGFβ1* +1632 (143). These studies suggest a minor role for TGF-β1 in disease pathogenesis.

Polymorphisms within *NOD2/CARD15* have been examined in AS patients due to the known association with Crohn's disease (144,145). In studies of AS patients no association has been noted between *NOD2/CARD15* and AS susceptibility (111,146–148). However, a marginal association has been observed in spondyloarthritis associated with ulcerative colitis, and a variant (Pro^{268} Ser) has been associated with disease severity; a microsatellite immediately adjacent to *NOD2/CARD15* is strongly linked with disease severity (146,149). AS complicating IBD tends to be more severe than primary AS, and the genetic findings support this being a clinically relevant subset with a worse outcome (150). However, the lack of association of variants of *NOD2/CARD15* with primary AS indicates that the terminal ileitis that is frequently present in this group is etiologically distinct from Crohn's disease, which is strongly genetically associated with *NOD2/CARD15* (144,145).

The *ank/ank* mouse develops ectopic calcium hydroxyapatite crystal deposition, leading to vertebral fusion resembling AS and chondrocalcinosis (151). This model has been investigated in the past due to the similarity to human AS, and it has been demonstrated that B27 carriage and immune suppression have no effect on the *ank/ank* phenotype (152,153). The defect gene has been identified, and the *ANK* gene is thought to be a membrane pyrophosphate transporter (154). In the *ank/ank* mouse dysfunction of the *ANK* gene results in an increase in intracellular inorganic pyrophosphate (PPi) and reduction of extracellular PPi. In humans a gain of function mutation of the human homologue *ANKH* is thought to result in an increase in extracellular PPi and subsequent calcium pyrophosphate deposition disease (CPPD) chondrocalcinosis (155). Studies of the role of *ANKH* in AS have been contradictory. One study demonstrated no association with *ANKH* variants and either susceptibility to or severity of disease, but another study showed weak linkage and association of the *ANKH* locus with disease susceptibility (156,157). Thus, it remains possible that *ANKH* variants may play a minor role in AS, although on the basis of its known function, it is unlikely to be involved in disease susceptibility.

REFERENCES

1. Gran JT, Husby G, Hordvik M. Prevalence of ankylosing spondylitis in males and females in a young middle-aged population of Tromso, Northern Norway. Ann Rheum Dis 1985; 44(6):359–367.
2. Gofton JP, Chalmers A, Price GE, Reeve CE. HL-A 27 and ankylosing spondylitis in B.C. Indians. J Rheumatol 1984; 11(5):572–573.
3. Boyer GS, Templin DW, Cornoni-Huntley JC, et al. Prevalence of spondyloarthropathies in Alaskan Eskimos. J Rheumatol 1994; 21(12):2292–2297.
4. Chalmers IM. Ankylosing spondylitis in African Blacks. Arthritis Rheum 1980; 23(12): 1366–1370.
5. Stein M, Davis P, Emmanuel J, West G. The spondyloarthropathies in Zimbabwe: a clinical and immunogenetic profile. J Rheumatol 1990; 17(10):1337–1339.
6. Adebajo AO. Spondyloarthropathies in sub-Saharan Africa. J Rheumatol 1991; 18(7): 1115.
7. Roberts-Thomson RA, Roberts-Thomson PJ. Rheumatic disease and the Australian aborigine. Ann Rheum Dis 1999; 58(5):266–270.
8. Dawkins RL, Owen ET, Cheah PS, Christiansen FT, Calin AA, Gofton JP. Prevalence of ankylosing spondylitis and radiological abnormalities of the sacroiliac joints in HLA-B27 positive individuals. J Rheumatol 1981; 8(6):1025–1026.
9. van der Linden S, Valkenburg H, Cats A. The risk of developing ankylosing spondylitis in HLA-B27 positive individuals: a family and population study. Br J Rheumatol 1983; 22(4 suppl 2):18–19.

10. Calin A, Marder A, Becks E, Burns T. Genetic differences between B27 positive patients with ankylosing spondylitis and B27 positive healthy controls. Arthritis Rheum 1983; 26(12):1460–1464.

11. Kaipiainen-Seppanen O, Aho K, Heliovaara M. Incidence and prevalence of ankylosing spondylitis in Finland. J Rheumatol 1997; 24(3):496–499.

12. Braun J, Bollow M, Remlinger G, et al. Prevalence of spondylarthropathies in HLA-B27 positive and negative blood donors. Arthritis Rheum 1998; 41(1):58–67.

13. Will R, Edmunds L, Elswood J, Calin A. Is there sexual inequality in ankylosing spondylitis? A study of 498 women and 1202 men. J Rheumatol 1990; 17(12):1649–1652.

14. Kennedy LG, Will R, Calin A. Sex ratio in the spondyloarthropathies and its relationship to phenotypic expression, mode of inheritance and age at onset. J Rheumatol 1993; 20(11):1900–1904.

15. Taylor AL, Balakrishnan C, Calin A. Reference centile charts for measures of disease activity, functional impairment, and metrology in ankylosing spondylitis. Arthritis Rheum 1998; 41(6):1119–1125.

16. Amor B, Santos RS, Nahal R, Listrat V, Dougados M. Predictive factors for the long-term outcome of spondyloarthropathies. J Rheumatol 1994; 21(10):1883–1887.

17. Brophy S, Calin A. Ankylosing spondylitis: interaction between genes, joints, age at onset, and disease expression. J Rheumatol 2001; 28(10):2283–2288.

18. Ward MM. Predictors of the progression of functional disability in patients with ankylosing spondylitis. J Rheumatol 2002; 29(7):1420–1425.

19. Gran JT, Skomsvoll JF. The outcome of ankylosing spondylitis: a study of 100 patients. Br J Rheumatol 1997; 36(7):766–771.

20. Roussou E, Kennedy LG, Garrett S, Calin A. Socioeconomic status in ankylosing spondylitis: relationship between occupation and disease activity. J Rheumatol 1997; 24(5):908–911.

21. Brown MA, Kennedy LG, MacGregor AJ, et al. Susceptibility to ankylosing spondylitis in twins: the role of genes, HLA, and the environment. Arthritis Rheum 1997; 40(10): 1823–1828.

22. Taurog JD, Richardson JA, Croft JT, et al. The germfree state prevents development of gut and joint inflammatory disease in HLA-B27 transgenic rats. J Exp Med 1994; 180(6):2359–2364.

23. Myllykangas-Luosujarvi R, Seuri M, Husman T, Korhonen R, Pakkala K, Aho K. A cluster of inflammatory rheumatic diseases in a moisture-damaged office. Clin Exp Rheumatol 2002; 20(6):833–836.

24. Risch N. Linkage strategies for genetically complex traits. I. Multilocus Models. Am J Hum Genet 1990; 46:222–228.

25. Brown MA, Laval SH, Brophy S, Calin A. Recurrence risk modelling of the genetic susceptibility to ankylosing spondylitis. Ann Rheum Dis 2000; 59(11):883–886.

26. Calin A, Brophy S, Blake D. Impact of sex on inheritance of ankylosing spondylitis: a cohort study. Lancet 1999; 354(9191):1687–1690.

27. Hoyle E, Laval SH, Calin A, Wordsworth BP, Brown MA. The X-chromosome and susceptibility to ankylosing spondylitis. Arthritis Rheum 2000; 43(6):1353–1355.

28. Hamersma J, Cardon LR, Bradbury L, et al. Is disease severity in ankylosing spondylitis genetically determined? Arthritis Rheum 2001; 44(6):1396–1400.

29. Brown MA, Brophy S, Bradbury L, et al. Identification of major loci controlling clinical manifestations of ankylosing spondylitis. Arthritis Rheum 2003; 48(8):2234–2239.

30. Brewerton DA, Hart FD, Nicholls A, Caffrey M, James DCO, Sturrock RD. Ankylosing spondylitis and HL-A27. Lancet 1973; 1:904–907.

31. Schlosstein L, Terasaki PI, Bluestone R, Pearson CM. High association of an HL-A antigen, w27, with ankylosing spondylitis. N Engl J Med 1973; 288:704–706.

32. Khan MA, van der Linden SM, Kushner I, Valkenburg HA, Cats A. Spondylitic disease without radiologic evidence of sacroiliitis in relatives of HLA-B27 positive ankylosing spondylitis patients. Arthritis Rheum 1985; 28(1):40–43.

33. Hill AV, Allsopp CE, Kwiatkowski D, Anstey NM, Greenwood BM, McMichael AJ. HLA class I typing by PCR: HLA-B27 and an African B27 subtype. Lancet 1991; 337: 640–642.

34. D'Amato M, Fiorillo MT, Carcassi C, et al. Relevance of residue 116 of HLA-B27 in determining susceptibility to ankylosing spondylitis. Eur J Immunol 1995; 25(11):3199–3201.

35. Lopez-Larrea C, Sujirachato K, Mehra NK, et al. HLA-B27 subtypes in Asian patients with ankylosing spondylitis. Evidence for new associations. Tissue Antigens 1995; 45:169.

36. Lopez-Larrea C, Gonzalez S, Martinez-Borra J. The role of HLA-B27 polymorphism and molecular mimicry in spondylarthropathy. Mol Med Today 1998:540–549.

37. Ren EC, Koh WH, Sim D, Boey ML, Wee GB, Chan SH. Possible protective role of HLA-B*2706 for ankylosing spondylitis. Tissue Antigens 1997; 49(1):67–69.

38. Kanga U, Mehra NK, Larrea CL, Lardy NM, Kumar A, Feltkamp TE. Seronegative spondyloarthropathies and HLA-B27 subtyes: a study in Asian Indians. Clin Rheumatol 1996; 15(suppl 1):13–18.

39. Brown MA, Jepson A, Young A, Whittle HC, Greenwood BM, Wordsworth BP. Ankylosing spondylitis in West Africans—evidence for a non-HLA-B27 protective effect. Ann Rheum Dis 1997; 56(1):68–70.

40. Rubin LA, Amos CI, Wade JA, et al. Investigating the genetic basis for ankylosing spondylitis. Arthritis Rheum 1994; 37(8):1212–1220.

41. Reveille JD, Suarez Almazor ME, Russell AS, et al. HLA in ankylosing spondylitis: is HLA-B27 the only *MHC* gene involved in disease pathogenesis? Semin Arthritis Rheum 1994; 23(5):295–309.

42. Laval SH, Timms A, Edwards S, et al. Whole-genome screening in ankylosing spondylitis: evidence of non-MHC genetic-susceptibility loci. Am J Hum Genet 2001; 68(4):918–926.

43. Park YH, Huang GS, Taylor JA, et al. Patterns of vertebral ossification and pelvic abnormalities in paralysis: a study of 200 patients. Radiology 1993; 188(2):561–565.

44. Hammer RE. Spontaneous inflammatory disease in transgenic rats expressing HLA-B27 and human beta 2m: an animal model of HLA-B27-associated human disorders. Cell 1990; 63:1099–1112.

45. Taurog JD, Maika SD, Simmons WA, Breban M, Hammer RE. Susceptibility to inflammatory disease in HLA-B27 transgenic rat lines correlates with the level of B27 expression. J Immunol 1993; 150:4168–4178.

46. Taurog JD, Hammer RE. Experimental spondyloarthropathy in HLA-B27 transgenic rats. Clin Rheumatol 1996; 15(suppl 1):22–27.

47. Khare SD, Hansen J, Luthra HS, David CS. HLA-B27 heavy chains contribute to spontaneous inflammatory disease in B27/human beta2-microglobulin (beta2m) double transgenic mice with disrupted mouse beta2m. J Clin Invest 1996; 98(12):2746–2755.

48. Kingsbury DJ, Mear JP, Witte DP, Taurog JD, Roopenian DC, Colbert RA. Development of spontaneous arthritis in beta2-microglobulin-deficient mice without expression of HLA-B27: association with deficiency of endogenous major histocompatibility complex class I expression. Arthritis Rheum 2000; 43(10):2290–2296.

49. Weinreich S, Eulderink F, Capkova J, et al. HLA-B27 as a relative risk factor in ankylosing enthesopathy in transgenic mice. Hum Immunol 1995; 42(2):103–115.

50. Rehakova Z, Capkova J, Stepankova R, et al. Germ-free mice do not develop ankylosing enthesopathy, a spontaneous joint disease. Hum Immunol 2000; 61(6):555–558.

51. Khare SD, Luthra HS, David CS. Spontaneous inflammatory arthritis in HLA-B27 transgenic mice lacking beta 2-microglobulin: a model of human spondyloarthropathies. J Exp Med 1995; 182(4):1153–1158.

52. Weinreich SS, Hoebe-Hewryk B, van der Horst AR, Boog CJ, Ivanyi P. The role of MHC class I heterodimer expression in mouse ankylosing enthesopathy. Immunogenetics 1997; 46(1):35–40.

53. Shi S, Ciurli C, Cartman A, Pidoux I, Poole AR, Zhang Y. Experimental immunity to the G1 domain of the proteoglycan versican includes spondylitis and sacroiliitis, of a kind seen in human spondylarthropathies. Arthritis Rheum 2003; 48(10):2903–2915.

54. Jones EY. MHC class I and class II structures. Curr Opin Immunol 1997; 9(1):75–79.
55. Rammensee HG. Chemistry of peptides associated with MHC class I and class II molecules. Curr Opin Immunol 1995; 7(1):85–96.
56. Hermann E, Yu DT, Meyer zum Buschenfelde KH, Fleischer B. HLA-B27-restricted CD8 T cells derived from synovial fluids of patients with reactive arthritis and ankylosing spondylitis. Lancet 1993; 342(8872):646–650.
57. Kuon W, Holzhutter HG, Appel H, et al. Identification of HLA-B27-restricted peptides from the Chlamydia trachomatis proteome with possible relevance to HLA-B27-associated diseases. J Immunol 2001; 167(8):4738–4746.
58. Ugrinovic S, Mertz A, Wu P, Braun J, Sieper J. A single nonamer from the Yersinia 60-kDa heat shock protein is the target of HLA-B27-restricted CTL response in Yersinia-induced reactive arthritis. J Immunol 1997; 159(11):5715–5723.
59. Fiorillo MT, Maragno M, Butler R, Dupuis ML, Sorrentino R. CD8(+) T-cell autoreactivity to an HLA-B27-restricted self-epitope correlates with ankylosing spondylitis. J Clin Invest 2000; 106(1):47–53.
60. Archer JR, Whelan MA, Badakere SS, McLean IL, Archer IV, Winrow VR. Effect of a free sulphydryl group on expression of HLA-B27 specificity. Scand J Rheumatol suppl 1990; 87:44–50.
61. Dangoria NS, DeLay ML, Kingsbury DJ, et al. HLA-B27 misfolding is associated with aberrant intermolecular disulfide bond formation (dimerization) in the endoplasmic reticulum. J Biol Chem 2002; 277(26):23,459–468.
62. Colbert RA. HLA-B27 misfolding: a solution to the spondyloarthropathy conundrum? Mol Med Today 2000; 6(6):224–230.
63. Mear JP, Schreiber KL, Munz C, Zhu X, et al. Misfolding of HLA-B27 as a result of its B pocket suggests a novel mechanism for its role in susceptibility to spondyloarthropathies. J Immunol 1999; 163(12):6665–6670.
64. Tran TM, Satumtira N, Dorris ML, Taurog JD. HLA-B27 heavy chain homodimers in HLA-B27 transgenic rats. Arthritis Rheum 2003; 28(suppl 9):S657.
65. Allen RL, O'Callaghan CA, McMichael AJ, Bowness P. Cutting edge: HLA-B27 can form a novel beta 2-microglobulin-free heavy chain homodimer structure. J Immunol 1999; 162(9):5045–5048.
66. Bird LA, Peh CA, Kollnberger S, Elliott T, McMichael AJ, Bowness P. Lymphoblastoid cells express HLA-B27 homodimers both intracellularly and at the cell surface following endosomal recycling. Eur J Immunol 2003; 33(3):748–759.
67. Wang J, Yu DT, Fukazawa T, et al. A monoclonal antibody that recognizes HLA-B27 in the context of peptides. J Immunol 1994; 152(3):1197–1205.
68. Purcell AW, Kelly AJ, Peh CA, Dudek NL, McCluskey J. Endogenous and exogenous factors contributing to the surface expression of HLA B27 on mutant APC. Hum Immunol 2000; 61(2):120–130.
69. Peh CA, Burrows SR, Barnden M, et al. HLA-B27-restricted antigen presentation in the absence of tapasin reveals polymorphism in mechanisms of HLA class I peptide loading. Immunity 1998; 8(5):531–542.
70. Benjamin RJ, Madrigal JA, Parham P. Peptide binding to empty HLA-B27 molecules of viable human cells. Nature 1991; 351(6321):74–77.
71. Khare SD, Lee S, Bull MJ, Hanson J, Luthra HS, David CS. Spontaneous inflammatory disease in HLA-B27 transgenic mice does not require transporter of antigenic peptides. Clin Immunol 2001; 98(3):364–369.
72. Zhou M, Sayad A, Simmons WA, et al. The specificity of peptides bound to human histocompatibility leukocyte antigen (HLA)-B27 influences the prevalence of arthritis in HLA-B27 transgenic rats. J Exp Med 1998; 188(5):877–886.
73. Kollnberger S, Bird L, Sun MY, et al. Cell-surface expression and immune receptor recognition of HLA-B27 homodimers. Arthritis Rheum 2002; 46(11):2972–2982.
74. Witter K, Lau M, Zahn R, Scholz S, Albert ED. Identification of a novel HLA-B*2722 allele from a Filipino cell. Tissue Antigens 2001; 58(4):263–268.

75. Garcia-Fernandez S, Gonzalez S, Mina Blanco A, et al. New insights regarding HLA-B27 diversity in the Asian population. Tissue Antigens 2001; 58(4):259–262.

76. Alvarez I, Lopez de Castro JA. HLA-B27 and immunogenetics of spondyloarthropathies. Curr Opin Rheumatol 2000; 12(4):248–253.

77. Khan MA. Update: the twenty subtypes of HLA-B27. Curr Opin Rheumatol 2000; 12(4):235–238.

78. Brown MA, Jepson A, Young A, Whittle HC, Greenwood BM, Wordsworth P. Ankylosing spondylitis in West Africans—evidence for a non-HLA-B27 protective effect. Ann Rheum Dis 1997; 56:68–70.

79. Khan MA. HLA-B27 polymorphism and association with disease. J Rheumatol 2000; 27(5):1110–1114.

80. Khan MA. HLA-B27 and its subtypes in world populations. Curr Opin Rheumatol 1995; 7:263–269.

81. Lopez-Larrea C, Sujirachato K, Mehra NK, et al. HLA-B27 subtypes in Asian patients with ankylosing spondylitis. Evidence for new associations. Tissue Antigens 1995; 45(3): 169–176.

82. Taurog JD. HLA-B27 subtypes, disease susceptibility, and peptide binding specificity. In: Calin A, Taurog JD, eds. The Spondylarthritides. Oxford: Oxford University Press, 1998:267–273.

83. Armas JB, Gonzalez S, Martinez-Borra J, et al. Susceptibility to ankylosing spondylitis is independent of the Bw4 and Bw6 epitopes of HLA-B27 allele. Tissue Antigens 1999; 53:237–253.

84. Gonzalez-Roces S, Alvarez MV, Gonzalez S, et al. HLA-B27 polymorphism and world-wide susceptibility to ankylosing spondylitis. Tissue Antigens 1997; 49(2):116–123.

85. Nasution AR, Mardjuadi A, Kunmartini S, et al. HLA-B27 subtypes positively and negatively associated with spondyloarthropathy. J Rheumatol 1997; 24(6):1111–1114.

86. Olivieri I, Padula A, Cianco G, et al. The HLA-B*2709 subtype in a patient with undifferentiated spondarthritis. Ann Rheum Dis 2000; 59(8):654–655.

87. Olivieri I, Ciancio G, Padula A, et al. The HLA-B*2709 subtype confers susceptibility to spondylarthropathy. Arthritis Rheum 2002; 46(2):553–554.

88. Brown MA, Pile KD, Kennedy LG, et al. HLA class I associations of ankylosing spondylitis in the white population in the United Kingdom. Ann Rheum Dis 1996; 55(4): 268–270.

89. Gonzalez-Roces S, Brautbar C, Pena M, et al. Molecular analysis of HLA-B27 haplotypes in Caucasoids. Frequencies of B27-Cw in Jewish and Spanish populations. Hum Immunol 1994; 41(2):127–134.

90. Breur-Vriesendorp BS, de Waal LP, Ivanyi P. Different linkage disequilibria of HLA-B27 subtypes and HLA-C locus alleles. Tissue Antigens 1988; 32(2):74–77.

91. Martinez-Borra J, Gonzalez S, Lopez-Vazquez A, et al. HLA-B27 alone rather than B27-related class I haplotypes contributes to ankylosing spondylitis susceptibility. Hum Immunol 2000; 61:131–139.

92. Sesma L, Montserrat V, Lamas JR, Marina A, Vazquez J, Lopez De Castro JA. The peptide repertoires of HLA-B27 subtypes differentially associated to spondyloarthropathy (B*2704 and B*2706) differ by specific changes at three anchor positions. J Biol Chem 2002; 277(19):16,744–749.

93. Ramos M, Paradela A, Vazquez M, Marina A, Vazquez J, Lopez de Castro JA. Differential association of HLA-B*2705 and B*2709 to ankylosing spondylitis correlates with limited peptide subsets but not with altered cell surface stability. J Biol Chem 2002; 277(32):28,749–756.

94. Schwimmbeck PL, Oldstone MB. Molecular mimicry between human leukocyte antigen B27 and Klebsiella. Consequences for spondyloarthropathies. Am J Med 1988; 85(6A):51–53.

95. Ebringer A. The cross-tolerance hypothesis, HLA-B27 and ankylosing spondylitis. Br J Rheumatol 1983; 22(4 suppl 2):53–66.

96. Benjamin R, Parham P. HLA-B27 and disease: a consequence of inadvertent antigen presentation? Rheum Dis Clin North Am 1992; 18(1):11–21.

97. Benjamin R, Parham P. Guilt by association: HLA-B27 and ankylosing spondylitis. Immunol Today 1990; 11(4):137–142.

98. Fiorillo MT, Greco G, Maragno M, et al. The naturally occurring polymorphism Asp116→His116, differentiating the ankylosing spondylitis-associated HLA-B*2705 from the non-associated HLA-B*2709 subtype, influences peptide-specific CD8 T cell recognition. Eur J Immunol 1998; 28(8):2508–2516.

99. Ramos M, Alvarez I, Sesma L, Logean A, Rognan D, Lopez de Castro JA. Molecular mimicry of an HLA-B27-derived ligand of arthritis-linked subtypes with chlamydial proteins. J Biol Chem 2002; 277(40):37,573–37,581.

100. Robinson WP, van der Linden SM, Khan MA, et al. HLA-Bw60 increases susceptibility to ankylosing spondylitis in HLA-B27+ patients. Arthritis Rheum 1989; 32(9): 1135–1141.

101. Hohler T, Schaper T, Schneider PM, Meyer zum Buschenfelde K-H, Marker-Hermann E. Association of different tumor necrosis factor α promoter allele frequencies with ankylosing spondylitis in HLA-B27 positive individuals. Arthritis Rheum 1998; 41(8):1489–1492.

102. McGarry F, Walker R, Sturrock R, Field M. The -308.1 polymorphism in the promoter region of the tumor necrosis factor gene is associated with ankylosing spondylitis independent of HLA-B27. J Rheumatol 1999; 26(5):1110–1140.

103. Milicic A, Lindheimer F, Laval S, et al. Interethnic studies of TNF polymorphisms confirm the likely presence of a second MHC susceptibility locus in ankylosing spondylitis. Genes Immun 2000; 1(7):418–422.

104. Rudwaleit M, Siegert S, Yin Z, et al. Low T cell production of TNFalpha and IFNgamma in ankylosing spondylitis: its relation to HLA-B27 and influence of the TNF-308 gene polymorphism. Ann Rheum Dis 2001; 60(1):36–42.

105. Brown MA, Rudwaleit M, Pile KD, et al. The role of germline polymorphisms in the T-cell receptor in susceptibility to ankylosing spondylitis. Br J Rheumatol 1998; 37(4): 454–458.

106. Nahal R, Gautreau C, Amor B. Genetic Investigations in familial SpA with focus on HLA region using TDT test. Arthritis Rheum 1996; 39:S122.

107. Satsangi J, Welsh KI, Bunce M, et al. Contribution of genes of the major histocompatibility complex to susceptibility and disease phenotype in inflammatory bowel disease. Lancet 1996; 347(9010):1212–1217.

108. Roussomoustakaki M, Satsangi J, Welsh K, et al. Genetic markers may predict disease behavior in patients with ulcerative colitis. Gastroenterology 1997; 112(6): 1845–1853.

109. Orchard TR, Thiyagaraja S, Welsh KI, Wordsworth BP, Hill Gaston JS, Jewell DP. Clinical phenotype is related to HLA genotype in the peripheral arthropathies of inflammatory bowel disease. Gastroenterology 2000; 118(2):274–278.

110. Laval SH, Bradbury L, Darke C, Brophy S, Calin A, Brown MA. The role of HLA-DR genes in ankylosing spondylitis complicating inflammatory bowel disease. Rheumatology 2000; 39(abstr suppl 1):64 (# 115).

111. Miceli-Richard C, Zouali H, Lesage S, et al. CARD15/NOD2 analyses in spondylarthropathy. Arthritis Rheum 2002; 46(5):1405–1406.

112. Sanmarti R, Ercilla MG, Brancos MA, Cid MC, Collado A, Rotes-Querol J. HLA class II antigens (DR, DQ loci) and peripheral arthritis in ankylosing spondylitis. Ann Rheum Dis 1987; 46(7):497–500.

113. Aaron S, Miller ML, Howard J, et al. Complementation with HLA-A and HLA-D locus alleles in ankylosing spondylitis with peripheral arthritis. J Rheumatol 1985; 12(3): 553–557.

114. Armstrong RD, Panayi GS, Welsh KI. Histocompatibility antigens in psoriasis, psoriatic arthropathy, and ankylosing spondylitis. Ann Rheum Dis 1983; 42(2):142–146.

115. Sakkas LI, Loqueman N, Bird H, Vaughan RW, Welsh KI, Panayi GS. HLA class II and T cell receptor gene polymorphisms in psoriatic arthritis and psoriasis. J Rheumatol 1990; 17(11):1487–1490.

116. Monowarul Islam SM, Numaga J, Fujino Y, et al. HLA-DR8 and acute anterior uveitis in ankylosing spondylitis. Arthritis Rheum 1995; 38(4):547–550.

117. Maksymowych WP, Jhangri GS, Gorodezky C, et al. The LMP2 polymorphism is associated with susceptibility to acute anterior uveitis in HLA-B27 positive juvenile and adult Mexican subjects with ankylosing spondylitis. Ann Rheum Dis 1997; 56(8):488–492.

118. Maksymowych WP, Adlam N, Lind D, Russell AS. Polymorphism of the LMP2 gene and disease phenotype in ankylosing spondylitis: no association with disease severity. Clin Rheumatol 1997; 16(5):461–465.

119. Maksymowych WP, Russell AS. Polymorphism in the LMP2 gene influences the relative risk for acute anterior uveitis in unselected patients with ankylosing spondylitis. Clin Invest Med 1995; 18(1):42–46.

120. Maksymowych WP, Suarez-Almazor M, Chou CT, Russell AS. Polymorphism in the LMP2 gene influences susceptibility to extraspinal disease in HLA-B27 positive individuals with ankylosing spondylitis. Ann Rheum Dis 1995; 54(4):321–324.

121. Maksymowych WP, Tao S, Vaile J, Suarez-Almazor M, Ramos-Remus C, Russell AS. LMP2 polymorphism is associated with extraspinal disease in HLA-B27 negative caucasian and mexican mestizo patients with ankylosing spondylitis. J Rheumatol 2000; 27(1):183–189.

122. Burney RO, Pile KD, Gibson K, et al. Analysis of the MHC class II encoded components of the HLA class I antigen processing pathway in ankylosing spondylitis. Ann Rheum Dis 1994; 53:58–60.

123. Westman P, Partanen J, Leirisalo-Repo M, Koskimies S. TAP1 and TAP2 polymorphism in HLA-B27-positive subpopulations: no allelic differences in ankylosing spondylitis and reactive arthritis. Hum Immunol 1995; 44:236–242.

124. Fraile A, Collado MD, Mataran L, Martin J, Nieto A. TAP1 and TAP2 polymorphism in Spanish patients with ankylosing spondylitis. Exp Clin Immunogenet 2000; 17(4):199–204.

125. Ricci-Vitiani L, Vacca A, Potolicchio I, et al. MICA gene triplet repeat polymorphism in patients with HLA-B27 positive and negative ankylosing spondylitis from Sardinia. J Rheumatol 2000; 27(9):2193–2197.

126. Tsuchiya N, Shiota M, Moriyama S, et al. MICA allele typing of HLA-B27 positive Japanese patients with seronegative spondylarthropathies and healthy individuals: differential linkage disequilibrium with HLA-B27 subtypes. Arthritis Rheum 1998; 41(1):68–73.

127. Westman P, Partanen J, Leirisalo-Repo M, Koskimies S. HSP70-Hom NcoI polymorphism and HLA-associations in the Finnish population and in patients with ankylosing spondylitis or reactive arthritis. Eur J Immunogenet 1994; 21(2):81–90.

128. Fraile A, Nieto A, Mataran L, Martin J. HSP70 gene polymorphisms in ankylosing spondylitis. Tissue Antigens 1998; 51(4 pt 1):382–385.

129. Vargas-Alarcon G, Londono JD, Hernandez-Pacheco G, et al. Heat shock protein 70 gene polymorphisms in Mexican patients with spondyloarthropathies. Ann Rheum Dis 2002; 61(1):48–51.

130. Brown MA, Pile KD, Kennedy LG, et al. A genome-wide screen for susceptibility loci in ankylosing spondylitis. Arthritis Rheum 1998; 41(4):588–595.

131. Laval SH, Timms A, Edwards S, et al. Whole-genome screening in ankylosing spondylitis: evidence of non-MHC genetic-susceptibility loci. Am J Hum Genet 2001; 68(4):918–926.

132. Lander E, Kruglyak L. Genetic dissection of complex traits: guidelines for interpreting and reporting linkage results. Nat Genet 1995; 11(3):241–247.

133. Miceli-Richard C, Hugot J-P, Said-Nahal R, Lesage S, Zouali H, Breban M. Genome-wide screen for susceptibility genes in French multiplex spondyloarthropathy families. J Rheumatol 2000; 27(suppl 59):4.

134. Zhang G, Luo J, Bruckel J, et al. Genetic studies in familial ankylosing spondylitis susceptibility. Arthritis Rheum 2004; 50(7):2246–2254.

135. Miceli-Richard C, Zouali H, Said-Nahal R, et al. Significant linkage to spondyloarthropathy on 9q31-34. Hum Mol Genet 2004; 13(15):1641–1648.

136. Beyeler C, Armstrong M, Bird HA, Idle JR, Daly AK. Relationship between genotype for the cytochrome P450 CYP2D6 and susceptibility to ankylosing spondylitis and rheumatoid arthritis. Ann Rheum Dis 1996; 55:66–68.

137. van der Paardt M, Crusius JB, Garcia-Gonzalez MA, et al. Interleukin-1beta and interleukin-1 receptor antagonist gene polymorphisms in ankylosing spondylitis. Rheumatology (Oxford) 2002; 41(12):1419–1423.

138. McGarry F, Neilly J, Anderson N, Sturrock R, Field M. A polymorphism within the interleukin 1 receptor antagonist (IL-1Ra) gene is associated with ankylosing spondylitis. Rheumatology (Oxford) 2001; 40(12):1359–1364.

139. Djouadi K, Nedelec B, Tamouza R, et al. Interleukin 1 gene cluster polymorphisms in multiplex families with spondylarthropathies. Cytokine 2001; 13(2):98–103.

140. Maksymowych WP, Reeve JP, Reveille JD, et al. High-throughput single-nucleotide polymorphism analysis of the IL1RN locus in patients with ankylosing spondylitis by matrix-assisted laser desorption ionization-time-of-flight mass spectrometry. Arthritis Rheum 2003; 48(7):2011–2018.

141. Timms AE, Crane AM, Sims AM, et al. The interleukin 1 gene cluster contains a major susceptibility locus for ankylosing spondylitis. Am J Hum Genet 2004; 75(4):587–595.

142. McGarry F, Cousins L, Sturrock RD, Field M. A polymorphism within the transforming growth factor beta 1 gene is associated with ankylosing spondylitis (AS). Rheumatology (Oxford) 2001; 41(suppl 1):16.

143. Jaakkola E, Crane AM, Laiho K, et al. The effect of transforming growth factor {beta}1 gene polymorphisms in ankylosing spondylitis. Rheumatology 2003; 30:30.

144. Hugot J-P, Chamaillard M, Zouali H, et al. Association of NOD2 leucine-rich repeat variants with susceptibility to Crohn's disease. Nature 2001; 411:599–603.

145. Ogura Y, Bonen DK, Inohara N, et al. A frameshift mutation in NOD2 associated with susceptibility to Crohn's disease. Nature 2001; 411(6837):603–606.

146. Crane AM, Bradbury L, van Heel DA, et al. Role of NOD2 variants in spondylarthritis. Arthritis Rheum 2002; 46(6):1629–1633.

147. Ferreiros-Vidal I, Amarelo J, Barros F, Carracedo A, Gomez-Reino JJ, Gonzalez A. Lack of association of ankylosing spondylitis with the most common NOD2 susceptibility alleles to Crohn's disease. J Rheumatol 2003; 30(1):102–104.

148. D'Amato M. The Crohn's associated NOD2 3020InsC frameshift mutation does not confer susceptibility to ankylosing spondylitis. J Rheumatol 2002; 29(11):2470–2471.

149. Brown MA, Brophy S, Bradbury L, et al. Identification of major loci controlling clinical manifestations of ankylosing spondylitis. Arthritis Rheum 2003; 48(8):2234–2239.

150. Edmunds L, Elswood J, Kennedy LG, Calin A. Primary ankylosing spondylitis, psoriatic and enteropathic spondyloarthropathy: a controlled analysis. J Rheumatol 1991; 18(5):696–698.

151. Sampson HW. Spondyloarthropathy in progressive ankylosis (ank/ank) mice: morphological features. Spine 1988; 13(6):645–659.

152. Krug HE, Wietgrefe MM, Ytterberg SR, Taurog JD, Mahowald ML. Murine progressive ankylosis is not immunologically mediated. J Rheumatol 1997; 24(1):115–122.

153. Krug HE, Taurog JD. HLA-B27 has no effect on the phenotypic expression of progressive ankylosis in ank/ank mice. J Rheumatol 2000; 27(5):1257–1259.

154. Ho AM, Johnson MD, Kingsley DM. Role of the mouse *ank* gene in control of tissue calcification and arthritis. Science 2000; 289:265–270.

155. Williams CJ, Zhang Y, Timms A, et al. Autosomal dominant familial calcium pyrophosphate dihydrate deposition disease is caused by mutation in the transmembrane protein ANKH. Am J Hum Genet 2002; 71(4):985–991.

156. Timms AE, Zhang Y, Bradbury L, Wordsworth BP, Brown MA. Investigation of the role of ANKH in ankylosing spondylitis. Arthritis Rheum 2003; 48(10):2898–2902.

157. Tsui FW, Tsui HW, Cheng EY, et al. Novel genetic markers in the 5′-flanking region of ANKH are associated with ankylosing spondylitis. Arthritis Rheum 2003; 48(3): 791–797.

3

Clinical Aspects of Ankylosing Spondylitis

Irene E. van der Horst-Bruinsma
Department of Rheumatology, VU University Medical Center, Amsterdam, The Netherlands

DISEASE CHARACTERISTICS OF ANKYLOSING SPONDYLITIS

Definition of the Disease

Ankylosing spondylitis (AS) is a relatively common chronic inflammatory disorder that more often manifests in young males than in females. The disease presents with low back pain and morning stiffness due to a chronic inflammation of the sacroiliac (SI) joints and vertebral column. This inflammatory process can result in destruction of the vertebral column leading to postural deformities, like ankylosis of the cervical spine and kyphosis of the thoracic spine. Extraspinal manifestations of the disease consist of arthritis of the peripheral joints (especially knees, shoulders, and hips), resulting in joint destruction that sometimes necessitates joint replacement, anterior uveitis, enthesitis, and cardiac and pulmonary complications (1,2).

The diagnosis of definite AS requires fulfillment of the modified New York criteria: obligatory are signs of a bilateral sacroiliitis grade 2–4 or unilateral sacroiliitis grade 3 or 4 plus at least one criterion out of three (inflammatory back pain, limited lumbar spinal motion in sagittal and frontal planes, and decreased chest expansion relative to normal) (3).

The onset of complaints is often gradual and the mean delay is eight years to the time of diagnosis (2). Until recently, the prevalence was estimated at 0.2% in the Caucasian population but later a prevalence up to 0.9% and even 1.4% in northern Norwegians was reported (4,5).

AS belongs to a group of diseases which are referred to as spondyloarthropathies (SpA). The group of SpA includes rheumatoid factor negative patients with inflammatory back pain and/or asymmetrical synovitis, like psoriatic arthritis, arthritis accompanying inflammatory bowel disease (IBD) (e.g., Crohn's disease), and reactive arthritis. The prevalence of SpA is estimated at 1% in the Caucasian population, which equals the prevalence of rheumatoid arthritis (RA) (5). SpA is diagnosed according to the criteria of the European Spondyloarthropathy Study Group (ESSG), which requires inflammatory spinal pain or synovitis plus a positive family history of psoriasis, IBD, alternate buttock pain, enthesiopathy, or sacroiliitis (6).

Etiology

The cause of AS is multifactorial, as in many autoimmune diseases, and based on endogenous factors, such as the very strong genetic influences of human leukocyte antigen (HLA)-B27 and exogenous factors, such as bacterial infections.

Endogenous Factors

The etiology of this chronic, familial disease is unknown. Heredity does play a major role. Familial recurrence of the disease is high and many patients belong to multi-case families.

Twin studies suggest that up to 97% of the susceptibility to AS can be attributed to genetic factors (7). The main genetic component is the increased prevalence of the HLA-B27 gene, located at chromosome 6. More than 95% of the primary Caucasian AS patients are HLA-B27 positive, whereas HLA-B27 is only present in 8% in most of the Caucasian populations (8). HLA-B27 positive first-degree relatives of patients with AS have been estimated to be 10 times more at risk to develop AS than B27-positive individuals without such family history (8).

However, genome scanning has shown that the major histocompatibility complex (MHC), including HLA-B27, contributes less than 40% to the recurrence risk ratio in AS (9).

Other potential candidates for genetic influences are the genes that encode for the production of proinflammatory cytokines, like interleukin 1 (located at chromosome 2q14), a *Interleukin 1* α and β polymorphisms, as well as the polymorphisms of its functional antagonist the *interleukin 1 receptor antagonist* gene (10). Another gene, CARD15, which plays an important role in the susceptibility to Crohn's disease, a disease which is clinically related to AS, and the gene encoding for the human transforming growth factor β1 (TGFβ1) is interesting because this cytokine is a regulator of osteoblast proliferation and plays a role in the development of osteoporosis and fibrosis, two manifestations of long standing AS (11–16).

Exogenous Factors

Apart from genetic factors, environmental factors also seem to play a role in the multifactorial causes of AS. The innate immunity could be disturbed, like in some polymorphisms of the *TLR4* and *CD14* genes, and make individuals prone to abnormal reactions after bacterial infections. The pathogenetic role of bacteria can be illustrated by the onset of another subtype of SpA, reactive arthritis. In this disease the symptoms manifest after bacterial infections, especially gastrointestinal (with Salmonella, Shigella, Yersinia, or Campylobacter) or urogenital (with *Chlamydia trachomatis*). These infections provoke the onset of reactive arthritis, but their role in the onset of AS is still under debate. However, it was suggested that HLA-B27 interferes with the elimination of bacteria and might support the onset of persistent infection (17).

The role of one of these bacteria, *C. trachomatis*, in the pathogenesis of AS is interesting. This microorganism was detected in 15–20% of the urethra swabs of male, German AS patients although a recent study did not reveal an increased prevalence of *C. trachomatis* infections in Dutch AS males compared with a group of healthy men (18,19).

Clinical Characteristics

Age at Onset

Most often the disease begins in late adolescence or early adulthood with an average age of onset at 28 years, but also occurs in children (juvenile onset) (20). The juvenile presentation is dominated by peripheral arthritis. Onset after the age of 45 years is very uncommon. The minority of patients is diagnosed after 40 years of age (6%) (21). However, at an early stage the diagnosis can be difficult because the complaints in AS are often gradual. This results in a mean delay of eight years from the first symptoms to the time of diagnosis (2). A survey of 3000 German AS patients also confirmed that the majority (90%) had the first spondylitis symptoms between 15 and 40 years (21). A small subset of patients (15%) have a juvenile onset (before age of 16 years), but in developing countries this form of AS is more common (40%) (22).

Male vs. Female Pattern

The disease is more common in males than females with a male-to-female ratio of approximately 3:1 (23,24). The age of onset might be slightly higher in females than males but the initial complaints are the same (25). Overall disease manifestations in men are most commonly located in the spine and pelvis, whereas women have more symptoms in the peripheral joints and pelvis (26–28).

The disease tends to be more severe in men. In men, a higher incidence of uveitis was observed, which lasted longer and more often resulted in visual loss than women (27). Also complete obliteration of the SI joints occurs more often in men than in women as well as an extensive spinal ankylosis (25,29). In females, radiological changes of the cervical spine are more commonly reported than in men, as well as symphysitis (29). Although a more benign disease outcome in females is often quoted, the results are contradictory.

Fertility in females with AS did not differ from the fertility rate of healthy controls (30). Pregnancy was reported as a precipitating factor for AS with a disease onset related to pregnancy until six months after delivery in 21% of the females (30).

Disease activity during pregnancy improved in only 30% of the patients, which is in contradiction with RA in which more than 70% of the patients show an improvement of the disease during pregnancy (31). Episodes of knee joint arthritis and acute anterior uveitis occurred, especially during the first and second trimester and within 4 to 12 weeks postpartum in 87% of patients. Pregnancy outcome, like complications during pregnancy and delivery, and fetal outcome, like stillbirth and spontaneous abortion, were not worse compared with healthy controls (30,32). Drugs used during pregnancy included intra-articular corticosteroid injections, low dose prednisone, nonsteroidal anti-inflammatory drugs (NSAIDs) until gestational week 32, and sulfasalazine (33).

Spinal vs. Extraspinal Manifestations

The clinical features of AS can be divided into spinal and extraspinal features. The spinal characteristics include sacroiliitis and spondylitis and skeletal complications like vertebral fractures, pseudoarthrosis, etc. The extraspinal manifestations comprise peripheral arthritis, enthesitis, uveitis, cardiovascular and pulmonary involvement, cauda equina syndrome, enteric mucosal lesions, amyloidosis, and others.

Spinal Features

The spinal involvement results in complaints of chronic inflammatory back pain (as is defined later in this chapter) with morning stiffness. This morning stiffness lasts at least one hour, but often many hours, and improves with exercise but is not relieved by rest. The low back pain is caused by inflammation of the SI joints and vertebral column. Sacroiliitis, the most important characteristic of AS, can be detected by a conventional radiograph of the pelvis which shows blurring of the distal part of the SI joints, progressing to joint space narrowing and finally sclerosis of the joints (Figs. 1 and 2). At an early stage of the disease magnetic resonance imaging (MRI) or computed tomography (CT) is more sensitive to reveal signs of SI-inflammation compared with conventional radiographs (34,35).

Pain at the cervical region and of the thoracic spine, especially with chest expansion, is caused by involvement of the cervical and costovertebral joints (Fig. 3).

The spinal inflammation coincides with the formation of syndesmophytes (Fig. 4) and squaring of the vertebrae, sometimes evolving into the classical bamboo spine (Fig. 5), which can lead to spinal ankylosis with a limited chest expansion, limited neck motion, flattening of the lumbar spine, and thoracic kyphosis. These deformities, which often evolve after more than 10 years of the disease, result in a characteristic stooped forward posture and difficulties in looking forward (36).

In a progressed disease, atlanto-axial subluxation might occur due to erosions of the transverse ligaments or other cervical structures, such as the odontoid process, resulting in neurological complaints due to myelum compression with quadriplegia even after a minor trauma of the neck (37,38).

Another possible complication of the spine is due to the decreased bone mineral density, in which case the osteoporotic spine is prone to fractures, especially

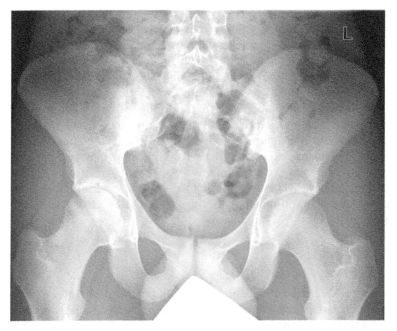

Figure 1 Sacroiliitis grade III bilaterally in a 20-year-old male with ankylosing spondylitis and joint space narrowing of the hips.

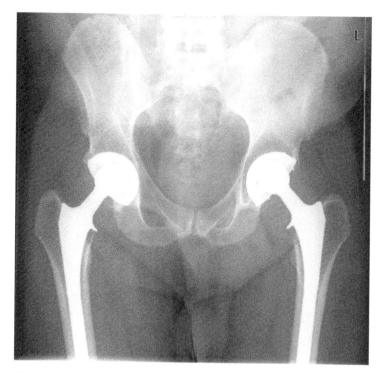

Figure 2 Sacroiliitis grade III on the right side and grade IV on the left side in combination with a total hip joint replacement on both sides in a 44-year-old male with ankylosing spondylitis. Ossification of ligamentous attachments, called "whiskering" is observed at the ischial tuberosities and at the pubic symphysis.

of the cervical spine, even after a minor trauma (39,40). Osteoporosis is more common in patients with syndesmophytes, cervical fusion, and peripheral joint involvement. Studies on bone mass density (BMD) measurement in AS focus on the generalized loss of bone measured in the lumbar spine or femoral neck, with incidence between 18% and 62% of the AS patients (41). BMD measurement at the hip is more reliable in AS because the interpretation of the BMD measured at the anteroposterior lumbar spine is difficult because of the para spinal ossification and syndesmophyte formation in more advanced diseases (42,43). Most AS patients, even after a short disease duration, show a decreased BMD, which might be explained by the chronic inflammation that could be an important determinant of bone mass loss due to the effect of osteolytic cytokines. In contrast, women with AS seem to show less severe losses of bone mass compared with male AS patients, which could be explained by protective hormonal influences in cases of premenopausal women or a lower disease activity (44,45).

Apart from the increased risk of osteoporosis, AS patients also have an increased risk of vertebral fractures (standard morbidity ratio of 7.6) (46–48). The risk of a vertebral compression fracture occurring over a 30 year period following the diagnosis of AS is 14% compared with 3.4% for population controls (41). The increased risk of a vertebral fracture seems to be related to a longer disease duration (46).

On the other hand, the risk of limb fractures, such as the hip, distal forearm, proximal humerus, and pelvis, was not significantly increased in association with AS (48).

The vulnerability of the spine in AS can be partly due to the low bone mass, but also to the rigidity of the spine which makes it prone to a fracture even after

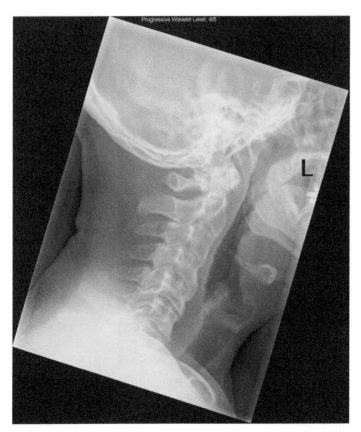

Figure 3 Lateral view of the cervical spine (in a 44-year-old male) showing ossification of the anterior ligaments and ankylosis of the facet joints of C2–C3, C3–C4, and C4–C5.

a minor trauma. Important to note is that vertebral fractures may occur silently and that the diagnosis of fractures can sometimes be difficult because the extra spinal bone formation may obscure them. Together with the possible neurological complications due to dislocation, like complete spinal cord lesions, incomplete lesions of the acute cervical central cord syndrome type, root lesion, and an incomplete quadriplegia, these fractures may result in a poor outcome (48).

Patients should be aware of this risk and adapt their lifestyle by avoiding dangerous activities. Osteoporosis should be treated in AS, even despite the male predominance and relatively young age of the patients. The treatment should be considered including exercise and the prescription of bisphosphonates, despite the fact that proper placebo-controlled trial of the efficacy on bisphosphonates in AS are missing (41).

Physicians should be aware of the increased risk of fractures even after a minor trauma and radiography of the spine should be performed at an early stage to detect these fractures and treat them adequately. Apart from conventional radiography, CT scanning and MRI are advised in case of a neck trauma because otherwise cord contusion and epidural hematoma can be missed (49).

Another spinal complication is noninfectious spondylodiscitis (Andersson lesion), which occurs in approximately 8% of AS patients, predominantly at the lumbar and thoracic level, but multiple level lesions are not uncommon. Occasionally,

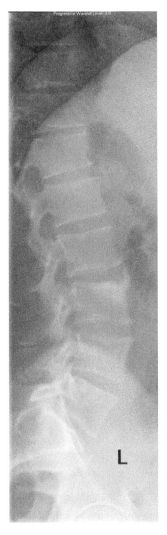

Figure 4 The lumbar spine with a syndesmophyte of the anterior site of the L3 typical for AS (40-year-old male).

a cervical discitis was described presenting with cervical pain in a previously quiescent, long-standing disease without a history of a preceding trauma (50). This sterile, destructive process in one intervertebral disc and the adjoining vertebral bodies, must be discriminated from an infectious discitis or osteomyelitis (51,52). The symptoms are renewed spinal pain, usually sharply localized and exacerbated by exercise, but most patients do not report symptoms localized to the lesion (52). In case of suspicion of spondylodiscitis, MRI scanning can detect the lesions. Important to realize is that bacterial cultures of this process should be obtained in order to exclude an infection and confirm the diagnosis of a sterile spondylodiscitis.

Extraspinal Features

Arthritis. Peripheral arthritis occurs in approximately one third of the patients, especially in the knees, hips, and shoulders (53). Hip involvement is usually

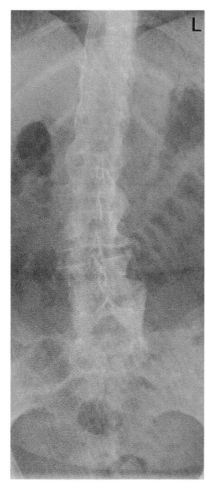

Figure 5 Bamboo spine of the thoracolumbar column in a 44-year-old female with ankylosing spondylitis, with a scoliosis, multiple syndesmophytes, and ankylosis of the SI joints (grade IV sacroiliitis). *Abbreviation*: SI, sacroiliac.

bilateral, very common in juvenile onset AS, and occurs mainly in the first 10 years of the disease. The hip joints are prone to a flexion contracture and destruction which might make total joint replacement necessary at a relatively young age (Fig. 2) (22). The shoulders are also frequently involved. Arthritis of more peripheral joints is often located in the knees, wrists, elbows, and feet, usually in an asymmetrical pattern. The radiographic features of the inflamed joints can be similar to RA, showing erosions, but in AS bony ankylosis of the wrists, tarsal bones, hips, and small joints of the fingers and toes more often occurs.

Enthesitis.   Many patients suffer from pain due to enthesitis, an extra-articular bony tenderness caused by local inflammation. Many sites can be involved, like costosternal junctions, spinous processes, iliac crests, great trochanters, ischial tuberosities, tibial tubercles, or tendons insertions, like the Achilles tendons (54). Recently, a feasible and validated enthesitis score was published, the Maastricht Ankylosing Spondylitis Enthesitis Score (MASES), which included 13 numbers of enthesis: the left and right first and seventh costochondral joints, anterior and posterior superior iliac spine, iliac crest, and proximal insertion of the Achilles tendon and the fifth lumbar spinous process (Fig. 2) (55). This MASES score (range 0–13) was at least as reliable as the older Mander enthesitis index, which included 66 sites, and more feasible in clinical practice and follow-up of clinical trials.

Ocular. Acute anterior uveitis (previously called "iridocyclitis") occurs in 25–30% of the patients and can be the first presenting symptom of the disease. In a recent study among 433 patients with different types of uveitis, 44 cases (almost 10%) of SpA were detected, whereas others showed a number of 50% of previously undiagnosed cases of SpA among uveitis patients (56–58).

The occurrence of acute anterior uveitis is increased in the HLA-B27 positive population, with a lifetime cumulative incidence of 0.2% in the general population compared with 1% in the HLA-B27 positive population (59).

The attacks of uveitis are unilateral and recurrent and cause sudden ocular pain with redness and photophobia. These attacks might lead to inflammatory debris accumulating in the anterior chamber which may cause papillary and lens dysfunction and blurring of vision. In some cases glaucoma and even blindness may occur if adequate treatment is delayed, but most of the time the uveitis subsides spontaneously within three months. It can be treated by local corticosteroids or tumor necrosis factor (TNF)-blocking agents, like infliximab, which seems to be successful in refractory uveitis (60–62). The efficacy of etanercept, another TNF-blocking agent, on uveitis seems to be controversial, because it does not seem to prevent a relapse in combination with methotrexate and it was suggested that this drug might even trigger an attack of uveitis (63,64). However, a comparison of three randomized studies with etanercept in AS showed a lower number of cases with uveitis in the etanercept-treated patients compared with placebo (65).

Gastrointestinal. Asymptomatic IBD is described in a high percentage of patients with SpA (60%) and can be detected by endoscopy of the colon and terminal ileum (66,67). These lesions can be divided into acute lesions, resembling acute bacterial infections, and chronic lesions that bear features of IBD. The chronic lesions are more often seen in association with AS, and although most of the time these enteric mucosal lesions are clinically silent, patients with chronic lesions experience significantly more episodes of diarrhea (68). During follow up studies it appeared that up to 25% of these AS patients with peripheral arthritis and chronic gut inflammation eventually develop Crohn's disease (69). On the other hand, Crohn's disease and ulcerative colitis (IBD) can manifest with sacroiliitis and peripheral arthritis, resembling AS.

Cardiovascular. Cardiac involvement can occur in long standing AS with aortic valve incompetence, due to aortitis of the ascending aorta and conduction abnormalities, caused by involvement of the atrioventricular node. Conduction disturbances in AS are due to inflammation and fibrosis of the membranous portion of the interventricular septum, thereby affecting the atrioventricular node (70). The latter sometimes requires pacemaker implantation in cases of a complete heart block. The occurrence of conduction disturbances in patients with AS varies from 1% to 33%, of aortic insufficiency from 1% to 10%, and increases with age, disease duration, and presence of peripheral arthritis (71,72). Aortic insufficiency develops because the aortic inflammatory process affects the aortic wall directly behind and above the sinuses of Valsava. This leads to scarred, fibrotic thicket, shortened aortic valve cusps, inward rolling of the edges of the cusps, and also to a dilated aortic root resulting in aortic regurgitation (73–75). Aortic regurgitation and/or variable degrees of atrioventricular or bundle branch block occur in approximately 5% of the patients. Mitral regurgitation also occurs but less often (76). The course of aortic valve incompetence often leads to heart failure in several years and the only effective therapy is valvular replacement (77,78). The incidence of atrioventricular or bundle branch block is increased among the HLA-B27 positive population, independently of the diagnosis of AS (79,80).

Other less common cardiovascular manifestations associated with AS are pericarditis, cardiomyopathy, and mitral valve disease (81).

Besides these characteristic cardiovascular lesions associated with AS, myocardial involvement may also occur, especially left ventricular dysfunction. Left ventricular dilatation, as well as a poorly contracting left ventricle and abnormal systolic time intervals, were reported in five of 28 patients with AS, and diastolic function of the left ventricle was significantly more often disturbed in AS compared with healthy controls (82,83). These findings were confirmed at necropsy in another group of AS patients, which reported an excess of connective tissue in the myocardium (73).

In conclusion, AS is associated with well-known characteristic cardiovascular manifestations, particularly conduction disturbances and aortic insufficiency. Moreover, there are some suggestions for a higher prevalence of left ventricular dysfunction and ischemic heart disease in AS.

Pulmonary. Pulmonary complications are infrequent and can be caused by rigidity of the chest wall and apical pulmonary fibrosis. In a retrospective study, an incidence of apical pulmonary fibrosis in AS was reported in 7%, based on plain radiography (84,85). This complication occurs, on average, two decades after the onset of AS, but recent studies with high resolution computed tomography (HRCT) detected interstitial lung disease in 50–70% of the patients with early AS, defined as a duration of <10 years (86–89). The changes detected with HRCT, in a small study of 26 outpatients with AS without respiratory symptoms, included signs of interstitial lung disease ($n = 16$) and a few showed signs of emphysema (four patients), apical fibrosis (two cases), or a mycetoma ($n = 1$). Plain radiography was abnormal in only four of these patients (88).

Cavities in these fibrotic parts can be infected by bacteria and fungi such as Aspergillus (90–93). These cavitations may mimic tuberculosis in one-third of the patients. Chronic Aspergillus colonization is reported in 50–65% of patients with AS, whereas 10–30% develop an aspergillosis infection (91). Treatment is based on the administration of antifungal drugs in combination with surgical resection of the cavity and removal of the fungal ball (Fig. 6) (94–97).

The inflammation of costovertebral and costotransverse joints do not seem to reduce the pulmonary function (98). The total lung and vital capacities are seldom reduced in AS patients, despite the diminished chest expansion, because the diaphragmatic function is not impaired. Therefore, the exercise tolerance is not reduced in most patients if the patients are encouraged to maintain cardiorespiratory fitness (99,100).

Renal. The incidence of renal abnormalities varies between 10% and 18% (101,102). Secondary renal amyloidosis is the most common cause of renal involvement in AS (62%), followed by Immunoglobin A (IgA)-nephropathy (30%), mesangioproliferative glomerulonephritis (5%), as well as membranous nephropathy (1%), focal segmental glomerulosclerosis (1%), and focal proliferative glomerulonephritis (1%) (103,104). However, renal amyloidosis is a very rare complication of AS (1–3% in European patients), but should be considered in case of proteinuria and/or renal failure in AS (105,106). In 7% of unselected AS patients, amyloid can be found in abdominal fat or rectal biopsies, but most do not develop clinically significant disease (107–109). Proteinuria or impaired renal function can indicate IgA-nephropathy,

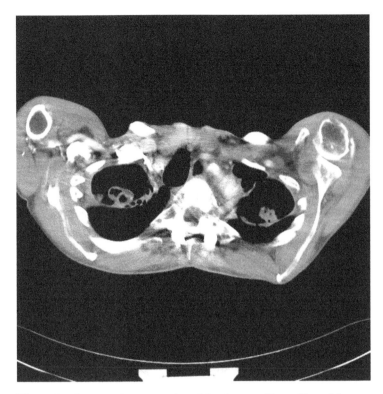

Figure 6 Computed tomography of the thorax with cavities of the upper lobes of both lungs and a parietal Aspergilloma on both sides (44-year-old male with AS).

which is interesting because of the increased serum IgA levels in AS patients (102,110,111). Also, cases of IgA multiple myeloma have been reported (112).

Neurological. Vertebral fractures, especially of the cervical spine, and cervical spine dislocations can cause neurological deficits after minor trauma, as was mentioned previously.

A slowly progressive cauda equina syndrome might occur late in the disease course as a rare complication, first described by Browie and Hauge in 1961 (113,114). The symptoms are a sensory loss in the lumbar and sacral dermatomes, less often weakness and pain in the legs, and loss of urinary and rectal sphincter tone (115,116). MRI can demonstrate arachnoiditis, with characteristic enlarged dural sacs and arachnoid diverticula, and exclude causes of myelopathies (117). One study with CT scan also showed dural calcification (118). Treatment with NSAIDs or corticosteroids alone is inappropriate to improve the neurological deficit, and often surgical treatment of the dural ectasia, by lumboperitoneal shunting or laminectomy, is necessary (119).

Hormonal. The elevated susceptibility for AS in men compared with women did suggest an etiological role for sex steroids in AS. In male patients, elevated serum testosterone and in premenopausal females lower 17β-estradiol levels were reported (120,121). It was even suggested that antiandrogenic treatment would be beneficial for AS patients (122). However, more recent studies revealed that serum testosterone levels are not elevated in male AS patients, but previously found elevations might be explained due to the use of phenylbutazone (123). Therefore, no basis is provided for antiandrogenic treatment. Also, the 17β-estradiol levels in later studies did not differ between AS patients and controls (124,125).

The influence of hormones like prolactin and growth hormone, which might have a proinflammatory effect, was recently studied in men with AS and RA. No unregulated responses of these hormones were found after stimulation with insulin hypoglycemia, in comparison with healthy controls (126).

Diagnostic Procedures

Symptoms

An important clue to the diagnosis of AS is a positive family history of AS or other associated spondylarthropathies. Familial aggregation of AS has been known for many years and a positive family history can be found in 15% to 20% of the cases (2,127,128). A positive family history is one of the important clues to detect early cases of spondylarthritis in patients with inflammatory back pain (Table 1) (128).

One of the major symptoms is typical pain in the buttock and lower lumbar region which is accompanied by a few hours morning stiffness and improves with activity. The worst complaints are often at night and early in the morning. The inflammatory back pain can be insidious at onset but usually becomes persistent within a few months. Inflammatory back pain is defined as: onset before 40 years of age, insidious onset, duration of the back pain longer than three months, morning stiffness, and improvement of the symptoms with exercise.

Sacroiliitis causes unilateral pain in the buttock that sometimes radiates down the thighs but not below the knee. Impaired movement of the back and neck occurs later in the disease.

In other patients bone pain, caused by enthesitis, is the first symptom which often presents in heel pain, due to inflammation at the Achilles tendon insertion to the calcaneus. Other enthesitis lesions are the plantar fascia, sternal and costochondral sites, and the large tendon insertions of extremities.

Thoracic pain, increased by deep breathing, coughing, or laughter, can be caused by inflammation of the costovertebral joints. Thoracic spine involvement can also cause anterior chest pain with a shortness of breath on activity, caused by a limited respiratory excursion in a progressed disease.

In patients with severe involvement and rigidity of the spine, spinal fractures can occur even after a minor trauma, due to osteoporosis of the spine. The signs of this fracture can be acute pain in the vertebral column or increased mobility of a previously immobilized spine. The spinal fracture can also result in neurological deficit with long-tract signs, including quadriplegia.

Asymmetrical pain and swelling of the knee, hip, ankle, or shoulder or metatarsal joints often occur, caused by oligoarthritis. Sometimes the temporomandibular joints may be affected, leading to a reduced mouth opening and discomfort on chewing, but this is more common in patients with RA. Dactylitis, with pain and a sausage-like swelling of a finger or toe, can be caused by an inflammation of the proximal interphalangeal (PIP) and distal interphalangeal (DIP) joints and can be found in AS but is more common in psoriatic arthritis.

Fatigue is common and is partly caused by a disturbed sleep pattern due to pain and stiffness. Other constitutional features include fever and weight loss.

Ocular features can present as attacks of acute pain, redness of the eye, and blurred vision in case of acute anterior uveitis, which occur in one-third of the patients.

Altered bowel habits with diarrhea and abdominal distension require investigation, because 60% of AS patients suffers from subclinical inflammatory changes

Table 1 Diagnostic Procedures of Ankylosing Spondylitis

Symptoms
Positive family history of ankylosing spondylitis
Inflammatory back pain
Thoracic pain
Fractures of the spine after minor trauma
Oligoarthritis
Anterior uveitis
Diarrhea
Shortness of breath
Physical examination
Blood pressure
Pulse rate
Skin: psoriatic lesions?
Eyes: redness, irregular pupil?
Heart: murmur?
Lungs
Abdomen
Costovertebral, costotransverse and manubriosternal joints
Cervical spine: flexion, extension, rotation, occiput to wall distance
Thoracic spine: chest expansion
Lumbar spine; Schober's test, fingers–floor distance, lateral flexion
Peripheral joints: arthritis?
Enthesitis lesions?
Laboratory tests
Erythrocyte sedimentation rate or C-reactive protein
Blood count
HLA-B27 antigen (in case of doubt of diagnosis)
Urine: erythrocytes, protein?
Radiology
Pelvis: sacroiliitis, hip involvement?
Cervical, thoracic, lumbar spine

Abbreviation: HLA, human leukocyte antigen.

of the small or large bowel and NSAIDs will be less well tolerated because they can also induce bowel inflammation (66).

Shortness of breath on exertion can, apart from thoracic stiffness, also be caused by cardiac or pulmonary complications of AS. Cardiovascular involvement includes cardiac conduction abnormalities or aortitis with dilatation of the aortic valve ring. Pulmonary involvement, with progressive upper lobe fibrosis, can also cause breathlessness.

Physical Examination

Physical examination should include measurement of the blood pressure to exclude hypertension in case of renal involvement (or aortic insufficiency) and pulse frequency to detect bradycardia in case of atrioventricular conduction disturbances.

The skin and nails should be examined to detect psoriatic lesions, especially in the ears, scalp, natal region, extension surfaces of the elbows and knees, and pitting lesions of the nails. The eyes should be inspected to detect redness, which might be caused by conjunctivitis or even an attack of acute anterior uveitis, in case of pain and blurred vision. An irregular pupil could be the result of an attack of uveitis in the past with synechiae to the cornea or lens, which might cause glaucoma in the long run.

Examination of the heart can detect a murmur caused by aortic insufficiency or bradycardia due to conduction abnormalities. The chest might show signs of a limited chest expansion and signs of apical fibrosis, although these lung deformities often can only be detected by radiographic procedures. The abdomen should also be examined, but signs of IBD are detected most often only with ileocolonoscopy.

Physical examination of the spine involves the cervical, thoracic, and lumbar region. Cervical involvement, which often occurs late in the disease, can result in a limited flexion, extension, rotation, or lateral flexion, but limitation in several directions often occurs. The stooping of the neck can be measured by the occiput-to-wall distance. The patient stands with the back and heels against the wall and the distance between the back of the head and the wall is measured. Another method is the tragus–wall test which measures the distance between the tragus of the ear and the wall. Loss of lateral rotation also occurs and eventually the neck may lose all motion and become fixed in a flexed position.

The thoracic spine can be tested by chest expansion, which normally exceeds 5 cm, but is age- and sex-dependent, with lower expansion in females compared with males and decreasing with age. It is measured at the fourth intercostal space and in women just below the breasts. The patient should be asked to force a maximal inspiration and expiration and the difference in chest expansion is measured. A chest expansion of less than 5 cm is suspicious and < 2.5 cm is abnormal and raises the possibility of AS unless there is another reason for it, like emphysema. In progressed AS, the anterior chest wall becomes flattened, shoulders become stooped, the abdomen becomes protuberant, and the breathing diaphragmatic. The normal thoracic kyphosis of the dorsal spine becomes accentuated.

The costovertebral, costotransverse, and manubriosternal joints should be palpated to detect inflammation, which causes pain on palpitation.

The lumbar spine can be tested by the ability of the patient bending forward to touch the floor with the fingertips with the knees fully extended. However, this test can be less reliable in case of limitations in the motion of the hips. A more appropriate test to detect limitation of the forward flexion of the lumbar spine is the Schober's test. This is performed by making a mark between the posterior superior iliac spines ("dimples of Venus") at the fifth lumbar spinous process. A second mark is placed 10 cm above the first one and the patient is asked to bend forward with extended knees. The distance between the two marks increases from 10 to at least 15 cm in normal people, but only to 13 cm or less in case of AS. Lumbar lateral flexion can be tested by the patient standing erect with the arms along side the body and by moving laterally with the fingers over the lateral side of the leg. The distance between the fingertips and the floor can be measured and the measurement can be repeated on the other side.

Tests to detect active sacroiliitis by palpation or other maneuvers, like hyperextension of the lumbar spine or hyperextension of one hip joint, are not very specific because the pain caused by these tests could also result from enthesitis or arthritis of the hip, and therefore are not recommended.

All peripheral joints should be investigated to look for signs of synovitis (pain, tenderness, swelling, and limited motion). The hips and shoulder are most often involved, in one-third of the patients, and any limitations in function should be recorded early in the disease in order to detect progression later. Other joints often involved are the knees, wrists, elbows, and feet. The presentation is usually asymmetric and often monoarticular or oligoarticular.

Enthesitis lesion can be detected by palpation of the locations described above in the MASES-index.

Laboratory Tests

Only 50% to 70% of the patients with an active disease show an elevated erythrocyte sedimentation rate (ESR) or a raised C-reactive protein (CRP) (129–131). These acute phase reactants seem to show a higher correlation with peripheral involvement of AS than with spinal disease activity.

In contrast with RA, these acute phase reactants do not have a high correlation with the disease activity of AS, and elevation is more often observed in case of extra-spinal manifestations than in case of more axial involvement. Therefore, their value as an outcome parameter for disease activity in therapeutic trials in AS is limited.

The platelet count may also be slightly elevated and a mild normochromic, normocytic anemia, due to a chronic disease, is common in 15% of the patients.

Positive tests for the rheumatoid factor and antinuclear antibodies (ANA) do not occur more often than in healthy controls (2,132).

The HLA-B27 antigen is present in the majority of the AS patients, but this test is inappropriate to confirm the diagnosis, which is primarily based on history, physical examination, and radiographic evidence of sacroiliitis. In adolescent patients, where the radiographic confirmation of sacroiliitis can be difficult, HLA-B27 testing could be helpful to establish the diagnosis.

Raised alkaline phosphatase, primarily derived from bone, and serum IgA levels are common in AS. The urine might show protein or erythrocytes in case of renal involvement.

Radiology

The radiograph of the pelvis is necessary to assess the SI joints, which might show signs of sacroiliitis, an obligatory sign for the diagnosis of AS. The severity of this sacroiliitis can be graded from 0 (no abnormalities) to grade IV (complete ankylosis of the SI joints) I (Figs. 1, 2 and 5). At early stages of the disease, signs of sacroiliitis can be detected with CT and MRI before the abnormalities are present at the plain radiograph of the pelvis (34,35).

Also, the vertebral column often shows characteristic changes, like bony sclerosis with squaring of the vertebral bodies and ossification of the annulus fibrosis with syndesmophytes (Figs. 3–5). This might lead to fusion of the vertebral column with a classical bamboo spine aspect on the radiograph of the lumbar region.

Involvement of the hip and shoulder joints with joint space narrowing can be detected by conventional X-rays.

Differential Diagnosis

The diagnosis of AS can be confirmed by the modified New York criteria as mentioned above. AS belongs to the group of diseases called SpA, which have inflammatory back pain as a common feature and are defined by the ESSG-criteria, as described previously. The other types of SpA include psoriatic arthritis, IBD such as ulcerative colitis and Crohn's disease, reactive arthritis, juvenile SpA, and a group of undifferentiated SpA (Table 2). The majority of affected individuals with SpA possess the HLA-B27 antigen.

Table 2   Differential Diagnosis of Ankylosing Spondylitis

Other types of spondyloarthropathy
Psoriatic arthritis
Inflammatory bowel disease: ulcerative colitis or Crohn's disease
Reactive arthritis
Juvenile spondyloarthropathy
Other types of arthritis
Rheumatoid arthritis
Other causes of back pain
Noninflammatory back pain
Fibromyalgia
Spine diseases: prolapsed intervertebral disc, spinal tumors, bone tumors
Infections: tuberculosis, and others
Metabolic diseases
Diffuse idiopathic skeletal hyperosthosis (DISH or Forestier'disease)
Other causes of sacroiliitis
Osteitis condensans ilii, septic sacroiliitis, paraplegia, Paget's disease, dialysis associated
   spondylarthropathy, hyperparathyroidism, etc.

Psoriatic arthritis occurs in 5% to 7% of the people with psoriasis. The psoriatic arthritis can present as a mono- or oligoarthritis, resembling the reactive arthritis pattern, or as a symmetrical polyarthritis, resembling RA, but with involvement of the DIP joints (instead of the PIP joints in RA) and without a positive rheumatoid factor. Axial disease occurs in about 5% of the psoriasis patients. Axial involvement may occur independent from peripheral arthritis and is often asymptomatic, but symptoms of inflammatory back pain or chest wall pain may be present. Sacroiliitis is observed in one-third of the patients and frequently asymmetric. Spondylitis may occur without sacroiliitis and may result in fusion of the spine. Enthesitis is common, especially in the oligoarticular form of the disease. The radiographic features of the spine in case of psoriatic spondylitis show more or less random syndesmophyte formation, whereas in AS, syndesmophytes form in a more ascending fashion (133).

In 10% to 20% of patients with IBD, like ulcerative colitis and Crohn's disease, peripheral arthritis occurs (134). Most often the knees, ankles, and feet are affected. Large-joint effusions, especially of the knee, are common. In 10% of the patients with IBD, sacroiliitis or spondylitis occurs and is often asymptomatic (134). The course of the spondylitis is independent of the active bowel inflammation.

Reactive arthritis refers to a mono- or oligoarthritis, which occurs after an infection of the genitourinary (with *C. trachomatis*), gastrointestinal tract (with Salmonella, Shigella, Yersina, or Campylobacter bacteria), or sometimes after a respiratory infection with *Chlamydia pneumoniae*. The arthritis usually occurs two to four weeks after the primary infection, presenting as an urethritis or a period of diarrhea. Conjunctivitis, with crusting of the eyelids in the morning, can accompany the urethritis, but an acute anterior uveitis might also occur. The combination of arthritis, conjunctivitis and urethritis is also known as Reiter's syndrome. The joint involvement is asymmetrical and located predominantly in the knees, ankles, and small joints of the feet, but joints of the upper extremities (wrists, elbows, and hand joints) can also be affected. The large joints show signs of synovitis whereas the small joints of the hands and feet present as sausage digits or dactylitis. The course of reactive arthritis is self limiting with 3 to 12 months in the majority of the patients, and the treatment consists of nonsteroidal anti-inflammatory drugs (NSAIDs) whereas antibiotic treatment is not indicated.

RA can manifest with a mono- or oligoarticular onset, but has most often a symmetrical polyarthritis. RA can be distinguished from AS by the absence of inflammatory back pain, the presence of the positive rheumatoid factor, in 60% to 70% of the patients, and because it is more often associated with an increased ESR or CRP. The radiological features of RA, with erosions of the small joints of hands and feet, differ from AS.

Juvenile SpA applies to a diagnosis made before the age of 16 and belongs to the group of juvenile idiopathic arthritis (JIA). Most patients are boys and HLA-B27 positive and the tests for the rheumatoid factor and ANA are usually negative. The symptoms mainly involve arthritis of the large joints of the lower extremities, especially the hip joint, which predicts a severe course of the disease. Enthesitis is common, as well as lower back or buttock pain. Acute anterior uveitis occurs in 5% to 10% of the patients. Plain radiographs of the SI joints and the lumbar spine often do not show abnormalities for many years. Treatment is based on NSAIDs and sulfasalazine is added in case of persistent arthritis (135,136).

Diagnoses resembling the complaints of AS are other syndromes or diseases that affect the spine, like a prolapsed intervertebral disc, fibromyalgia, spinal tumors like chordoma or ependymoma, bone tumors like osteoid osteoma, plasmacytoma, bone metastases, or leukemic infiltration, and infections of the spinal or SI joints like tuberculosis and brucellosis. Metabolic bone diseases like osteomalacia, hypophosphatemia, and rickets can also cause back pain. The noninflammatory back pain is, in most cases, aggravated by activity and relieved by rest and is not associated with a limited chest expansion or a limited lateral flexion of the lumbar spine.

Diffuse idiopathic skeletal hyperostosis (DISH or Forestier's disease) can resemble AS because of the stiffness of the spine due to hyperostosis of the anterior longitudinal ligaments and bony attachments of the tendons. Occasionally the SI joints show hyperostotic changes resembling sacroiliitis, but in most cases of DISH, this feature is absent. However, in contrast with AS, the onset of the disease is at a later age (over 50), there is no association with HLA-B27 and there are more flowing ligamentous ossifications but less syndesmophyte formations.

Radiographic signs of sacroiliitis must be distinguished from osteitis condensans ilii, which consists of a symmetric sclerosis on the iliac sides of both SI joints without erosions seen in women who have borne children (53).

DISEASE OUTCOME

In many cases the disease outcome is favorable, but approximately one-third of the patients develop disabling deformities (2). A few studies showed that the outcome of AS can be predicted by several disease characteristics during the first 10 years of AS (137–140). Predictors of a severe outcome are hip arthritis, an increased erythrocyte sedimentation rate (ESR > 0 mm/hr), peripheral arthritis and a juvenile onset (≤16 years). The rate of radiological progression appears to be constant during the several decades of the disease duration and is not higher in the first decade as was previously thought (141). However, most patients who have mild spinal restriction after the first decade of their disease do not progress to severe spinal involvement during later years. Because AS starts at a young age, the socioeconomic consequences are high. Apart from the physical complaints, many patients struggle with work disability.

This subject was recently studied by Boonen in the Netherlands (142). The age- and sex-adjusted risk of work withdrawal was three times higher in AS compared with the figures of the general Dutch population.

The stage of the disease at the time of diagnosis and the delay of appropriate treatment also influence the outcome of the disease. Women appear to have a later age of onset and a milder disease compared with men (24–30).

The majority of AS patients possess the HLA-B27 antigen (>95%), which is found to be associated with the onset of the disease. The relationship of this antigen with disease severity of AS is less obvious. In HLA-B27 negative patients, a later age of onset, and less frequent occurrence of acute anterior uveitis and less familial aggregation, was described (143). Also, HLA-B27 homozygous individuals seem to develop a more severe disease compared with HLA-B27 heterozygotes (144).

There are conflicting data regarding mortality in patients with AS. One population-based study showed no difference in mortality between males with AS and the general male population (145). Other studies indicated that mortality in AS, patients seen at referral centers was higher than expected with standardized mortality ratios (SMR) of approximately 1.7 (range 1.5–1.9) (146–149). This might be due to a linear relation observed between disease severity and mortality as well as associations found between disease duration and mortality (149–151). Among older patients, X-ray treatment, which was used until 1960, might be a factor in the increased mortality risk of 4.8 due to leukemia and other types of cancer among these patients (151).

TREATMENT

NSAIDs and physical therapy seem to improve the long-term outcome of AS (152,153). However, the effect of disease modifying antirheumatic drugs (DMARDs) is less impressive compared with their effect in RA. In placebo-controlled trials, sulfasalazine showed some improvement of disease activity, especially in SpA patients with peripheral arthritis (154,155). Altogether the number of therapeutic options for AS is limited and other drugs, such as methotrexate, leflunomide, or thalidomide, will be explored further in placebo-controlled trials (156).

However, the therapeutic possibilities in AS have changed since the introduction of biologicals, especially drugs that block the effect of the proinflammatory cytokine TNFα. After a few successful pilot studies with antiTNF therapy (infliximab and etanercept) in AS, large placebo-controlled trials confirmed the efficacy of the biologicals in these patients in disease activity, as well as in regression of MRI changes (157–159). These new therapies will undoubtedly change the outcome and prognosis of AS dramatically in the forthcoming years.

REFERENCES

1. Zeidler H, Schumacher HR. Spondylarthropathies. Baillieres Clin Rheumatol 1998; 12(4):551–583, 695–715.
2. Calin A, Taurog JD. The Spondylarthritides. Oxford: Oxford University Press, 1998.
3. van der Linden S, Valkenburg HA, Cats A. Evaluation of the diagnostic criteria for ankylosing spondylitis; a proposal for the modification of the New York criteria. Arthritis Rheum 1984; 27:361–368.

4. Gran JT, Husby G, Hordvik M. Prevalence of ankylosing spondylitis in males and females in a young middle–aged population of Tromso, northern Norway. Ann Rheum Dis 1985; 44:359–367.

5. Braun J, Bollow M, Remlinger G, et al. Prevalence of spondylarthropathies in HLA-B27 positive and negative blood donors. Arthritis Rheum 1998; 41:58–67.

6. Dougados M, van der Linden S, Juhlin R, et al. The European spondylarthropathy study group preliminary criteria for the classification of spondylarthropathy. Arthritis Rheum 1991; 34:1218–1227.

7. Brown MA, Kennedy LG, MacGregor AJ, et al. Susceptibility to ankylosing spondylitis. The role of genes, HLA and the environment. Arthritis Rheum 1997; 40:1823–1828.

8. van der Linden SM, Valkenburg HA, de Jongh BM, Cats A. The risk of developing ankylosing spondylitis in HLA-B27 positive individuals. A comparison of relatives of spondylitis patients with the general population. Arthritis Rheum 1984; 27(3):241–249.

9. Laval SH, Timms A, Edwards S, et al. Whole-genome screening in ankylosing spondylitis: evidence of non-MHC genetic-susceptibility loci. Am J Hum Genet 2001; 68(4): 918–926.

10. van der Paardt M, van der Horst-Bruinsma IE, Crusius JBA, et al. Interleukin-1 beta and interleukin-1 receptor antagonist gene polymorphisms in the susceptibility to ankylosing spondylitis. Rheumatology 2002; 41:1419–1423.

11. Hugot JP, Chamaillard M, Zouali H, et al. Association of NOD2 leucine-rich repeat variants with susceptibility to Crohn's disease. Nature 2001; 411(6837):599–603.

12. Ogura Y, Bonen DK, Inohara N, et al. A frameshift mutation in NOD2 associated with susceptibility to Crohn's disease. Nature 2001; 411(6837):603–606.

13. Hampe J, Cuthbert A, Croucher PJ, et al. Association between insertion mutation in NOD2 gene and Crohn's disease in German and British populations. Lancet 2001; 357(9272):1925–1928.

14. van der Paardt M, Crusius JBA, de Koning MHMT, et al. CARD 15 gene mutations are not associated with ankylosing spondylitis. Genes Immun 2003; 4:77–78.

15. Massague J. The transforming growth factor-beta family. Annu Rev Cell Biol 1990; 6:597–641.

16. van der Paardt M, Crusius JBA, García-González MA, Dijkmans BAC, Peña AS, van der Horst-Bruinsma IE. Susceptibility to ankylosing spondylitis: no evidence for the involvement of transforming growth factor B1 gene polymorphisms. Ann Rheum Dis 2005; 64(4):616–619.

17. Koehler L, Zeidler H, Hudson AP. Aetiological agents: their molecular biology and phagocyte–host interaction. Baillieres Clin Rheumatol 1998; 12(4):589–609.

18. Lange U, Berliner M, Weidner W, Schiefer HG, Schmidt KL, Federlin K. Ankylosing spondylitis and urogenital infection: diagnosis of urologic infection and correlation with rheumatologic findings. Z Rheumatol 1996; 55(4):249–255.

19. van der Paardt M, van Denderen JC, van den Brule AJC, et al. Prevalence of *Chlamydia trachomatis* in urine of male patients with ankylosing spondylitis is not increased. Ann Rheum Dis 2000; 59:300–303.

20. Brophy S, Calin A. Ankylosing spondylitis: interaction between genes, joints, age at onset, and disease expression. J Rheumatol 2001; 28:2283–2288.

21. Feldtkeller E. Age at disease onset and delayed diagnosis of spondylarthropathies. Z Rheumatol 1999; 58:21–30.

22. Burgos-Vargas R, Vazquez-Mellado J. The early clinical recognition of juvenile onset ankylosing spondylitis and its differentiation from juvenile rheumatoid arthritis. Arthritis Rheum 1995; 38:835–844.

23. Calin A, Fries JF. Striking prevalence of ankylosing spondylitis in "healthy" w27 positive males and females. A controlled study. N Engl J Med 1975; 293:835–839.

24. Will R, Edmunds L, Elswood J, Calin A, et al. Is there a sexual inequality in ankylosing spondylitis? A study of 498 women and 1202 men. J Rheumatol 1990; 17:1649–1652.

25. Gran JT, Ostensen M, Husby G, et al. A clinical comparison between males and females with ankylosing spondylitis. J Rheumatol 1985; 12:126–129.

26. Braunstein EM, Martel W, Moidel R. Ankylosing spondylitis in men and women: a clinical and radiographic comparison. Radiology 1982; 144:91–94.

27. Jiminez-Balderas F, Mintz G. Ankylosing spondylitis: a clinical course in women and men. J Rheumatol 1993; 20:2069–2072.

28. Resnick D, Niwayama G. Ankylosing Spondylitis. In: Resnick D, ed. Diagnosis of bone and joint disorders. 3rd edition. Philadelphia: WB Saunders; 1995:1008–1074.

29. Ostensen M, Fuhrer L, Mathieu R, et al. A prospective study of pregnant patients with rheumatoid arthritis and ankylosing spondylitis using validated clinical instruments. Ann Rheum Dis 2004; 63:1212–1217.

30. Ostensen M, Ostensen H. Ankylosing spondylitis—the female aspect. J Rheumatol 1998; 25(1):120–124.

31. Ostensen M. The effect of pregnancy on ankylosing spondylitis, psoriatic arthritis, and juvenile rheumatoid arthritis. Am J Reprod Immunol 1992; 28:235–237.

32. Ostensen M, Romberg O, Husby G. Ankylosing spondylitis and motherhood. Arthritis Rheum 1982; 25(2):140–143.

33. Ostensen M, Fuhrer L, Mathieu R, Seitz M, Villiger PM. A prospective study of pregnant patients with rheumatoid arthritis and ankylosing spondylitis using validated clinical instruments. Ann Rheum Dis 2004; 63(10):1212–1217.

34. Oostveen J, Prevo R, den Boer J, et al. Early detection of sacroiliitis on magnetic resonance imaging and subsequent development of sacroiliitis on plain radiography. A prospective, longitudinal study. J Rheumatol 1999; 26:1953–1958.

35. Braun J, Bollow M, Eggens U, et al. Use of dynamic magnetic resonance imaging with fast imaging in the detection of early and advanced sacroiliitis in spondylarthropathy patients. Arthritis Rheum 1994; 37:1039–1045.

36. Khan MA. Ankylosing spondylitis: clinical aspects. In: Calin A, Taurog J, eds. The Spondylarthritides. Oxford: Oxford University Press, 1998.

37. Ramos-Remus C, Gomez-Vargas A, Guzman-Guzman JL, et al. Frequency of atlanto-axial subluxation and neurologic involvement in patients with ankylosing spondylitis. J Rheumatol 1995; 22:2120.

38. Thompson GH, Khan MA, Bilenker RM, et al. Spontaneous atlantoaxial subluxation as presenting manifestation of juvenile ankylosing spondylitis. Spine 1982; 7:78–79.

39. Gratacos J, Collado A, Pons F, et al. Significant loss of bone mass in patient with early, active ankylosing spondylitis: follow up study. Arthritis Rheum 1999; 42(11):2319–2324.

40. Toussirot E, Michel F, Wendling D. Bone density, ultrasound measurements and body composition in early ankylosing spondylitis. Rheumatology 2001; 40(8):882–888.

41. Bessant R, Keat A. How should clinicians manage osteoporosis in ankylosing spondylitis? J Rheumatol 2002; 29:1511–1519.

42. Dos Santos FP, Constantin A, Laroche M, et al. Whole body and regional bone mineral density in ankylosing spondylitis. J Rheumatol 2001; 28(3):547–549.

43. Singh A, Bronson W, Walker SE, Allen SH. Relative value of femoral and lumbar bone mineral density assessments in patients with ankylosing spondylitis. South Med J 1995; 88(9):939–943.

44. Juanola X, Mateo L, Nolla JM, Roig-Vilaseca D, Campoy E, Roig-Escofet D. Bone mineral density in women with ankylosing spondylitis. J Rheumatol 2000; 27:1028–1031.

45. Speden DJ, Calin AI, Ring FJ, Bhalla AK. Bone mineral density, calcaneal ultrasound, and bone turnover markers in women with ankylosing spondylitis. J Rheumatol 2002; 29(3):516–521.

46. Mitra D, Elvins DM, Speden DJ, Collins AJ. The prevalence of vertebral fractures in mild ankylosing spondylitis and their relationship to bone mineral density. Rheumatology (Oxford) 2000; 39(1):85–89.

47. Donnelly S, Doyle DV, Denton A, Rolfe I, McCloskey EV, Spector TD. Bone mineral density and vertebral compression fracture rates in ankylosing spondylitis. Ann Rheum Dis 1994; 53(2):117–121.

48. Ralston SH, Urquhart GD, Brzeski M, Sturrock RD. Prevalence of vertebral compression fractures due to osteoporosis in ankylosing spondylitis. Br Med J 1990; 300(6724): 563–565.

49. Nakstad PH, Server A, Josefsen R. Traumatic cervical injuries in ankylosing spondylitis. Acta Radiol 2004; 45:222–226.

50. Rasker JJ, Prevo RL, Lanting PJH. Spondylodiscitis in ankylosing spondylitis, inflammation or trauma? Scand J Rheumatol 1996; 25:52–57.

51. Dihlmann W, Delling G. Disco-vertebral destructive lesions (so-called Andersson lesions) associated with ankylosing spondylitis. Skeletal Radiol 1978; 3:10–16.

52. Kabaskal Y, Garrett SL, Calin A, et al. The epidemiology of spondylodiscitis in ankylosing spondylitis, a controlled study. Br J Rheum 1996; 35:660–663.

53. Resnick D, Niwayama G. Ankylosing spondylitis. In: Resnick D, ed. Diagnosis of Bone and Joint Disorders. 3rd ed. Philadelphia, PA: WB Saunders, 1995:1008–1074.

54. McGonagle D, Khan MA, Marzo-Ortega H, et al. Enthesitis in ankylosing spondylitis and related spondylarthropathies. Curr Opin Rheumatol 1999; 11:244–250.

55. Heuft-Dorenbosch L, Spoorenberg A, Tubergen A, et al. Assessment of enthesitis in ankylosing spondylitis. Ann Rheum Dis 2003; 62:127–132.

56. Linder R, Hoffmann A, Brunner R. Prevalence of the spondyloarthritides in patients with uveitis. J Rheumatol 2004; 31(11):2226–2229.

57. Monnet D, Breban M, Hudry C, Dougados M, Brezin AP. Ophthalmic findings and frequency of extraocular manifestations in patients with HLA-B27 uveitis: a study of 175 cases. Ophthalmology 2004; 111(4):802–809.

58. Pato E, Banares A, Jover JA, et al. Undiagnosed spondyloarthropathy in patients presenting with anterior uveitis. J Rheumatol 2000; 27(9):2198–2202.

59. Linssen A, Rothova A, Valkenburg HA, et al. The lifetime cumulative incidence of acute anterior uveitis in a normal population and its relation to ankylosing spondylitis and histocompatibility antigen HLA-B27. Invest Ophthalmol Vis Sci 1991; 32(9):2568–2578.

60. Kruithof E, Kestelyn P, Elewaut C, et al. Successful use of infliximab in a patient with treatment resistant spondyloarthropathy related uveitis. Ann Rheum Dis 2002; 61(5):470.

61. El-Shabrawi Y, Hermann J. Anti-tumor necrosis factor-alpha therapy with infliximab as an alternative to corticosteroids in the treatment of human leukocyte antigen B27-associated acute anterior uveitis. Ophthalmology 2002; 109(12):2342–2346.

62. Murphy CC, Ayliffe WH, Booth A, Makanjuola D, Andrews PA, Jayne D. Tumor necrosis factor alpha blockade with infliximab for refractory uveitis and scleritis. Ophthalmology 2004; 111(2):352–356.

63. Foster CS, Tufail F, Waheed NK, et al. Efficacy of etanercept in preventing relapse of uveitis controlled by methotrexate. Arch Ophthalmol 2003; 121(4):437–440.

64. Reddy AR, Backhouse OC. Does etanercept induce uveitis? Br J Ophthalmol 2003; 87(7):925.

65. Rosenbaum JT. Effect of etanercept on iritis in patients with ankylosing spondylitis. Arthritis Rheum 2004; 50(11):3736–3737.

66. Mielants H, Veys EM, Cuvelier C, De Vos M. Ileocolonoscopy and spondarthritis. Br J Rheumatol 2003; 27(2):163–164.

67. De Keyser F, Mielants H. The gut in ankylosing spondylitis and other spondyloarthropathies: inflammation beneath the surface. J Rheumatol 2003; 30(11):2306–2307.

68. Mielants H, Veys EM, Goemaere S, Goethals K, Cuvelier C, De Vos M. Gut inflammation in the spondyloarthropathies: clinical, radiologic, biologic, and genetic features in relation to the type of histology. A prospective study. J Rheumatol 1991; 18(10): 1542–1551.

69. Mielants H, Veys EM, Cuvelier C, et al. The evolution of spondyloarthropathies in relation to gut histology. II. Histological aspects. J Rheumatol 1995; 22(12):2273–2278.
70. Youssef W, Russell AS. Cardiac, ocular, and renal manifestations of seronegative spondyloarthropathies. Curr Opin Rheumatol 1990; 2:582–585.
71. O'Neill TW, Bresnihan B. The heart in ankylosing spondylitis. Ann Rheum Dis 1992; 51:705–706.
72. Peters MJ, van der Horst-Bruinsma IE, Dijkmans BAC, Nurmohamed MT. Cardiovascular risk profile of patients with spondylarthropathies, particularly ankylosing spondylitis and psoriatic arthritis. Semin Arthr Rheum 2004; 34:585–592.
73. Brewerton DA, Goddard DH, Moore RB, et al. The myocardium in ankylosing spondylitis: a Clinical, echocardiographic, and histopathological study. Lancet 1987; 1(8540): 995–998.
74. Gould BA, Turner J, Keeling DH, et al. Myocardial dysfunction in ankylosing spondylitis. Ann Rheum Dis 1992; 51:227–232.
75. Nagyhegyi G, Nadas I, Banyai F, et al. Cardiac and cardiopulmonary disorders in patients with ankylosing spondylitis and rheumatoid arthritis. Clin Exp Rheumatol 1988; 6:17–26.
76. Roberts MET, Wright V, Hill AGS, Mehra AC. Psoriatic arthritis: follow-up study. Ann Rheum Dis 1976; 35:206–212.
77. O'Neill TW, King G, Graham IM. Echocardiographic abnormalities in ankylosing spondylitis. Ann Rheum Dis 1992; 51:652–654.
78. Qaiyumi S, Hassan ZU, Toone E. Seronegative spondyoarthropathies in lone aortic insufficiency. Arch Intern Med 1985; 145:822–824.
79. Bergfeldt L, Edhag O, Vedin L, et al. Ankylosing spondylitis: an important cause of severe disturbances of the cardiac conduction system: prevalence among 223 pacemaker-treated men. Am J Med 1982; 73:187–191.
80. Peeters AJ, ten Wolde S, Sedney MI, et al. Heart conduction disturbance: an HLA-B27 associated disease. Ann Rheum Dis 1991; 50:348–350.
81. Bergfeldt L. HLA-B27-associated cardiac disease. Ann Intern Med 1997; 127:621–629.
82. Ribeiro P, Morley KD, Shapiro LM, et al. Left ventricular function in patients with ankylosing spondylitis and Reiter's disease. Eur Heart J 1984; 5:419–422.
83. Yildirir A, Aksoyek S, Calguneri M, et al. Echocardiographic evidence of cardiac involvement in ankylosing spondylitis. Clin Rheumatol 2002; 21:129–134.
84. Applerouth D, Gottlieb NL. Pulmonary manifestations of ankylosing spondylitis. J Rheumatol 1975; 2:446–453.
85. Rumancik WM, Firooznia H, Davis MS Jr, et al. Fibrobullous disease of the upper lobes: an extraskeletal manifestation of ankylosing spondylitis. J Comput Tomogr 1984; 8(3):225–229.
86. Kiris A, Ozgocmen S, Kocakoc E, Ardicoglu O, Ogur E. Lung findings on high resolution CT in early ankylosing spondylitis. Eur J Radiol 2003; 47(1):71–76.
87. Senocak O, Manisali M, Ozaksoy D, Sevinc C, Akalin E. Lung parenchyma changes in ankylosing spondylitis: demonstration with high resolution CT and correlation with disease duration. Eur J Radiol 2003; 45(2):117–122.
88. Casserly IP, Fenlon HM, Breatnach E, Sant SM. Lung findings on high-resolution computed tomography in idiopathic ankylosing spondylitis—correlation with clinical findings, pulmonary function testing and plain radiography. Br J Rheumatol 1997; 36(6):677–682.
89. El Maghraoui A, Chaouir S, Abid A, et al. Lung findings on thoracic high-resolution computed tomography in patients with ankylosing spondylitis. Correlations with disease duration, clinical findings and pulmonary function testing. Clin Rheumatol 2004; 23(2):123–128.
90. Zizzo G, Castriota-Scanderbeg A, Zarrelli N, Nardella G, Daly J, Cammisa M. Pulmonary aspergillosis complicating ankylosing spondylitis. Radiol Med (Torino) 1996; 91(6):817–818.

91. Pontier S, Bigay L, Doussau S, Recco P, Lacassagne L, Didier A. Chronic necrotizing pulmonary aspergillosis and ankylosing spondylarthritis. Rev Mal Respir 2000; 17(3): 683–686.

92. Hendrix WC, Arruda LK, Platts-Mills TA, Haworth CS, Jabour R, Ward GW Jr. Aspergillus epidural abscess and cord compression in a patient with aspergilloma and empyema. Survival and response to high dose systemic amphotericin therapy. Am Rev Respir Dis 1992; 145(6):1483–1486.

93. Hillerdal G. Ankylosing spondylitis lung disease-an underdiagnosed entity? Eur J Respir Dis 1983; 64(6):437–441.

94. Elliott JA, Milne LJ, Cumming D. Chronic necrotising pulmonary aspergillosis treated with itraconazole. Thorax 1989; 44(10):820–821.

95. Stiksa G, Eklundh G, Riebe I, Simonsson BG. Bilateral pulmonary aspergilloma in ankylosing spondylitis treated with transthoracic intracavitary instillations of antifungal agents. Scand J Respir Dis 1976; 57(4):163–170.

96. Massard G, Roeslin N, Wihlm JM, Dumont P, Witz JP, Morand G. Pleuropulmonary aspergilloma: clinical spectrum and results of surgical treatment. Ann Thorac Surg 1992; 54(6):1159–1164.

97. Babatasi G, Massetti M, Chapelier A, et al. Surgical treatment of pulmonary aspergilloma: current outcome. J Thorac Cardiovasc Surg 2000; 119(5):906–912.

98. Cerrahoglu L, Unlu Z, Can M, Goktan C, Celik P. Lumbar stiffness but not thoracic radiographic changes relate to alteration of lung function tests in ankylosing spondylitis. Clin Rheumatol 2002; 21(4):275–279.

99. Fisher LR, Cawley MI, Holgate ST. Relation between chest expansion, pulmonary function, and exercise tolerance in patients with ankylosing spondylitis. Ann Rheum Dis 1990; 49:921–925.

100. Seckin U, Bolukbasi N, Gursel G, et al. Relationship between pulmonary function and exercise tolerance in patients with ankylosing spondylitis. Clin Exp Rheumatol 2000; 18(4):503–506.

101. Jones DW, Mansell MA, Samuell CT, Isenberg DA. Renal abnormalities in ankylosing spondylitis. Br J Rheumatol 1987; 26:341–345.

102. Wall BA, Agudelo CA, Pisko EJ. Increased incidence of recurrent hematuria in ankylosing spondylitis: a possible association with IgA nephropathy. Rheumatol Int 1984; 4(1):27–29.

103. Strobel ES, Fritschka E. Renal diseases in ankylosing spondylitis: review of the literature illustrated by case reports. Clin Rheumatol 1998; 17:524–530.

104. Shu KH, Lian JD, Yang YF, et al. Glomerulonephritis in ankylosing spondylitis. Clin Nephrol 1986; 25:169–174.

105. Cruickshank B. Pathology of ankylosing spondylitis. Clin Orthop Relat Res 1971; 74: 43–58.

106. Kovacsovics-Bankowski M, Zufferey P, So AK, Gerster JC. Secondary amyloidosis: a severe complication of ankylosing spondylitis. Two case-reports. Joint Bone Spine 2000; 67:129–133.

107. Gratacos J, Collado A, Sanmarti R, Poch E, Torras A, Munoz-Gomez J. Coincidental amyloid nephropathy and IgA glomerulonephritis in a patient with ankylosing spondylitis. J Rheumatol 1993; 20:1613–1615.

108. Lehtinen K. Ankylosing spondylitis and renal amyloidosis. J Rheumatol 1991; 18:1639.

109. Lance NJ, Curran JJ. Amyloidosis in a case of ankylosing spondylitis with a review of the literature. J Rheumatol 1991; 18(1):100–103.

110. Lai KN, Li PK, Hawkins B, Lai FM. IgA nephropathy associated with ankylosing spondylitis: occurrence in women as well as in men. Ann Rheum Dis 1989; 48:435–437.

111. Krothapalli R, Neeland B, Small S, Duffy WB, Gyorkey F, Senekjian HO. IgA nephropathy in a patient with ankylosing spondylitis and a solitary kidney. Clin Nephrol 1984; 21:134–137.

112. Quinton R, Siersema PD, Michiels JJ, ten Kate FJ. Renal AA amyloidosis in a patient with Bence Jones proteinuria and ankylosing spondylitis. J Clin Pathol 1992; 45:934–936.
113. Browie EA, Glasgow GL. Cauda equina lesions associated with ankylosing spondylitis: a report of three cases. Br Med J 1961; 2:24–27.
114. Hauge T. Chronic rheumatoid arthritis and spondylarthritis associated with neurological symptoms and signs occasionally simulating an intraspinal expansive process. Acta Chir Scand 1961; 120:395–401.
115. Sant SM, O'Connell D. Cauda equina syndrome in ankylosing spondylitis: a case report and review of the literature. Clin Rheumatol 1995; 14(2):224–226.
116. Schroder R, Urbach H, Zierz S. Cauda equina syndrome with multiple lumbar diverticula complicating long-standing ankylosing spondylitis. Clin Invest 1994; 72:1056–1059.
117. Charlesworth CH, Savy LE, Stevens J, Twomey B, Mitchell R. MRI demonstration of arachnoiditis in cauda equina syndrome of ankylosing spondylitis. Neuroradiology 1996; 38:462–465.
118. Bilgen IG, Yunten N, Ustun EE, Oksel F, Gumusdis G. Adhesive arachnoiditis causing cauda equina syndrome in ankylosing spondylitis: CT and MRI demonstration of dural calcification and a dorsal dural diverticulum. Neuroradiology 1999; 41:508–511.
119. Ahn NU, Ahn UM, Nallamshetty L, et al. Cauda equina syndrome in ankylosing spondylitis (the CES-AS syndrome): meta-analysis of outcomes after medical and surgical treatments. J Spinal Disord 2001; 14:427–433.
120. Tapia-Serrano R, Jiminez-Balderas FJ, Murietta S, et al. Testicular function in active ankylosing spondylitis. Therapeutic response to human chorionic gonadotrophin. J Rheumatol 1991; 18:841–848.
121. Jiminez-Balderas FJ, Tapia-Serrano R, Madero-Cervera JI, et al. Ovarian function studies in active ankylosing spondylitis in women. Clinical response to estrogen treatment. J Rheumatol 1990; 17:497–502.
122. James WH. Might patients with HLA-B27 related diseases benefit from anti-androgenic treatment? (letter). Ann Rheum Dis 1995; 54:531–532.
123. Giltay EJ, Popp-Snijders C, van Denderen JC, van Schaardenburg D, Gooren LJ, Dijkmans BA. Phenylbutazone can spuriously elevate unextracted testosterone assay results in patients with ankylosing spondylitis. J Clin Endocrinol Metab 2000; 85(12):4923–4924.
124. Spector TD, Ollier W, Perry LA, et al. Free and serum testosteron levels in 276 males: a comparative study of rheumatoid arthritis, ankylosing spondylitis and healthy controls. Clin Rheumatol 1989; 8:37–41.
125. Straub RH, Struharova S, Scholmerich J, Harle P. No alterations of serum levels of adrenal and gonadal hormones in patients with ankylosing spondylitis. Clin Exp Rheumatol 2002; 20(6 suppl 28):S52–S59.
126. Rovensky J, Imrich R, Malis F, et al. Prolactin and growth hormone responses to hypoglycemia in patients with rheumatoid arthritis and ankylosing spondylitis. J Rheumatol 2004; 31:2418–2421.
127. van der Paardt M, Dijkmans BAC, Giltay E, van der Horst-Bruinsma IE. Dutch patients with familial and sporadic ankylosing spondylitis do not differ in disease phenotype. J Rheumatol 2002; 29:2583–2584.
128. Rudwaleit M, van der Heijde D, Khan MA, Braun J, Sieper J. How to diagnose axial spondylarthritis early. Ann Rheum Dis 2004; 64:535–543.
129. Laurent MR, Panayi GS. Acute-phase proteins and serum immunoglobulins in ankylosing spondylitis. Ann Rheum Dis 1983; 42:524–528.
130. Ruof J, Stucki G. Validity aspects of erythrocyte sedimentation rate and C-reactive protein in ankylosing spondylitis: a literature review. J Rheumatol 1999; 26:966–970.
131. Spoorenberg A, Van Der Heijde D, De Klerk E, et al. Relative value of erythrocyte sedimentation rate and C-reactive protein in assessment of disease activity in ankylosing spondylitis. J Rheumatol 1999; 26:980–984.

132. Khan MA. Five classical clinical papers on ankylosing spondylitis. In: Dieppe P, Wolheim FA, Schumacher HR, eds. Classical Papers in Rheumatology. London: Martin Dutz, 2002:118–133.
133. Khan MA. Clinical features of ankylosing spondylitis. In: Hochberg MC, Silman AJ, Weinblatt ME, Weisman MH, eds. Rheumatology. Vol. 2. Edinburg: Mosby, 2003: 1161–1181.
134. Palm O, Moum B, Ongre A, et al. Prevalence of ankylosing spondylitis and other spondylarthropathies among patients with inflammatory bowel disease: a population study. J Rheumatol 2002; 29:511–515.
135. Job-Deslandre C, Menkes CJ. Treatment of juvenile spondylarthropathies with sulphasalazine. Rev Rheum 1993; 60:489–491.
136. Van Rossum MA, Fiselier TJ, Franssen MJ, et al. Sulfasalazine in the treatment of juvenile chronic arthritis: a randomised, double blind, placebo-controlled, multicenter study. Dutch Juvenile Chronic Arthritis Study Group. Arthritis Rheum 1998; 41: 808–816.
137. Carette S, Graham D, Little H, Rubenstein J, Rosen P. The natural disease course of ankylosing spondylitis. Arthritis Rheum 1983; 26(2):186–190.
138. Gran JT, Skomsvoll JF. The outcome of ankylosing spondylitis: a study of 100 patients. Br J Rheumatol 1997; 36(7):766–771.
139. Amor B, Santos RS, Nahal R, Listrat V, Dougados M. Predictive factors for the long-term outcome of spondyloarthropathies. J Rheumatol 1994; 21(10):1883–1887.
140. Claudepierre P, Gueguen A, Ladjouze A, et al. Predictive factors of severity of spondyloarthropathy in North Africa. Br J Rheumatol 1995; 34(12):1139–1145.
141. Brophy S, Mackay K, Al-Saidi A, Taylor G, Calin A. The natural history of ankylosing spondylitis as defined by radiological progression. J Rheumatol 2002; 29(6):1236–1243.
142. Boonen A, Chorus A, Miedema H, et al. Withdrawal from labour force due to work disability in patients with ankylosing spondylitis. Ann Rheum Dis 2001; 60(11): 1033–1039.
143. Khan MA, van der Linden SM. Ankylosing spondylitis and other spondyloarthropathies. Rheum Dis Clin North Am 1990; 16(3):551–579.
144. Arnett FC Jr, Schacter BZ, Hochberg MC, Hsu SH, Bias WB. Homozygosity for HLA-B27. Impact on rheumatic disease expression in two families. Arthritis Rheum 1977; 20(3):797–804.
145. Carter ET, McKenna CH, Brian DD, Kurland LT. Epidemiology of ankylosing spondylitis in Rochester, Minnesota, 1935–1973. Arthritis Rheum 1979; 22(4):365–370.
146. Radford EP, Doll R, Smith PG. Mortality among patients with ankylosing spondylitis not given X-ray therapy. N Engl J Med 1977; 297(11):572–576.
147. Kaprove RE, Little AH, Graham DC, Rosen PS. Ankylosing spondylitis: survival in men with and without radiotherapy. Arthritis Rheum 1980; 23(1):57–61.
148. Smith PG, Doll R. Mortality among patients with ankylosing spondylitis after a single treatment course with x rays. Br Med J (Clin Res Ed) 1982; 284:449–460.
149. Lehtinen K. Mortality and causes of death in 398 patients admitted to hospital with ankylosing spondylitis. Ann Rheum Dis 1993; 52(3):174–176.
150. Khan MA, Khan MK, Kushner I. Survival among patients with ankylosing spondylitis: a life-table analysis. J Rheumatol 1981; 8(1):86–90.
151. Callahan LF, Pincus T. Mortality in the rheumatic diseases. Arthritis Care Res 1995; 8(4):229–241.
152. Dougados M, Behier JM, Jolchine I, et al. Efficacy of celecoxib, a cyclooxygenase 2-specific inhibitor, in the treatment of ankylosing spondylitis: a six-week controlled study with comparison against placebo and against a conventional nonsteroidal antiinflammatory drug. Arthritis Rheum 2001; 44(1):180–185.
153. Melian A, van der Heijde DM, James MK. Etoricoxib in the treatment of ankylosing spondylitis (AS). Arthritis Rheum 2002; 46:S432.

154. Nissila M, Lehtinen K, Leirisalo-Repo M, Luukkainen R, Mutru O, Yli-Kerttula U. Sulfasalazine in the treatment of ankylosing spondylitis. A twenty-six-week, placebo-controlled clinical trial. Arthritis Rheum 1988; 31(9):1111–1116.

155. Dougados M, vam der Linden S, Leirisalo-Repo M, et al. Sulfasalazine in the treatment of spondylarthropathy. A randomized, multicenter, double-blind, placebo-controlled study. Arthritis Rheum 1995; 38(5):618–627.

156. van der Horst-Bruinsma IE, Clegg DO, Dijkmans BA. Treatment of ankylosing spondylitis with disease modifying antirheumatic drugs. Clin Exp Rheumatol 2002; 20(6 suppl 28): S67–S70.

157. Braun J, Brandt J, Listing J, et al. Treatment of active ankylosing spondylitis with infliximab: a randomised controlled multicentre trial. Lancet 2002; 359(9313):1187–1193.

158. Gorman JD, Sack KE, Davis JC Jr. Treatment of ankylosing spondylitis by inhibition of tumor necrosis factor alpha. N Engl J Med 2002; 346(18):1349–1356.

159. Braun J, Baraliakos X, Golder W, et al. Magnetic resonance imaging examinations of the spine in patients with ankylosing spondylitis, before and after successful therapy with infliximab: evaluation of a new scoring system. Arthritis Rheum 2003; 48(4): 1126–1136.

4

Imaging in Ankylosing Spondylitis

Dennis McGonagle, Ai Lyn Tan, Richard Wakefield, and Paul Emery
Academic Unit of Musculoskeletal Disease, Chapel Allerton Hospital, Leeds, U.K.

INTRODUCTION

Ankylosing spondylitis (AS) is the disease entity on which the concept of the spondyloarthropathies (SpA) is based. The clinical, immunological, and imaging features of AS attest to the fact that its pathogenesis is fundamentally different from rheumatoid arthritis (RA) and that this disease is not indeed a form of RA or a "rheumatoid spondylitis" as once considered. After a brief description of the anatomical basis for AS, this chapter highlights the imaging of AS using radiography, ultrasonography, and concentrates mainly on magnetic resonance imaging (MRI), with a brief mention on computed tomography (CT) and bone scintigraphy.

Interpretation of the imaging findings of AS, and SpA in general, is best understood when one grasps the anatomical basis for inflammation in both types of inflammatory arthritis. RA primarily involves the synovium, and bone erosion is a secondary phenomenon (1–4). The primary site of disease in AS is at the enthesis. The enthesis forms part of a complex organ that involves the adjacent bone trabecular network; inflammation of the entheses is thus associated with adjacent osteitis (5). Also some structures, while themselves not insertions, including fibrocartilageneous joints—especially the sacroiliac joint (SIJ)—share the same biomechanics, histopathology, and imaging features as the enthesis proper and can be viewed as "functional entheses" (5). Unlike RA, where disease has an anatomical basis revolving around sites of synovitis, the anatomical basis for SpA revolves around the concept of the enthesis organ and related structures, and disease appears to have a unifying biomechanical basis occurring at sites of high shear and compressive forces—best exemplified at insertions. Furthermore, the clinical disease phenotype of polysynovitis in RA is associated with progressive radiographic joint destruction and osteoporosis, while prominent reparative processes are evident radiographically in AS and SpA in general.

While periarticular erosion is the most distinctive feature of RA and reflects cumulative damage due to synovitis, the classically described features of AS are more diverse and include bone sclerosis adjacent to fibrocartilages, bone erosions, and cyst formation at the same sites, normal bone mineralization, bone proliferation at insertions with bridging between adjacent vertebrae, and occasionally periostitis. These diverse pathologies represent inflammation at insertions proper and also in the adjoining tissues that form part of the enthesis organ (6).

Diagnostic imaging in AS has taken on a much greater importance in the last few years with the advent of biologic therapy, especially antitumor necrosis factor therapy, which has transformed the management of AS. Although multiple imaging modalities are available to evaluate AS including conventional radiography, CT, bone scintigraphy, ultrasonography, and now MRI, only the latter of these seems to be capable of diagnostic evaluation of early active disease and monitoring of therapy. In a short space of time MRI has become the diagnostic modality of choice both in the diagnosis of early axial AS involvement and for monitoring the disease.

Although rheumatologists have been slow to embrace MRI in comparison to orthopedic surgeons, a number of things have happened in the last decade to make MRI the modality of choice for the assessment of the SIJ and the spine in AS. Firstly, the widespread application of fat suppression MRI techniques has made it possible to visualize the osteitis process in the SIJ and spine. Secondly, MRI scanners are commonplace and although the capital costs of installation remain high, the cost of obtaining noncontrast enhanced sequences is acceptable. Also the MRI findings in AS are quite characteristic and often extensive, therefore, clinicians involved in the care of patients with AS can quickly learn to recognize the MRI features.

IMAGING OF THE SACROILIAC JOINTS

Conventional Radiography of the Sacroiliac Joints

Chronic AS is radiographically characterized by bilateral symmetrical SIJ disease with ankylosis, bone sclerosis, and sometimes cyst formation (Fig. 1), squaring of vertebral bodies, symmetric syndesmophytes, and entheseal new bone formation elsewhere including synovial joints and peripheral entheseal insertions. In contrast to this, axial psoriatic and reactive arthritis are characterized by more asymmetrical SIJ disease and bulky asymmetrical syndesmophyte formation.

AS invariably starts in the SIJ, which is considered one of the most difficult joints in the body to image. Even with optimal positioning and image interpretation by an experienced clinician or skeletal radiologist, it is often difficult to unequivocally diagnose early sacroiliitis on conventional radiography. Early radiographically detectable sacroiliitis is characterized by poor definition of the joint margin, subsequent subchondral erosion especially on the iliac side of the joint, apparent joint widening, and finally bony reaction with sclerosis. Ossification of the superior ligamentous part of the SIJ and other regions may eventually occur leading to joint fusion or ankylosis. The insensitivity of radiography for diagnosing early disease and its relative insensitivity to change over time has hampered its utility in the diagnosis of AS. Further, the intra- and interobserver variability in interpreting radiographic sacroiliitis is a significant problem (7,8). Somewhat surprisingly radiographic sacroiliitis remains the gold standard for the diagnosis of AS and forms part of the diagnostic and classification criteria of both AS and SpA (9,10).

Computed Tomography of the Sacroiliac Joints

Historically a delay of a decade in the diagnosis of AS was common because of the slow evolution of radiographic changes and difficulty in interpretation of images. This inability to define early disease radiographically is no longer acceptable as the need

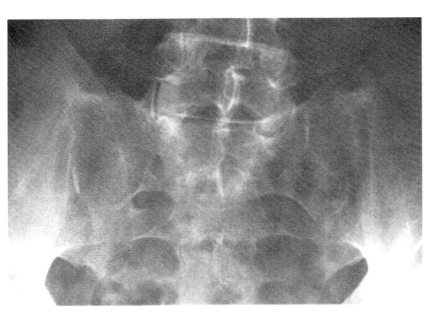

Figure 1 Conventional radiograph of chronic sacroiliac joints showing complete fusion in a 56-year-old male with ankylosing spondylitis for 33 years. Unfortunately, radiographic changes may take several years to appear in AS; so the changes, while characteristic, are not particularly common in early disease. *Abbreviation*: AS, ankylosing spondylitis.

to define disease early is imperative, especially since effective therapies have been developed. In the recent past CT was employed as it was superior for the detection of subchondral sclerosis, bone erosion, and bony bridging across the SIJ and indeed it briefly looked as if it could become the modality of choice for imaging in AS (11–13).

However, CT suffers from two major disadvantages—it requires ionizing radiation and more importantly it is not able to distinguish between active and inactive sacroiliitis. Bone scintigraphy can certainly diagnose sacroiliitis early but again the radiation usage, lack of specificity for sacroiliitis, and lack of suitability for serial monitoring of therapy has hindered its development in the assessment of disease (14,15).

Ultrasonography of the Sacroiliac Joints

The inaccessibility of the SIJ means that it is not a site that readily lends itself to assessment by ultrasonography. Only one study has shown the use of color and duplex Doppler sonography in identifying active sacroiliitis and its use in monitoring therapy (16). Clearly, further work to validate these findings is needed.

Magnetic Resonance Imaging of the Sacroiliac Joints

It is over a decade ago since the first MRI study demonstrating the importance of SIJ subchondral osteitis was first published and it was suggested that the disease commenced in the subchondral bone. A number of recent studies have used MRI in the diagnostic evaluation of AS and SpA. The most important study utilizing MRI in AS showed that an abnormal MRI at baseline predicted the subsequent development of radiographic sacroiliitis (17). Indeed other studies have shown that the MRI diagnosis of sacroiliitis precedes any radiographic changes (18,19). This has important implications and indicates that the gold standard for the diagnosis of AS, that is the presence of radiographic sacroiliitis, has been superseded by MRI. The SIJ is often imaged in the coronal oblique plane, which is most commonly used, or in the axial plane, which gives better visualization of the ligaments behind the joint cavity (Fig. 2). Fat suppression MRI techniques are used to demonstrate sites of inflammation, and with good quality fat suppression there is no need to use the MRI contrast agent gadolinium diethylenetriamine penta-acetic acid (20,21). Unlike radiography, where essentially there are only a couple of ways of obtaining the image, several different MRI sequences, imaging planes, and several potential artifacts complicate scoring and interpretation of the images and interested rheumatologists need to liaise closely with fellow radiologists.

Other studies have shown that the sacroiliitis pathology is widespread, encompassing inflammation of virtually every joint structure including insertions and bone adjacent to fibrocartilages reflecting the enthesis organ concept (22). While the MRI appearances of inflammatory sacroiliitis are characteristic, other causes of sacroiliitis need to be considered including infection, the latter often being associated with inflammation or abscess formation in the adjacent soft tissues.

In the last few years, MRI studies of the SIJ have been reported before and after biological therapy with etanercept, infliximab, and anakinra (21,23,24). All of these show good improvement of the osteitic process. It remains to be determined whether these excellent MRI responses correlate with subsequent retardation of

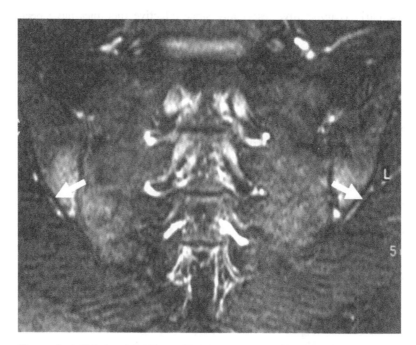

Figure 2   MRI showing bilateral sacroiliitis in an ankylosing spondylitis patient, represented by bone enhancement following gadolinium-DTPA administration (*arrows*) on the coronal oblique view of the postcontrast image indicating subchondral bone edema. Histological studies have confirmed that the bony changes in this joint represent osteitis. *Abbreviation*: MRI, magnetic resonance imaging.

radiographic cyst and erosion formation and joint fusion. Further work is therefore needed for international standardization for the early diagnosis of AS and for the monitoring of therapy using MRI.

IMAGING OF THE SPINE

Conventional Radiography of the Spine

Virtually all of the imaging changes in the spine in AS that are evident on plain radiographs are directly related to enthesitis related disease. The earliest radiographic changes in the spine are small erosions with adjacent repair at the corners of the vertebral bodies, resulting in a loss of the normal concave contour of the anterior border of the vertebral bodies leading to squaring of the vertebral bodies. The repair adjacent to the enthesis leads to a small focus of regional bone sclerosis or what is termed a "shiny corner," also known as a Romanus lesion. The spine has numerous insertions including the annulus of the intervertebral discs and longitudinal ligaments, which ossify with eventual bridging between adjacent insertions, leading to what are termed syndesmophytes with the extent of syndesmophyte formation in the spine leading to the characteristic radiographic bamboo spine of chronic AS (Fig. 3). The apophyseal joints are also commonly fused in AS, and based on CT studies it has been suggested that these are the first sites involved in the spine with subsequent ankylosis of other structures (25,26). In comparison to AS the spinal involvement in psoriatic arthritis is characterized by chunky syndesmophytes. A number of other radiographic features may also be evident in the spine in chronic AS including disc calcification, pseudoarthroses, fracture, and osteopenia.

Magnetic Resonance Imaging of the Spine

Until recently, both CT and MRI had a limited role in the assessment of spinal disease in AS including the evaluation of associated disk disease, fractures, dural ectasia, and spinal stenosis. However, analogous to the SIJ, the ability of fat suppression MRI techniques has transformed the assessment of spinal disease but little has been published on this to date. The abnormalities on spinal fat suppressed MRI basically mirror radiographic abnormalities with MRI Romanus lesions, spinous process lesions, facetal joint, enthesitis/osteitis, and costovertebral joint enthesitis (Fig. 4). However, these abnormalities can be seen at a stage when radiographs are normal. Importantly these lesions may regress completely following therapy with either etanercept or infliximab and may improve with anakinra (21,23,24).

To summarize this section, the axial skeleton is universally involved in AS and X-rays are insensitive for showing early disease. The inaccessibility of the axial skeleton for clinical assessment also renders ultrasonography of limited value at this site. The greatest potential for imaging axial disease rests with MRI and further validation work is needed in this regard.

IMAGING OF THE PERIPHERAL JOINTS

Conventional Radiography of the Peripheral Joints

Up to 20% of patients with AS may develop a peripheral synovitis; this may be the presenting feature in juvenile AS and can precede clinically manifested axial disease.

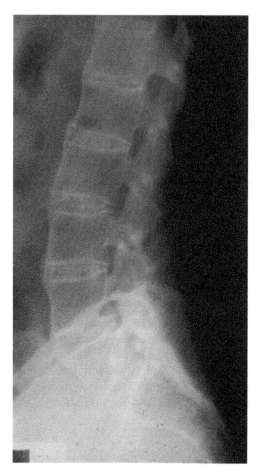

Figure 3 Plain radiograph of a "bamboo" spine of a patient with chronic ankylosing spondylitis showing syndesmophytes and squaring of the vertebra. The spine is totally fused. Like the sacroiliac joints, the use of radiography for the early diagnostic evaluation of early spinal AS and for monitoring of spinal changes has proved difficult. *Abbreviation*: AS, ankylosing spondylitis.

The synovial joints most typically involved in AS are curiously those in closest proximity with the axial skeleton, namely, the shoulders and the hips, but knee and other joint involvement are also common. That these joints are inflamed is comparatively easy to determine from clinical findings and thus imaging is less important than in the spine. Here the demonstration of enthesitis/osteitis on MRI is essential to make an accurate diagnosis, especially since the inflammatory response can be minimally abnormal in AS.

AS associated hip disease is thought to define a worst prognostic group (27). The hip involvement in AS, usually symmetrical, is most typically associated with capsular calcification emanating from insertions, which can culminate in joint fusion, and bridging in the face of relatively little intra-articular erosion can be seen. Occasionally, a normal femoral head and joint space may be observed through bone ankylosis, which can make joint replacement problematic. Likewise shoulder involvement in AS can be characterized by proliferative new bone formation adjacent to insertions.

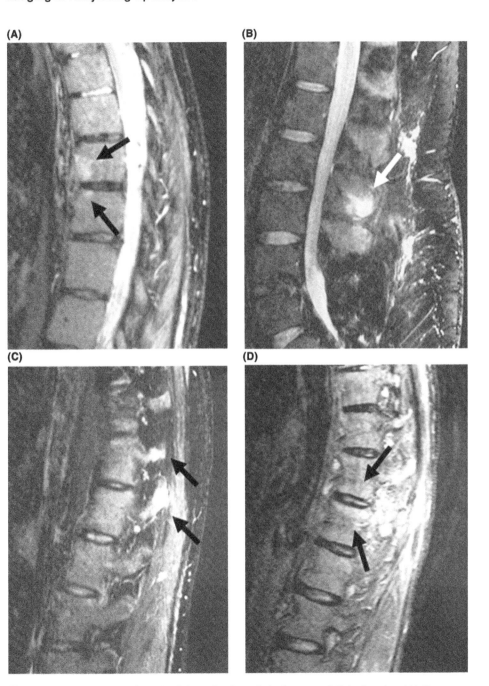

Figure 4 Fat suppressed MRI of the spine in ankylosing spondylitis showing (**A**) Romanus lesions, (**B**) spinous process edema, (**C**) facet joint enthesitis/osteitis, and (**D**) end-plate edema. *Abbreviation*: MRI, magnetic resonance imaging.

MRI of the Synovial Joints

A systematic evaluation of MRI in diseased synovial joints in early AS has not yet been reported. However, in patients presenting with knee synovitis, AS and SpA can sometimes be differentiated from RA based on the presence of MRI determined enthesitis and osteitis (28). In the case of SpA, capsular and entheseal changes are evident in the small joints of the hands in SpA (29). Whether enthesitis/osteitis evident in these diseased joints is prognostically relevant remains to be determined.

Ultrasonography of the Entheses

Isolated enthesitis not related to the spine, including the Achilles tendon and plantar fascia, is also a characteristic feature of AS. Again, the recognition of enthesitis at the plantar fascia or Achilles tendon does not require imaging as this clinical pattern of disease points toward AS and SpA, especially in the context of inflammatory back pain. On ultrasound, proliferative new bone can be occasionally seen in chronic enthesitis at the various sites of disease. Acute enthesitis is characterized by hypo-echoic thickening of insertions (Figs. 5 and 6). A number of unblinded studies have used sonography to assess the lower limbs for enthesopathy in patients with SpA and these showed that clinically unsuspected enthesitis was not uncommon and often missed by clinical examination (30,31). It is possible that clinically unrecognized enthesitis in the lower limbs may be of value in the diagnostic evaluation of AS but this awaits further controlled studies.

Recently power Doppler (PD) ultrasound has been used to assess enthesitis. In patients with SpA, a characteristic pattern is evident with increased PD signal adjacent to the bony insertion (32). Furthermore PD signal improvement was noted following therapy with infliximab (33).

CONCLUSION

The emphasis in imaging AS has now switched from the demonstration of interesting, chronic but irreversible radiographic abnormalities that is characteristic of late disease

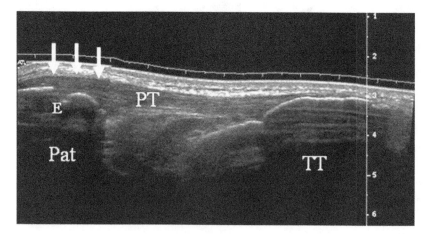

Figure 5 Longitudinal ultrasound image through the PT of a HLA-B27 positive patient with inflammatory low back pain and right knee pain. The image shows proximal enthesitis demonstrated by swelling, hypoechogenicity, and loss of normal fibrillar architecture (*arrows*) in addition to bone (E) on the Pat. *Abbreviations*: PT, patella tendon; E, erosin; Pat, patella; TT, tibial tuberosity.

(A)

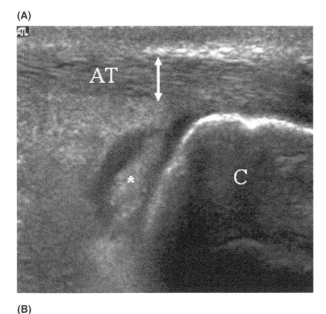

(B)

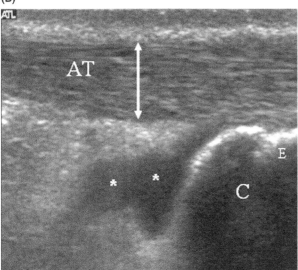

Figure 6 Longitudinal ultrasound image through the AT of a patient with ankylosing spondy-litis. The asymptomatic side (**A**) demonstrated a normal tendon, however, there was a small retro-calcaneal bursa (∗). The symptomatic side (**B**) revealed a thicker tendon and larger bursa compared to image (**A**). There is also mild bone irregularity of the C in image (**B**) probably repre-senting early bone E. *Abbreviations*: AT, achilles tendons; C, calcaneum; E, early bone erosion.

to the early diagnosis of AS using MRI. The abnormalities shown on MRI may predate radiographic abnormalities by years; they will help define the epidemiology of disease in the future and thus far have been shown to regress following biological therapy. The application of MRI early in the course of AS could lead to prompt effec-tive therapy. It remains to be determined whether this makes radiographically defined changes in AS an infrequent finding.

REFERENCES

1. Boers M, Kostense PJ, Verhoeven AC, van der Linden S. Inflammation and damage in an individual joint predict further damage in that joint in patients with early rheumatoid arthritis. Arthritis Rheum 2001; 44(10):2242–2246.
2. McGonagle D, Conaghan PG, O'Connor P, et al. The relationship between synovitis and bone changes in early untreated rheumatoid arthritis: a controlled magnetic resonance imaging study. Arthritis Rheum 1999; 42(8):1706–1711.
3. Østergaard M, Hansen M, Stoltenberg M, et al. Magnetic resonance imaging-determined synovial membrane volume as a marker of disease activity and a predictor of progressive joint destruction in the wrists of patients with rheumatoid arthritis. Arthritis Rheum 1999; 42(5):918–929.
4. Conaghan PG, O'Connor P, McGonagle D, et al. Elucidation of the relationship between synovitis and bone damage: a randomised magnetic resonance imaging study of individual joints in patients with early rheumatoid arthritis. Arthritis Rheum 2003; 48(1):64–71.
5. McGonagle D, Marzo-Ortega H, Benjamin M, Emery P. Report on the Second International Enthesitis Workshop. Arthritis Rheum 2003; 48(4):896–905.
6. Benjamin M, McGonagle D. The anatomical basis for disease localisation in seronegative spondyloarthropathy at entheses and related sites. J Anat 2001; 199(pt 5):503–526.
7. Hollingsworth PN, Cheah PS, Dawkins RL, Owen ET, Calin A, Wood PH. Observer variation in grading sacroiliac radiographs in HLA-B27 positive individuals. J Rheumatol 1983; 10:247–254.
8. van Tubergen A, Heuft-Dorenbosch L, Schulpen G, et al. Radiographic assessment of sacroiliitis by radiologists and rheumatologists: does training improve quality? Ann Rheum Dis 2003; 62(6):519–525.
9. van der Linden S, Valkenburg HA, Cats A. Evaluation of diagnostic criteria for ankylosing spondylitis. A proposal for modification of the New York criteria. Arthritis Rheum 1984; 27(4):361–368.
10. Dougados M, van der Linden S, Juhlin R, et al. The European Spondylarthropathy Study Group preliminary criteria for the classification of spondylarthropathy. Arthritis Rheum 1991; 34(10):1218–1227.
11. Lawson TL, Foley WD, Carrera GF, Berland LL. The sacroiliac joints: anatomic, plain roentgenographic, and computed tomographic analysis. J Comput Assist Tomogr 1982; 6:307–314.
12. Ryan LM, Carrera GF, Lightfoot RW Jr, Hoffman RG, Kozin F. The radiographic diagnosis of sacroiliitis: a comparison of different views with computed tomograms of the sacroiliac joints. Arthritis Rheum 1983; 26:760–763.
13. Fam AG, Rubenstein JD, Chin Sangh H, Leung FY. Computed tomography in the diagnosis of early ankylosing spondylitis. Arthritis Rheum 1985; 28:930–937.
14. Chase WF, Houk RW, Winn RE, Hinzman GW. The clinical usefulness of radionuclide scintigraphy in suspected sacro-iliitis: a prospective study. Br J Rheumatol 1983; 22(2):67–72.
15. Goldberg RP, Genant HK, Shimshak R, Shames D. Applications and limitations of quantitative sacroiliac joint scintigraphy. Radiology 1978; 128(3):683–686.
16. Arslan H, Sakarya ME, Adak B, Unal O, Sayarlioglu M. Duplex and color Doppler sonographic findings in active sacroiliitis. Am J Roentgenol 1999; 173(3):677–680.
17. Oostveen J, Prevo R, den Boer J, van de Laar M. Early detection of sacroiliitis on magnetic resonance imaging and subsequent development of sacroiliitis on plain radiography. A prospective, longitudinal study. J Rheumatol 1999; 26(9):1953–1958.
18. Bollow M, Braun J, Hamm B, et al. Early sacroiliitis in patients with spondyloathropathy: evaluation with dynamic gadolinium-enhanced MR imaging. Radiology 1195; 194: 529–536.

19. Yu W, Feng F, Dion E, Yang H, Jiang M, Genant HK. Comparison of radiography, computed tomography and magnetic resonance imaging in the detection of sacroiliitis accompanying ankylosing spondylitis. Skeletal Radiol 1998; 27:311–320.

20. Docherty P, Mitchell MJ, MacMillian L, et al. Magnetic resonance imaging in the detection of sacroiliitis. J Rheumatol 1992; 19:393–401.

21. Braun J, Baraliakos X, Golder W, et al. Magnetic resonance imaging examinations of the spine in patients with ankylosing spondylitis, before and after successful therapy with infliximab: evaluation of a new scoring system. Arthritis Rheum 2003; 48(4):1126–1136.

22. Muche B, Bollow M, Francois RJ, Sieper J, Hamm B, Braun J. Anatomic structures involved in early- and late-stage sacroiliitis in spondylarthritis: a detailed analysis by contrast-enhanced magnetic resonance imaging. Arthritis Rheum 2003; 48(5):1374–1384.

23. Marzo-Ortega H, McGonagle D, O'Connor P, Emery P. Efficacy of etanercept in the treatment of the entheseal pathology in resistant spondylarthropathy: a clinical and magnetic resonance imaging study. Arthritis Rheum 2001; 44(9):2112–2117.

24. Tan AL, Marzo-Ortega H, O'Connor P, Fraser A, Emery P, McGonagle DG. Efficacy of anakinra in active ankylosing spondylitis: a clinical and magnetic resonance imaging study. Ann Rheum Dis 2004; 63(9):1041–1045.

25. Russell AS, Jackson F. Computer assisted tomography of the apophyseal changes in patients with ankylosing spondylitis. J Rheumatol 1986; 13(3):581–585.

26. de Vlam K, Mielants H, Verstaete KL, Veys EM. The zygapophyseal joint determines morphology of the enthesophyte. J Rheumatol 2000; 27(7):1732–1739.

27. Brophy S, Calin A. Ankylosing spondylitis: interaction between genes, joints, age at onset, and disease expression. J Rheumatol 2001; 28(10):2283–2288.

28. McGonagle D, Gibbon W, O'Connor P, Green M, Pease C, Emery P. Characteristic magnetic resonance imaging entheseal changes of knee synovitis in spondylarthropathy. Arthritis Rheum 1998; 41(4):694–700.

29. Jevtic V, Watt I, Rozman B, Kos-Golja M, Demsar F, Jarh O. Distinctive radiological features of small hand joints in rheumatoid arthritis and seronegative spondyloarthritis demonstrated by contrast-enhanced (Gd-DTPA) magnetic resonance imaging. Skeletal Radiol 1995; 24(5):351–355.

30. Balint PV, Kane D, Wilson H, McInnes IB, Sturrock RD. Ultrasonography of entheseal insertions in the lower limb in spondyloarthropathy. Ann Rheum Dis 2002; 61(10): 905–910.

31. Lehtinen A, Taavitsainen M, Leirisalo-Repo M. Sonographic analysis of enthesopathy in the lower extremities of patients with spondylarthropathy. Clin Exp Rheumatol 1994; 12(2):143–148.

32. D'Agostino MA, Said-Nahal R, Hacquard-Bouder C, Brasseur JL, Dougados M, Breban M. Assessment of peripheral enthesitis in the spondyloarthropathies by ultrasonography combined with power doppler: a cross-sectional study. Arthritis Rheum 2003; 48(2):523–533.

33. D'Agostino MA, Breban M, Said-Nahal R, Dougados M. Refractory inflammatory heel pain in spondylarthropathy: a significant response to infliximab documented by ultrasound. Arthritis Rheum 2002; 46(3):840–841 (author reply 841–843).

5
Criteria and Outcome Assessment of Ankylosing Spondylitis

Désirée van der Heijde and Sjef van der Linden
Division of Rheumatology, Department of Internal Medicine, University Maastricht, Maastricht, The Netherlands

CRITERIA

Classification as a general term means separating certain issues into classes. Criteria are used to define those issues that belong to a specific class and those that do not belong to it. Classification, therefore, makes use of criteria and may address a whole spectrum of specific purposes. Examples are criteria for staging of severity or classification of separate diseases or related groups of diseases. In this latter field one encounters the terms diagnostic and classification criteria. Although the main purpose of both sets of criteria is to ensure comparability across patients or studies, it is important to keep in mind that diagnostic and classification criteria have quite distinct features. Diagnostic and classification criteria are examples of discriminative instruments. They are used, at a given point in time, to distinguish between patients or between groups of patients. Of course, both diagnostic and classification criteria must be insensitive to changes in disease activity. Apart from this, test characteristics such as sensitivity and specificity of both types of criteria might differ considerably.

Classification criteria apply to groups of patients. These groups should be homogeneous and not include many false positives, i.e., they should have high specificity (at a loss of sensitivity). Such criteria enable comparison and are mainly applied in clinical studies. Patients who do not fulfill a certain set of classification criteria will usually not be included in clinical trials assessing the efficacy or safety of a particular intervention. Of course, generalizability of study results to all patients in clinical practice with that particular disease might be limited if one applies classification criteria strictly.

Diagnostic criteria primarily apply not to groups, but to individual persons. Such criteria should have high sensitivity [especially for early cases of a particular disease, e.g., early ankylosing spondylitis (AS)]. This will result in lower specificity, i.e., more false positives might be expected as compared to classification criteria. Therefore, diagnostic criteria are mainly applied in clinical practice to individual patients. Clearly, patients who do not (yet) fulfill a certain set of diagnostic criteria should not be withheld appropriate treatment.

Classification criteria, although clearly not intended for diagnostic purposes, are frequently used in clinical practice as an aid to identify somewhat atypical or undifferentiated cases.

Classification Criteria for Spondyloarthritis

AS is the typical example of the group of spondyloarthritis (spondyloarthropathies; SpA). SpA is a family of interrelated and overlapping inflammatory rheumatic diseases of uncertain etiology. The basis of the concept lies in common epidemiology and similar clinical features and was first introduced by Moll and Wright (1). These overlapping clinical features include radiographic sacroiliitis with or without accompanying inflammation of the axial skeleton; peripheral arthritis usually in an asymmetrical pattern and predominantly of the lower legs, enthesitis, and dactylitis; association with chronic inflammatory bowel disease and psoriasis; acute anterior uveitis; increased familial incidence; lack of rheumatoid factor and absence of rheumatoid nodules; and strong association with HLA-B27. These symptoms may occur simultaneously or sequentially in the same patient or in a family. The various forms that are recognized as separate entities within SpA are: AS; reactive arthritis (including Reiter's syndrome); arthritis associated with psoriasis; arthritis associated with Crohn's disease or ulcerative colitis; a juvenile form of SpA; and undifferentiated SpA.

Two sets of classification criteria have been developed for SpA: Amor's criteria and the European Spondyloarthropathy Study Group (ESSG) criteria (Tables 1 and 2) (2,3). The main purpose of these is for use in studies to have clearly defined

Table 1 Amor's Classification Criteria for Spondyloarthritis

	Score
Clinical symptoms or past history of	
Lumbar or dorsal pain at night or morning stiffness of lumbar or dorsal pain	1
Asymmetrical oligoarthritis	2
Buttock pain	1
If alternate buttock pain	2
Sausage-like toe or digit	2
Heel pain or other well-defined enthesopathy	2
Iritis	1
Non-gonococcal urethritis or cervicitis within one month before the onset of arthritis	1
Acute diarrhea within one month before the onset of arthritis	1
Psoriasis, balanitis, or inflammatory bowel disease (ulcerative colitis or Crohn's disease)	2
Radiological findings	
Sacroiliitis (bilateral grade 2 or unilateral grade 3)	3
Genetic background	
Presence of HLA-B27 and/or family history of ankylosing spondylitis, reactive arthritis, uveitis, psoriasis or inflammatory bowel disease	2
Response to treatment	
Clear-cut improvement within 48 hr after NSAIDS intake or rapid relapse of the pain after their discontinuation	2

Note: A patient is considered as suffering from spondyloarthritis if the sumscore is ≥6.

Table 2 The European Spondylarthropathy Study Group Criteria: Classification Criteria for SpA

- Inflammatory back pain OR synovitis (asymmetric, predominantly in lower extremities)
- AND one or more of the following characteristics:
  - Family history: first- or second-degree relatives with ankylosing spondylitis, psoriasis, acute iritis, reactive arthritis, or inflammatory bowel disease
  - Past or present psoriasis, diagnosed by a physician
  - Past or present ulcerative colitis or Crohn's disease, diagnosed by a physician and confirmed by radiography or endoscopy
  - Past or present pain alternating between the two buttocks
  - Past or present spontaneous pain or tenderness at examination of the site of the insertion—the Achilles tendon or plantar fascia (enthesitis)
  - Episode of diarrhea occurring within one month before onset of arthritis
  - Non-gonococcal urethritis or cervicitis occurring within one month before onset of arthritis

---

Sensitivity 77% and specificity 89% for the presented criteria; if bilateral grade 2–4 sacroiliitis or unilateral grade 3 or 4 sacroiliitis [grades are 0, normal, 1, possible, 2, minimal, 3, moderate, 4, completely fused (ankylosed)] is added sensitivity increases to 87% with a specificity of 87%.

groups. However, they are also frequently used as guidance in making a diagnosis. However, one has to keep in mind that these criteria were developed in patients with established disease, and lack sensitivity in patients with early disease. Advantages of the list of signs and symptoms as, e.g., described by Amor, alerts the clinician that these features are interrelated, and helps to identify patients with incomplete (often developing) forms of SpA. Recently, it has been proposed to differentiate patients with SpA with axial involvement, in order to be able to recognize these earlier in the course of the disease, than patients with full-blown AS. Feasibility and validity of this concept is being investigated.

Classification Criteria for AS

A patient with classical AS is easy to recognize. However, early in the course of the disease this might be quite difficult. A delay of about eight years between symptom onset and diagnosis is still the average in many cohorts of patients. Modified New York criteria are developed as classification criteria to obtain homogeneous groups for research purposes (Table 3) (4). For making a diagnosis these criteria lack sensitivity, especially early in the disease at a time that radiographic sacroiliitis cannot be demonstrated yet. Also limitations of lumbar spine and of chest expansion are

Table 3 Modified New York Criteria for Classification of AS

---

1. Low back pain at least three month duration improved by exercise and not relieved by rest
2. Limitation of lumbar spine in sagittal and frontal planes
3. Chest expansion decreased relative to normal values for age and sex
4a. Unilateral sacroiliitis grade 3–4
4b. Bilateral sacroiliitis grade 2–4

Note: Definite ankylosing spondylitis if (4a or 4b) and any clinical criterion (1–3).
Abbreviation: AS, ankylosing spondylitis.

usually not early features and reflect more disease duration. With the availability of magnetic resonance imaging (MRI) to assess inflammation in sacroiliac joints, new possibilities become available to modify the existing criteria. At the moment, inflammation (and/or damage) on MRI is not yet included in the existing criteria, but work is ongoing to test the usefulness and validity of this concept.

OUTCOME ASSESSMENT OF AS

For most physicians it is obvious that for research purposes assessments need to be applied in a standardized and consequent manner to be able to describe the course and outcome of patients under study. However, similar recommendations can be given for use in daily clinical practice. Only by the use of measurements, we are able to judge and document truthfully if the patient is improving or worsening over time after the start of a new treatment or as the natural course of the disease. Many instruments applied in clinical research are also feasible for use in clinical practice. An international group of experts in the field of AS, the ASsessment in Ankylosing Spondylitis (ASAS) International Working Group (www.asas-group.org), defined domains with accompanying instruments for use in both clinical research and clinical record keeping (5,6). These so-called core sets for clinical research are different for evaluating efficacy of symptom modifying antirheumatic drugs (SMARDs) and physical therapy at one hand, and disease controlling antirheumatic therapy (DCART) at the other hand. The overview of the domains of the core sets is presented in Figure 1 and the instruments belonging to the domains in Table 4. Following a process of literature review, expert consultation, and a final large consensus meeting, recommendations were made under auspices of the Spondylitis Association of America (SAA) and ASAS on how to conduct clinical trials in AS (7).

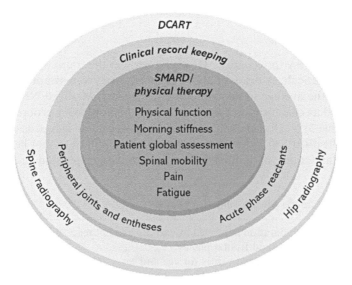

Figure 1 Domains included in the ASAS core set for evaluating Symptom Modifying Antirheumatid Drugs (SMARDs) and physical therapy (*inner circle*), Disease Controlling Antirheumatic Therapy (DCART) (*outer circle*), and clinical practice (*middle circle*).

Table 4   Domains and Instruments for All Three ASAS Core Sets

Domain	Recommended instrument
Physical function[a]	BASFI a patient oriented questionnaire of 10 questions that are averaged to yield a score between 0 and 10. As an alternative the Dougados functional index including 20 questions on a 5-point Likert scale (range 0–40) is acceptable.
Pain[a]	Two separate questions: (1) total pain in the spine due to AS, (2) pain at night in the spine due to AS.
Patient global of disease activity[a]	Patient global-visual analogue scale with 0 being no disease activity and 100 being severe disease activity.
Spinal mobility[a]	Four instruments: Occiput to wall distance Chest expansion Modified schober index Lateral lumbar flexion or BASMI[a]
Inflammation (spinal stiffness)[a]	Average of morning stiffness duration and intensity (e.g., BASDAI questions 5 and 6) or duration of morning stiffness only
Fatigue[a,d]	Fatigue question from the BASDAI
Peripheral joints and entheses[b]	Number of swollen joints (44 joint count) Validated entheses index (no preferred instrument)
Acute phase reactants[b]	ESR
Radiographs of spine and hips[c]	X-pelvis (SI joints and hips) Lateral lumbar spine and lateral cervical spine (mSASSS)

[a]Included in all three core sets for DCART, SMARD/physical therapy, and clinical record keeping.
[b]Included in core sets for DCART and clinical record keeping.
[c]Included in core set for DCART.
[d]Added in an update of the core set (ASAS Workshop Gent, Oct 2002).
Abbreviations: ASAS, ASsessment in Ankylosing Spondylitis international working group; AS, ankylosing spondylitis; BASFI, Bath ankylosing spondylitis functional index; BASMI, Bath ankylosing spondylitis meterology index; BASDAI, Bath ankylosing spondylitis disease activity index; DCART, disease modifying antirheumatic therapy; ESR, erythrocyte sedimemtation rate; SMARD, symptom modifying antirheumatic drug.
Source: From Ref. 6.

There are four groups of features that may be present in each patient with AS: axial involvement, peripheral joint involvement, entheseal involvement, and extra-articular/extra-spinal features. It is important to check all these four areas in every patient at every visit. The description of the assessment below follows these presentations.

Definition and Consequences of Axial Involvement

Not only sacroiliitis and spinal features but also the anterior chest wall and root joints (shoulders and hips) relate to the concept of axial involvement. Active inflammation of the sacroiliac joints causes pain and functional impairment. This inflammation of the sacroiliac joints may result in full ankylosis. At this stage the pain due to sacroiliitis usually disappears. Pain and loss of function are also consequences of inflammation elsewhere in the spine. But there are other possible consequences of spinal inflammation: abnormal posture, ankylosis of the spine (if complete often called bamboo spine), and fracture. Abnormal posture has often the greatest implications on physical functioning, even more than ankylosis of the spine. An important first sign is the loss of the physiological lumbar lordosis. This may be followed by all the other features of abnormal posture, including thoracic kyphosis. These features of abnormal posture should be detected as early as possible to consider appropriate treatment, in particular daily exercises and physiotherapy. Ankylosis is a consequence of spinal inflammation and is located in the ligaments, but at the thoracic level also in the vertebro-costal and sterno-costal joints. This ankylosis at the thoracic level may lead to reduced thoracic expansion and, thereafter, potentially to, although rarely, respiratory failure. The ankylosis in the lumbar and thoracic spine is not necessarily linked to severe physical limitations. However, ankylosis of the cervical spine has major physical consequences, as the patient will be unable to turn the head. There are two types of fractures: osteoporotic vertebral fractures and fractures of the rigid, ankylosed spine. Osteoporosis is present in a high percentage of patients with AS. Dual energy X-ray absorptiometry (DXA) scans of the spine might reveal falsely normal bone density due to the extra bone formation leading to ankylosis. The prevalence of osteoporotic fractures is high. It has been demonstrated that osteoporotic fractures of the thoracic spine contribute to the thoracic kyphosis and increased occiput to wall distance. Fractures in the ankylosed spine often occur after very minimal trauma.

Root joint involvement is important to check, as this is responsible for major disability. Hip involvement may lead to severe destruction necessitating total hip replacement.

Clinical Assessment of Axial Involvement

The domain spinal mobility comprises four instruments and is assessed as follows:

a. *Chest expansion.* Hands resting on or behind the head. Assess the difference between maximal inspiration and exspiration at the fourth intercostal level anteriorly (e.g., 4.4 cm). The better of two tries should be recorded.

b. *Modified Schober test.* Make a mark on the skin on the imaginary line between the two superior, posterior iliac spines. Make a second mark 10 cm higher than the first mark. Ask the patient to bend forward maximally. Measure the distance between the two marks on the skin. The increase above 10 cm should be noted (e.g., 3.4 cm). The better of two tries should be recorded.

c. *Occiput to wall test.* The patient should stand with the heels and back, with hips and knees as straight as possible, against the wall. The chin should be held at the usual carrying level. The patient should undertake the maximal effort to touch the head against the wall. The distance between the wall and the occiput is measured in centimeters (e.g., 9.2 cm). The better of two tries should be recorded.

d. *Lateral spinal flexion.* It is measured by fingertip to floor distance in full lateral flexion without flexing forward or bending the knees. The patient should stand as close to the wall as possible with shoulders at usual level. The distance between patient's middle fingertip and the floor is measured with a tape measure. The patient is asked to bend sideways without bending his knees or lifting his heels and attempting to keep his shoulders in the same place. A second reading is taken and the difference between the two is recorded. The better of two tries is recorded for left and right. The mean of left and right gives the final result for lateral spinal flexion (in cm to the nearest 0.1 cm).

A combined index to assess various aspects of spinal mobility and hip mobility is proposed by the group in Bath: the Bath Ankylosing Spondylitis Metrology Index (BASMI) (8). The usefulness of this combined index over separate domains still needs to be established.

Clinical Assessment of Peripheral Involvement

The 44 swollen joint count is included in the ASAS core set as an objective measure for quantitation of arthritis. Joints included in the 44 joint are: acromioclavicular joints, humeroscapular joints, sternoclavicular joints, elbows, wrists, metacarpophalangeal joints, proximal interphalangeal joints, knees, ankles, and metatarsophalangeal joints. In clinical practice it is important to check also for involvement of the manubriosternal, sterno-costal, and distal interphalangeal joints, as these might also be involved.

Clinical Assessment of Enthesitis

In clinical practice painful sites should be examined. Frequently involved are the plantar fascia (heel pain) and the Achilles tendon. In fact the attachments of all tendons can be involved. Common sites are the pelvis, symphysis, thorax, spine, and large joints. For clinical studies, a few validated enthesitis scores exist, but there is no information yet on the performance in clinical practice.

Clinical Assessment of Extra-Articular Features

There are no specific recommendations to assess extra-articular features. Presence of psoriasis should be actively looked for, especially in the umbilicus and intergluteal region, as patients are often not aware of this or do not mention this spontaneously. A search for inflammatory bowel disease and acute anterior uveitis should be mainly based on asking for symptoms and, if suspected, followed by appropriate investigations.

Clinical Assessment of Global Level of Disease Activity and Functioning

In addition to the four groups of specific features as discussed above, global information on disease activity and physical functioning are also important to know. The domains patient global assessment of disease activity, pain, morning stiffness, fatigue, and physical functioning are aimed at gaining this information. Physical functioning has a special position in this, as this is influenced by both disease activity and disease severity.

Many instruments are answered on a visual analogue scale (VAS). This is a horizontal line of 10 cm with two anchors: best situation represented at the left (0) and worst situation represented at the right (10). The patients are asked to put a vertical mark on the line that best represents their symptoms. The distance from the left until the vertical mark should be measured and presented with one decimal. Another answer modality is the numerical rating scale (NRS). This is a row of numbers from 0 to 10, and the patient is asked to cross one of the numbers. The anchors are identical to the VAS. The advantages of an NRS above a VAS are that the NRS is better understood by patients, results are immediately visible without measuring, and results can also be obtained by telephone. It has been proven in several studies that there is no loss of information by using an NRS instead of a VAS. Especially for clinical practice, the NRS is much more useful.

The various domains to assess the global level of disease activity and physical functioning are assessed as follows:

a. *Patient global*. The question is answered on a VAS or NRS. "How active was your spondylitis on average last week?"

b. *Pain*. There are two questions related to pain. Both ask patients to rate their pain as experienced "on average last week" and are answered on a VAS or NRS. The first question is: "How much pain of your spine due to AS did you have?" and the second "How much pain of your spine due to AS did you have at night?"

c. *Stiffness*. Assessed by the question: "How long did the morning stiffness of your spine last from the time you woke up on average last week?" This is recorded in minutes or on a VAS or NRS where the maximum score represents two hours or more.

d. *Fatigue*. There is one general question on the level of fatigue worded as: "How would you describe the overall level of fatigue/tiredness you have experienced?" and recorded on a VAS or NRS.

e. *Function*. To capture functional capacity, two disease-specific functional indexes are available: the Bath As Functional Index (BASFI) and the Dougados functional index (9,10). The BASFI consists of 10 questions, answered on a VAS or NRS. The final score is the average of the questions, ranging from 0 (no limitation) to 10 (maximal limitation in function). The Dougados functional index has 20 questions answered on a 3- or 5-point verbal rating scale and summed to get the total score. The answers are coded 0, 1, and 2 or 0, 0.5, 1, 1.5, and 2, respectively, to ensure the same range of the final score (0–40). Both functional indexes have shown to be valid and sensitive to differentiate between groups of patients with a different level and/or improvement in physical function. There seems to be little difference in sensitivity to change between the two instruments. The BASFI is the most frequently used index. As an alternative for clinical practice one VAS or NRS can be used to describe the overall level of functioning with the anchors "no physical limitations" and "very severe physical limitations." The accompanying wording would be: "How would you describe the overall level of physical limitations you have experienced?"

For the ASAS core set, only single variables have been selected. However, in recent years several combined instruments became available, especially from the Bath group in the United Kingdom. These are pooled instruments developed to assess the various aspects of the disease process. The Bath Ankylosing Spondylitis Disease Activity Index (BASDAI) is a measure to assess signs and symptoms of disease activity such as morning stiffness (duration and severity), several aspects of pain, and fatigue (11). The BASDAI is used to assess disease activity when starting and monitoring patients on tumor necrosis factor (TNF)-blocking agents (12).

Laboratory and Imaging Assessments

Except for acute phase reactants, laboratory tests are of little value in assessing AS. Both the erythrocyte sedimentation rate (ESR) after one hour according to Westergren and C-reactive protein (CRP) are equally good in following the patient. The ASAS group advised to follow patients by one of the acute phase reactants, preferably the ESR. Absence of an increased ESR or CRP is the rule in patients with AS and does not rule out inflammation or active inflammation.

Radiographs of the pelvis are important in making a diagnosis of sacroiliitis. However, this provides little information in following the patients. A recent study showed that progression of any structural damage in the spine is present in about 40% of the patients after two years of follow-up and in about 60% of the patients after four years of follow-up (13). For clinical trials, various scoring methods are available to quantify radiographic damage, of which the modified Stoke Ankylosing Spondylitis Spinal Score (mSASSS) is preferred for use in clinical trials (13). The Bath Ankylosing Spondylitis Radiology Index (BASRI) is less sensitive to change, but due to its simplicity could be more useful for application in clinical practice (14). At the moment it is unknown how frequent radiographs should be taken in clinical practice, but more frequent than every two years seems inappropriate. Recent data show that spinal inflammation can be quantified on MRI very well (15). For clinical research this is a very useful tool, but the usefulness in daily practice still needs to be established.

RESPONSE CRITERIA

Mostly, studies are analyzed on a group level. However, these results are difficult to translate to an effect for the individual patient. Therefore, response criteria have been developed to assess the response to nonsteroidal anti-inflammatory drug (NSAID) therapy in AS. These so-called ASAS20 response criteria are presented

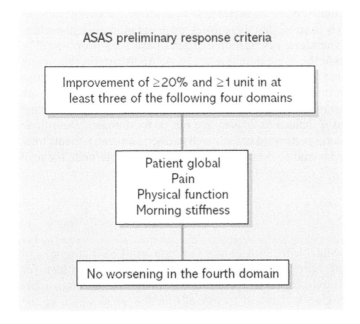

ASAS preliminary response criteria

Improvement of ≥20% and ≥1 unit in at least three of the following four domains

Patient global
Pain
Physical function
Morning stiffness

No worsening in the fourth domain

Figure 2 ASAS20 response criteria.

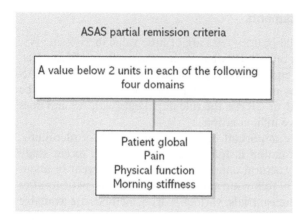

Figure 3 ASAS partial remission criteria.

in Figure 2 (16). These include the following four instruments: BASFI or Dougados FI (domain function), morning stiffness (domain inflammation), patient global of disease activity on a VAS (domain patient global), and overall pain on a VAS (domain pain). In summary, three out of four domains should improve by at least 20% and a minimum of 1 unit on a 10-point scale, and there should be no worsening of 20% and a minimum of 1 unit in the remaining domain. Besides the response criteria, a proposal was made for a state of "partial remission" as an indication of very low disease activity (Fig. 3). Partial remission is defined as a value below 2 (on a 10-point scale) in all four domains (function, inflammation, patient global, and pain). By applying the response and partial remission criteria to clinical trials, more information is available on the percentage of patients benefiting from therapy. With the introduction of TNF-blockers, high percentages of ASAS20 responders were achieved. It was felt that the hurdle should be higher: in a quantitative way and/or in a qualitative way, quantitatively, to be better able to describe the effectiveness of these drugs, and qualitatively to stress that these drugs are doing more than just relieving signs and symptoms. Therefore, new response criteria have been proposed (17). The ASAS40 criteria include the same domains as the ASAS20 criteria but now a 40% improvement is required with a minimum of 2 units in three out of four domains with no worsening at all in the fourth domain. The qualitatively different criteria are the ASAS5/6 criteria that have two extra domains: acute phase reactants and spinal mobility. The improvement is defined as 20% in five out of six domains. Both these ASAS40 and ASAS5/6 criteria performed equally well in discriminating patients treated with TNF-blocking agents and placebo. Further research will determine the final place of these criteria.

SUMMARY

Classification criteria are available for SpA (Amor's criteria and ESSG criteria) and for AS (modified New York criteria). These are suitable for classifying patients for participation in clinical research. However, these lack sensitivity to be useful to apply in clinical practice for making a diagnosis, especially in the early stages of the disease. Lists with signs and symptoms such as the Amor criteria are thought to be helpful in identifying patients with (early and/or incomplete) forms of SpA.

There are four groups of features that may be present in each patient with AS: axial involvement, peripheral joint involvement, entheseal involvement, and extra-articular features. For the first three, assessments have been defined for application in both clinical research and daily clinical practice. In addition, measures are in place to describe global disease activity and physical functioning. Acute phase reactants are the only useful laboratory assessments to monitor patients with AS. Both for radiographs and for MRI of the spine, scoring methods are available which are valuable in evaluating clinical trials. Usefulness in daily practice still needs to be ascertained.

Response criteria to evaluate signs and symptoms and criteria to define partial remission have been published for use in clinical trials. Such assessments are helpful to delineate the clinical achievements of the new, powerful treatment modalities, the so-called biologicals that have become available in recent years.

REFERENCES

1. Moll JM, Haslock I, Macrae IF, Wright V. Associations between ankylosing spondylitis, psoriatic arthritis, Reiter's disease, the intestinal arthropathies and Behçet's syndrome. Medicine (Baltimore) 1974; 53:343–364.
2. Amor B, Dougados M, Listrat V, et al. Are classification criteria for spondyloarthropathy useful as diagnostic criteria? Rev Rhum Engl Ed 1995; 62(1):10–15.
3. Dougados M, van der Linden S, Juhlin R, et al. The European Spondyloarthropathy Study Group preliminary criteria for the classification of spondyloarthropathy [see comments]. Arthritis Rheum 1991; 34:1218–1227.
4. van der Linden S, Valkenburg HA, Cats A. Evaluation of diagnostic criteria for ankylosing spondylitis. A proposal for modification of the New York criteria. Arthritis Rheum 1984; 27(4):361–368.
5. van der Heijde D, van der Linden S, Bellamy N, Calin A, Dougados M, Khan MA. Which domains should be included in a core set for endpoints in ankylosing spondylitis? Introduction to the ankylosing spondylitis module of OMERACT IV. J Rheumatol 1999; 26(4):945–947.
6. van der Heijde D, Calin A, Dougados M, Khan MA, van der Linden S, Bellamy N. Selection of instruments in the core set for DC-ART, SMARD, physical therapy, and clinical record keeping in ankylosing spondylitis. Progress report of the ASAS Working Group. Assessments in ankylosing spondylitis. J Rheumatol 1999; 26(4):951–954.
7. van der Heijde D, Dougados M, Davis J, et al. ASAS/SAA recommendations for conducting clinical trials in ankylosing spondylitis. Arthritis Rheum. 2005; 52:386–394.
8. Jenkinson TR, Mallorie PA, Whitelock HC, Kennedy LG, Garrett SL, Calin A. Defining spinal mobility in ankylosing spondylitis (AS). The Bath AS Metrology Index. J Rheumatol 1994; 21(9):1694–1698.
9. Calin A, Garrett S, Whitelock H, Kennedy LG, OH J, Mallorie P, Jenkinison T. A new approach to defining functional ability in ankylosing spondylitis: the development of the bath ankylosing spondylitis functional index. J Rheumatol 1994; 21:2281–2285.
10. Dougados M, Gueguen A, Nakache JP, Nguyen M, Mery C, Amor B. Evaluation of a functional index and an articular index in ankylosing spondylitis. J Rheumatol 1988; 15:302–307.
11. Garrett S, Jenkinson T, Kennedy LG, Whitelock H, Gaisford P, Calin A. A new approach to defining disease status in ankylosing spondylitis: the Bath Ankylosing Spondylitis Disease Activity Index. J Rheumatol 1994; 21:2286–2291.
12. Braun J, Pham T, Sieper J, et al. International ASAS consensus statement for the use of anti-tumour necrosis factor agents in patients with ankylosing spondylitis. Ann Rheum Dis 2003; 62(9):817–824.

13. Wanders A, Landewé R, Spoorenberg A, et al. What is the most appropriate radiological scoring method for ankylosing spondylitis? A comparison of the available methods based on the Outcome Measures in Rheumatology Clinical Trials filter. Arthritis Rheum 2004; 50(8):2622–2632.
14. Calin A, Mackay K, Santos H, Brophy S. A new dimension to outcome: application of the Bath Ankylosing Spondylitis Radiology Index. J Rheumatol 1999; 26(4):988–992.
15. Braun J, Baraliakos X, Golder W, et al. Magnetic resonance imaging examinations of the spine in patients with ankylosing spondylitis, before and after successful therapy with infliximab: evaluation of a new scoring system. Arthritis Rheum 2003; 48(4):1126–1136.
16. Anderson JJ, Baron G, van der Heijde D, Felson DT, Dougados M. Ankylosing spondylitis assessment group preliminary definition of short-term improvement in ankylosing spondylitis. Arthritis Rheum 2001; 44(8):1876–1886.
17. Brandt J, Listing J, Sieper J, Rudwaleit M, Van Der Heijde D, Braun J. Development and preselection of criteria for short-term improvement after anti-TNFα therapy in ankylosing spondylitis. Ann Rheum Dis 2004; 63(11):1438–1444.

6
Patient's Perspective[*]

Muhammad Asim Khan
Division of Rheumatology, Department of Medicine, MetroHealth Medical Center, Case Western Reserve University, Cleveland, Ohio, U.S.A.

On a recent visit to New York City, as I was taking a 15-block walk in midtown Manhattan, I was thinking about how fortunate I have been. In 1998 I underwent a transluminal coronary angioplasty with stent placement and subsequently I received anticoagulant therapy, which resulted in painless hematuria. This led to the discovery of renal-cell carcinoma, for which I had a radical nephrectomy. This experience has prompted me to share with you my perspective as a patient for 44 years, now facing the added uncertainty that a cancer patient has to live with.

You see, I have had arthritis since age 12, and my physician at that time, the chief of orthopedic surgery at the local university hospital, treated me with frequent bed rests and hospitalizations. There were no rheumatologists in Pakistan in those days. He at one point prescribed one full year of antituberculous treatment (streptomycin injections, isoniazid, and para-aminosalicylic acid), without any resultant clinical benefit. Later on, he treated me intravenously with honey imported from West Germany. By then I was 16 years old and had just become a medical student.

Two years later, during my first clinical rotation in medical school, I spoke to my teacher, a professor in the department of medicine, about my symptoms. He examined me and diagnosed my disease as ankylosing spondylitis. It primarily involved my back, hip joints, and, to a lesser extent, my neck and shoulders. He prescribed phenylbutazone, a nonsteroidal anti-inflammatory drug, to relieve my pain and stiffness, and it worked effectively.

Soon after, I graduated from medical school in 1965, at the age of 21 years. Pakistan at that time was attacked by its neighbor, and I decided to enlist in the Pakistan Army Medical Corps. In my zeal to serve the nation in its hour of need, a nation that had accepted me as a three-year-old refugee, and had provided me with almost free medical education, I did not reveal my illness. My service in the Pakistani Armed Forces was a great experience.

In 1967, when I had just left the army, I received a call for assistance from the very professor from medical school who had diagnosed my ankylosing spondylitis. This professor wanted me to treat his best friend, a prominent local

---

[*] This is the reproduction of the article published in 2000; 133(3):233–235 in the Annals of Internal Medicine, and is reproduced here with the permission of the American College of Physicians.

95

businessman, who had just experienced an acute myocardial infarction. I provided the necessary care, including, later that day, successfully resuscitating the patient when he experienced cardiac arrest. (He went on to live for another 28 years and helped build a hospital for the needy, but that is another story entirely.)

I arrived in London in the summer of 1967 to begin my postgraduate medical studies despite my arthritis, which never ceased to plague me. In an effort to pursue my goal of an academic career in medicine, cardiology was my initial choice for a medical subspecialty, but I felt that the anticipated progressive decrease of my spinal mobility, as well as having limited chest expansion due to my ankylosing spondylitis, might one day impair my ability to resuscitate patients. During the required one year of residency training, I chose orthopedics as my surgical elective. While assisting the surgeons in various orthopedic procedures, including total hip arthroplasty, I was keenly aware that the tables would someday be turned and I would be the one at the receiving end of the operation.

I came to the United States in the summer of 1969 and have successfully pursued an academic career in rheumatology. Knowing what it feels like to be an arthritis sufferer and therefore having a special empathy for patients with this condition, my choice of subspecialty was an easy one to make. Not surprisingly, my primary research interests have included ankylosing spondylitis and related spondyloarthropathies, along with the associated genetic marker HLA-B27.

Inevitably, the tables did turn, and I experienced the following: bilateral total hip joint replacement; revision hip arthroplasty; fracture of the cervical spine; nonunion of the fracture, despite five months of wearing a halo with vest immobilization; surgical fusion of the fracture and another three months of immobilization; recurrent episodes of acute anterior uveitis; hypertension and coronary artery disease; coronary transluminal balloon angioplasties on three separate occasions; and, most recently, right radical nephrectomy. Perhaps you will agree that my many encounters as a patient serve as sufficient "qualifications," if we can call them that, to assert my own view point. I am very grateful to modern medicine for keeping me going. In some ways, I consider myself a "bionic man." My ankylosing spondylitis, however, has resulted in a complete fusion of my whole spine, including the neck. I cannot turn or even nod my head, and I have to bend at my hip joints to give an impression of a nod. I need to grab onto something to pull myself up from a squatting position. I have virtually no chest expansion. One can imagine what might happen to me if I were to have the misfortune of being in an accident or needing cardiac resuscitation; the probability would be high that, inadvertently, my death would be hastened because of a possible neck fracture or broken ribs.

Although I have always sought the best care possible for myself, I have been unlucky on many occasions in not receiving optimum medical care. However, being a perpetual optimist, I am thankful that I am still alive. I sometimes like to give the analogy of the old Timex watch commercial, because I keep on ticking. But if my personal experiences as a patient were extrapolated to the population at large, they would unfortunately highlight many deficiencies in the current practices of medicine, even here in the United States: the unreceptive receptionists, the allied health professionals who lack empathy for their "clients," and the physicians for whom time is such a precious commodity that they start looking at their wrist watches just minutes into the history-taking to signal their impatience.

We physicians frequently do not acquire the skills of a good communicator, and we often neglect patient education. The word "doctor," as I understand it, means an educator or communicator. Yet some physicians apparently lack the traits required to be a good communicator, and some claim that they simply have no time for it, anyway. In such situations, an allied health professional, such as a nurse practitioner, could better handle communications with the patients. Better physician–patient communication is certainly needed.

I underwent bilateral hip arthroplasty as a single surgical procedure at a hospital that specializes in such surgeries. A few years later, I had to undergo a revision hip arthroplasty. Before I left the hospital, I noticed that one leg was now shorter than the other by about a half inch, but my surgeon would not acknowledge this. I still, to this day, wear a shoe lift to minimize my limp.

My first transluminal coronary angioplasty resulted in an extensive intimal tear. When I subsequently had restenosis of the involved artery, I was advised by an independent consultant to have a stent inserted at the time of the revision angioplasty. I had my second angioplasty performed at a highly rated medical center and, although I had requested a stent placement, none was given, and my angina symptoms recurred shortly thereafter.

When I fractured my neck, I was treated with the placement of a halo and a vest to immobilize the fracture. I pointed out to my surgeon on numerous occasions that the fracture was not fully immobilized, as was most noticeable when I leaned back or tried to lie on my back. I voiced my concern that the back plate of the vest was not properly conforming to my thoracic kyphosis, but the surgeon repeatedly reassured me that everything was fine. I had to sleep sitting upright. After three months, a radiograph revealed nonunion of the fracture. Subsequently, the vest was changed, but precious time had already been wasted; because months of further immobilization did not heal the fracture, I ultimately needed a surgical fusion.

I have never sued anyone. My forgiving and nonlitigious nature tells me that as patients we should always give our physicians the benefit of the doubt, just as we physicians, likewise, should always show respect for our patients and give them some degree of latitude. But in our current health care system, there is an obvious need for a more open dialogue between physicians and their patients.

During the seven-month period in which I wore a halo that was screwed into my skull and attached to a vest that surrounded my chest (just imagine trying to sleep at night wearing all that hardware!), I continued to care for my patients. I found myself in ever greater awe at the power we, as physicians, hold as healers. On one occasion, a new patient came to see me, and after our initial handshake, I noticed that his face was turning pale. I immediately had him lie down on the examination table just before he fainted. When he felt better the patient started to laugh, and said, "Doc, I had been hurting and waiting to see you for two weeks, but with one look at you all my pains are gone!"

One morning, a few days later, I was walking by the emergency room on my way to the office and had not yet donned my white coat. A young child noticed my halo and asked, "What happened?"

"I had an accident," I replied.

Having surmised that I was en route to the emergency room for acute medical attention, the child inquired "Is that the steering wheel of your car that is stuck around your head?"

I have enjoyed every bit of my life, with all its humor, hardships, hurdles, and dramatics that could even appeal to the Hollywood movie moguls. And I continue to enjoy my walks. After all, my doctor has instructed me to get daily exercise.

7

Bone Mineral Density and Osteoporosis in Ankylosing Spondylitis

Jean Francis Maillefert
University of Burgundy and Department of Rheumatology, Dijon University Hospital, Hôpital Général, Dijon, France

Christian Roux
Department of Rheumatology, René Descartes University and Institut de Rhumatologie, Cochin Hospital, Paris, France

Ankylosing spondylitis (AS) is characterized by sacroiliac and spine inflammation, and by extraosseous calcifications, leading in some patients to vertebral ankylosis. Generalized bone loss and osteoporosis were not considered in the past as important features of the disease and actually are currently underestimated by numerous rheumatologists (1). However, in the recent years, several studies have established that bone mineral density (BMD) is decreased, and that the prevalence of osteoporosis is increased, in AS compared to general population. In this chapter, we will present the current knowledge on BMD and bone metabolism in AS, discuss the clinical manifestations and the pathophysiology of bone loss and osteoporosis in AS, and discuss the management in clinical practice.

BONE MINERAL DENSITY IN AS

Bone Mineral Density

Numerous techniques are available to assess bone density. Dual energy X-ray absorptiometry (DXA) has been proved to be safe, convenient, accurate, and reproducible, and is currently the most widely used technique. BMD, as measured by DXA, is a well-known predictor of fracture, with an increased risk of 1.5- to 3-fold or more for each standard deviation decrease in postmenopausal women (2–6). DXA-measured BMD forms the basis of the definition of osteoporosis proposed by a World Health Organization (WHO) study group (7).

Bone Mineral Density in AS

Numerous studies have shown that the lumbar, hip, or total body BMD are reduced in AS in comparison to controls (Table 1) (8–15). According to the WHO definition,

Table 1 Bone Mineral Density (BMD), and Bone Mineral Content (BMC) in Ankylosing Spondylitis (AS) Patients

Reference	Patients	Design	Results: bone mineral density
8	19 AS men, mean age = 50.5 yr, mean disease duration = 25.2 yr; 19 controls	Cross-sectional	Decrease in total hip (−14%) and L3 on lateral projection (−21%) BMD in patients compared to controls. No difference in vertebral BMD using posteroanterior approach Osteopenia in the total hip in 72% patients and 10.5% controls (WHO definition), no patient with osteoporosis
9	62 AS men, men age = 43.5 yr, mean disease duration = 16.3 yr; 25 AS women, mean age = 44.8 yr, mean disease duration = 16.6 yr	Cross-sectional	Femoral neck BMD reduced in mild, moderate, and severe AS (defined using the Schober's test), lumbar BMD reduced in mild and moderate, but not in severe AS No difference between patients with and without associated bowel disease or psoriatic arthritis No difference between patients with and without peripheral joint involvement Lower lumbar and whole body BMD in male than in female, trend toward a lower femoral neck BMD in male
10	Patients with AS (30), psoriatic arthritis (23), and reactive arthritis (10); 41 controls	Cross-sectional	Decrease in femoral neck, but not in lumbar BMD in AS patients compared to controls Osteoporosis (WHO definition) in 47% of AS patients Normal BMD at both sites in patients with psoriatic arthritis
11	27 men, 3 women, mean age and disease duration = 37 and 17 yr; 30 controls	Cross-sectional	Osteopenia and osteoporosis (WHO definition) in 55% and 31% (total proximal femur) and in 23% and 27% of patients (lumbar spine) 10% and 21% decrease in lumbar and proximal femur BMD in patients compared to controls
12	16 men with mild AS (syndesmophyte scores of 0 and 1) mean age and disease duration = 36.6 and 8.7 yr; 11 men with advanced AS (syndesmophyte score of 4), mean age and disease duration = 42.5 and 11.7 yr; 6 women with mild AS, mean age and disease duration = 36.7 and 6.8 yr; 41 controls	Cross-sectional	Men with mild AS: 9% and 13% reduction of lumbar and femoral neck BMD compared to controls Men with advanced AS: 10% increase in lumbar BMD, and no difference in femoral neck BMD compared to controls Women: 17% reduction of lumbar spine and no significant difference in femoral neck BMD compared to controls
13	39 AS men, mean age and disease duration = 39 and 15.4 yr, with no syndesmophyte; 39 controls	Cross-sectional	12% decrease in lumbar spine BMD in patients compared to controls. No statistically significant difference between patients and controls in pelvis BMD

14	71 early AS patients (49 male, 22 female), mean age = 39 yr, mean disease duration = 10.6 yr; 71 controls	Cross-sectional	8.5% and 6.7% decrease in lumbar spine and femoral neck BMD in patients compared to controls. Osteoporosis (WHO definition) in 14.1% (lumbar spine) and 4.3% (femoral neck) of patients, and in 0% and 0% of controls. Osteopenia in 32.4% (lumbar spine) and 22.5% (femoral neck) of patients and in 23.9% and 14.1% of controls
15	25 AS men, mean age and disease duration = 33 and 11.5 yr, mobile lumbar spine, X-ray scores for hip and lumbar spine ≤2 on a five-point scale; 25 controls	Cross-sectional	10% decrease in lumbar spine and femoral neck BMD in patients compared to controls
16	80 patients (52 men, 22 premenopausal women, 6 menopausal women), mean age = 36.7 yr, mean disease duration = 12.3 yr	Cross-sectional	18.7% of patients with osteoporosis (WHO definition) at the lumbar spine and 31.2% with osteopenia (WHO definition). 13.7% of patients with osteoporosis at the femoral neck and 41.2% with osteopenia. Positive correlation between spinal T-score and total fat mass percentage and disease duration. No significant correlation between femoral T-score and any evaluated parameter
17	66 AS women, mean age = 43.4 yr, mean disease duration = 21.1 yr, including 50 premenopausal and 16 postmenopausal women; 132 controls	Cross-sectional	Premenopausal women: 5% reduction in total hip BMD compared to controls. Postmenopausal women: 9.6% reduction in total hip BMD compared to controls. No difference in lumbar BMD. Total hip BMD: osteoporosis in 4% of patients and 1% of controls, osteopenia in 35% of patients and 23% of controls
18	7 men with early AS, no syndesmophytes, mean age and disease duration = 33 and 5.4 yr; 7 men with late AS, vertebral calcifications, mean age and disease duration = 54 and 27 yr	Longitudinal (15 mo follow-up)	Reduced baseline axial BMD measured by QCT: mean Z-scores = −1.8 and −3.8 in early and late disease, respectively. Baseline lumbar BMD reduced in early but not in late disease (mean Z-scores = −1.08 and +0.79). Hip BMD not different from predicted values in early disease and decreased in late disease. Longitudinal evaluation: lumbar BMD stable in late disease and increase compared to baseline in early disease. No change in hip BMD, nor in lumbar BMD measured by QCT

(Continued)

Table 1 Bone Mineral Density (BMD), and Bone Mineral Content (BMC) in Ankylosing Spondylitis (AS) Patients (*Continued*)

Reference	Patients	Design	Results: bone mineral density
19	66 men with mild AS (mobile lumbar spine and syndesmophyte score 0 or 1), median age and disease duration = 37 and 9.8 yr; 39 controls aged 50–60 yr	Cross-sectional	Mean lumbar and femoral T-scores = -0.97 ± 0.14 and -0.82 ± 0.12. No relationship between BMD and disease duration
20	35 men, 19 women, mean age = 37.3 yr, mean disease duration = 12.4 yr	Longitudinal (2 yr follow-up)	No change in lumbar BMD at 2 yr compared to baseline. 1.6% decrease in femoral neck BMD at 2 yr compared to baseline. Significant bone loss at 2 yr compared to baseline (defined as greater than 2.8× measurement precision) in 21% and 20% patients, at the lumbar spine and the femoral neck
21	60 men, mean age = 39 yr, mean disease duration = 15 yr, 10 premenopausal women, mean age = 35 yr, mean disease duration = 13 yr	Cross-sectional; longitudinal (mean follow-up = 3.4 yr) in 19 patients	Radius: no statistically difference between patients and controls. Lumbar spine: BMC lower in AS men with syndesmophyte score of 0 or 1 than in controls. No difference between other AS population and controls. QCT: BMD lower in patients than controls. Longitudinal analysis: mean increase in lumbar BMC of 1.3% per year
22	20 men and 2 premenopausal women, mean age and disease duration = 36.8 and 9.8 yr	Cross-sectional	BMD not related to disease duration. Lumbar BMD related to the syndesmophyte score (diminished in grade 2 compared to grades 0 and 1, increased in grades 3 and 4 compared to grades 0, 1, and 2). Femoral neck BMD decreased in radiological grade 2 AS compared to grades 0 and 1
23	18 premenopausal AS women, mean age = 37 yr, mean disease duration = 15 yr, no syndesmophytes on x-rays	Cross-sectional	Lumbar spine and femoral neck Z-scores not different from general population. Osteopenia and osteoporosis (WHO definition) in 11.1% and 5.6% of patients, respectively

Syndesmophyte score: 0, no syndesmophyte; 1, incipient syndesmophyte; 2, syndesmophytes bridging 1 or 2 intervertebral disc space; 3, syndesmophytes producing an undulating vertebral contour; 4, "trolley track sign."
World Health Organization (WHO) definition of osteoporosis: osteoporosis defined as T-score<-2.5, ostopenia defined as T-score between -1 and -2.5 (7).
Abbreviation: QCT, quantitative computer tomography.

osteopenia and osteoporosis are frequent in AS. The prevalence of osteopenia in patients (*T*-score between −1 and −2.5) ranges from 22% to 72% at the hip and from 18% to 32% at the lumbar spine, while the prevalence of osteoporosis (*T*-score less than −2.5) ranges from 0% to 31% at the hip and from 5% to 27% at the lumbar spine (8,11,14,16,17).

In the absence of long-standing longitudinal studies, there are only indirect data regarding the course of BMD in AS. Bone loss occurs early in the disease history, and can be demonstrated in patients with a mean disease duration of only five years (12,18,19). It seems likely that bone mass continues to decrease thereafter, although some studies have not found any relationship between BMD and disease duration. The course of BMD can be assessed by DXA, at least at the hip (20). On the contrary, in some patients with advanced disease, DXA is unable to demonstrate any decrease in lumbar BMD, which can be found normal or increased, because of new bone formation, i.e., syndesmophytes, interapophyseal joint and interpedicular ankylosis, leading to apparently preserved or increased lumbar bone mass on DXA (8,9,12,18, 21,22). This overestimation of lumbar trabecular bone mass can be overridden by techniques that isolate the vertebral bodies from the peripheral layers, such as DXA in lateral projection, or quantitative computer tomography (8,18,21).

Due to the overestimation of lumbar bone mass in advanced diseases, it is difficult to know whether the rate of bone loss is site-dependent or not. Some studies in patients with early AS, or without syndesmophytes on X-ray, suggest that the loss of trabecular bone might be higher at the lumbar spine than at the femoral neck, but confirmation is needed (13,18).

Determinants of Bone Mineral Density in AS

Although numerous studies have evaluated the determinants of bone loss, convincing data on that point are lacking. Substantial evidence indicates, however, that inflammation is involved in bone loss. Most cross-sectional studies failed to demonstrate a correlation between BMD and clinical or laboratory inflammatory parameters (Table 2) but BMD measurement reflects bone loss over several years whereas inflammatory parameters reflects inflammation at the time of measurement (11,14,16,17,22). Thus, longitudinal follow-ups are needed to assess the relationship. Such studies were conducted and demonstrated an increased bone loss in AS patients with persistent systemic inflammation. In the first one, 34 patients with AS of less than 10 years duration were followed up for a mean of 19 months (24). The patients were rated as active or inactive AS on the basis of determination of erythrocyte sedimentation rate (ESR) and C-reactive protein (CRP) during the follow-up. BMD, evaluated at baseline and at endpoint, decreased only in the active group, with a mean loss during follow-up of 5% at the lumbar spine (0.2% in the inactive group) and 3% at the femoral neck (0.6% in the inactive group). In the second study, in which 54 patients were followed up for two years, the decrease in femoral neck BMD was higher in patients with persistent systemic inflammation, defined using mean ESR determinations during the follow-up, compared to other patients (−4.1% vs. −1.2%) (20).

Other potential determinants of bone mass in AS have been discussed. Cross-sectional studies suggested that bone loss is more pronounced in males than in females, but changes in BMD were not related to gender in a two years longitudinal study (9,20,21). Conflicting results have been published on the spondyloarthropathies disease subtypes (9,10,20). The decrease in spine mobility may play a role in the occurrence of vertebral bone loss.

Table 2 Correlations Between Clinical Activity, Inflammatory Parameters, or Cytokines, and BMD or Bone Markers in AS Patients

Reference	Patients	Results
10	See Table 1	Psoriatic arthritis: CTx correlated to ESR and CRP, D-PYR correlated with ESR
		Reactive arthritis: D-PYR and CTx correlated with ESR
		AS: no relationship between bone markers and ESR nor CRP
		No correlation between bone formation markers or osteoprotegerin and ESR nor CRP
11	See Table 1	No correlation between lumbar and total proximal femur BMD with regard to AS activity
13	See Table 1	When artificially rating patients as low or normal lumbar BMD (Z-score $<$ or ≥ 1.5), significant increase in ESR and CRP in patients with low lumbar BMD (ESR $= 29.4 \pm 23$ vs. 12.1 ± 10.8 mm/hr; CRP $= 24.8 \pm 18$ vs. 12.7 ± 14.2 mg/L)
14	See Table 1	No correlation between BASDAI, ESR, CRP, and BMD
16	See Table 1	BMD not related to clinical indices of disease severity
		Positive relationship between urinary D-PYR and CTx concentrations and CRP
		Trend toward increased ESR and CRP levels in patients with osteoporosis (defined as T-score <2.5), compared to others
17	See Table 1	Femoral neck BMD not related to clinical severity and CRP
20	See Table 1	24-mo percentage changes in lumbar and femoral neck BMD not related to baseline ESR, CRP, or clinical parameters of disease severity
		24-mo percentage changes in femoral neck BMD increased in patients with persistent systemic inflammation (defined as mean ESR during the follow-up ≥ 28 mm/hr), compared to other patients ($-4.1 \pm 5.7\%$ vs. $-1.2 \pm 3.9\%$)
21	See Table 1	No correlation between lumbar BMC and ESR nor CRP
22	See Table 1	BMD not related to clinical severity, ESR, and CRP
24	14 patients with active, 20 with inactive disease, mean age $= 33$ and 31 yr, mean disease duration $= 7.5$ and 5.3 yr	After 19 mo follow-up, increased bone loss in patients with active, compared to inactive disease (-5 vs. -0.2% at the lumbar spine; -3% vs. -0.6% at the femoral neck)
		No difference in PTH and 25OHvitD between patients with active or inactive disease
		Interleukin 6 increased in patients with active compared to inactive disease
26	56 AS men with mild disease; 52 controls	ESR and CRP positively correlated to serum bone alkaline phosphatase, urinary pyridinoline, and urinary D-PYR, and negatively to serum osteocalcin
27	49 AS men and 13 AS women, mean age $= 41$ and 40 yr, mean disease duration $= 13$ yr; 50 controls	No correlation between total and bone alkaline phosphatase, nor osteocalcin and ESR or CRP
		Positive relationship between urinary pyridinoline and ESR and CRP

28	32 AS patients (23 men, 9 women), mean age and disease duration = 37 and 6 yr; 25 controls	Urinary free D-PYR significantly increased in patients with raised ESR (>15 mm/hr) compared to other patients. No difference between groups in free pyridinoline and β-CTx. Osteocalcin not correlated to ESR
29	22 men, 7 women, median age and disease duration = 46 and 20 yr	No correlation between lumbar or femoral BMD and ESR. Urinary pyridinoline and D-PYR positively correlated with CRP, but not ESR. C-terminal propeptide of type 1 collagen negatively correlated with ESR, but not with CRP
30	48 men, 22 women, mean age and disease duration = 38 and 17 yr; 45 controls	Negative correlation between PTH, 1–25(OH)2vitD, and CRP. Positive correlation between urinary pyridinium crosslinks and CRP

Abbreviations: BMD, bone mineral density; ESR, erythrocyte sedimentation rate; CRP, C-reactive protein; D-PYR, deoxypyridinoline; CTx, C-telopeptide; BASDAI, bath ankylosing spondylitis disease activity index.

BONE REMODELING AND CALCIUM METABOLISM IN AS

Bone Remodeling

Conflicting results have been published in this area (Table 3). Serum osteocalcin, a bone formation parameter, was found to be decreased or normal (8,13,17,18, 25–28,31). Bone-specific alkaline phosphatases, another bone formation marker, were found decreased, normal, or increased (8,17,26,27,32). The bone resorption markers were reported to be increased or normal (8,10,26–28,32).

All these differences in results might be due to patient selection and, particularly, patients' inflammatory status, since bone resorption markers are positively related to laboratory inflammatory parameters in AS (Table 2) (10,16,26–29,32). The relationship between bone formation markers and inflammation is less clear (10,26,27,29).

All these results suggest that bone remodeling is normal in inactive AS, and is characterized by an uncoupling of bone resorption to bone formation, with at least an increase in resorption, in active AS (as reported in another rheumatic disorder, rheumatoid arthritis). Such uncoupling was not confirmed by two histomorphometric studies, which failed to demonstrate an increased bone resorption (18,33). However, the ESR was normal in all patients included in the first study (not stated in the second one), and the results of the second study are difficult to interpret, since the patients were compared to a control population of different geographic area, ethnic composition, and physical activity (18,33).

Calcium Metabolism

The dietary calcium intake appears as normal (13). Serum calcium and phosphorus and urinary calcium have been found within the normal values in most studies (Table 3) (8,13,16,26,28,31,32). The serum levels of 25-hydroxyvitamin D (25OHvit D) were found normal in all studies except one (8,18,26,28,30–32). The serum 1,25-dihydroxyvitamin D [1,25(OH)2vitD] levels were normal in one study, increased by 22% compared to controls in another one, and decreased by 25% in a third one, in which serum 1,25(OH)2vitD was found to be negatively correlated with laboratory inflammatory parameters (18,25,30). Interestingly, the ESR was normal in all patients, or in all patients except two, in the other studies evaluating 1,25(OH)2vitD. The serum parathyroid hormone (PTH) levels were found normal in all studies except one in which a 35% decrease in mean serum level compared to controls, and a negative relationship between PTH and laboratory inflammatory parameters was demonstrated (8,13,16,24,28,30,31).

Taken together, all these results suggest that serum calcium, phosphorus, 25OHvitD, and urinary calcium are not modified in AS. The results are less clear for 1,25(OH)2vitD and for PTH. The discrepancies between studies might be due in part to differences in study populations, and to statistical power. These parameters might be slightly decreased in biologically active AS. Other studies including a sufficient number of patients are needed to address this question.

OSTEOPOROTIC FRACTURES IN AS

Prevalence of Osteoporotic Fractures

Osteoporosis is a systemic skeletal disease characterized by low BMD and microarchitectural deterioration of bone tissue, leading to bone fragility and increased

Table 3 Histomorphometry, Calcium Metabolism and Bone Markers in AS Patients

Reference	Patients	Design	Results: calcium metabolism and bone markers
8	See Table 1	See Table 1	No difference between patients and controls in serum calcium, phosphorus, PTH Slight increase in 25OHvitD in patients compared to controls 42% increase in ICTP in patients compared to controls, 32% and 24% increase in pyridinoline and D-PYR ($p < 0.06$)
10	See Table 1	See Table 1	42–45% increase in CTx, and 44–86% increase in D-PYR in patients compared to controls; no difference between patients' groups 24% increase in BALP in psoriatic arthritis, 24% increase in osteocalcin in AS compared to controls 26–35% increase in osteoprotegerin in patients compared to controls, with no difference between patients' groups
13	See Table 1	See Table 1	No difference in calcium intake between patients and controls Mean values of serum calcium, phosphorus, 25OHvitD, PTH, bone formation markers within the normal ranges When artificially rating patients as low or normal lumbar BMD (Z-score < or ≥1.5), no differences between groups in all evaluated parameters
16	See Table 1	See Table 1	Normal values of serum calcium, phosphorus, and urinary calcium Increased and decreased osteocalcin in 23.8% and 12.7% of patients Increased urinary D-PYR and CTx in 40% and 40% of patients Positive relationship between urinary D-PYR and CTx concentrations and CRP and Larsen radiological hip score, and negative correlation with Schober's score
17	See Table 1	See Table 1	13% and 22% decrease in BALP and in osteocalcin, trend toward an increase in D-PYR, in patients compared to controls Correlation between osteocalcin and femoral neck and total hip BMD Correlation between D-PYR and C-reactive protein

(Continued)

Table 3 Histomorphometry, Calcium Metabolism and Bone Markers in AS Patients (*Continued*)

Reference	Patients	Design	Results: calcium metabolism and bone markers
18	See Table 1	See Table 1	Normal urinary calcium at baseline Normal 25OHvitD, 1,25(OH)2vitD, PTH, osteocalcin, and urinary hydroxyproline Histomorphometry: low bone volume and trabecular width in many cases, no change in bone turnover, no osteomalacia
21	See Table 1	See Table 1	No correlation between radiographic changes or lumbar BMC and fasting urinary calcium or hydroxyproline ratios
25	38 patients with mild or moderate AS; 13 women and 25 men, mean age = 37 and 42 yr; 52 controls	Cross-sectional	47% (men) and 74% (women) decrease in serum osteocalcin in patients compared to controls 18% increase in alkaline phosphatase in patients compared to controls Nonsignificant increase in 25OHvitD and PTH in patients compared to controls 22% increase in 1,25(OH)2vitD compared to controls (unknown statistical significance)
26	See Table 2	Cross-sectional	Increased BALP (+27%) and decreased osteocalcin (−18%) in patients compared to controls No difference between patients and controls in PTH, 25OHvitD, urinary pyridinoline, and D-PYR Bone markers not related to the presence of fractures or to BMD
27	See Table 2	Cross-sectional	No difference in total and bone alkaline phosphatase, osteocalcin between patients and controls Increased urinary pyridinoline (+51%) in patients compared to controls Urinary pyridinoline not related to age, sex, disease duration, treatment with NSAIDs
28	See Table 2	Cross-sectional	No difference in urinary free pyridinium cross-links, βCTx, and osteocalcin in patients compared to controls Lumbar BMD not related to resorption bone markers

31	16 men, 14 women with AS, mean age and disease duration = 36 and 4 yr; 30 age and sex-matched controls	Cross-sectional	No difference between patients and controls
33	16 AS men, mean age = 34 yr, mean disease duration = 11 yr	Cross-sectional	Lumbar and femoral BMD decreased compared to controls Decreased trabecular bone mass, wall thickness, and plate Increased relative osteoid volume and thickness. Decreased mineral apposition rate, and doubly labeled trabecula With mineralization lag time increased compared to normal values 14 patients with osteopenia, 10 mineralization defects, and 3 with osteomalacia. Normal bone resorption markers No correlation between histomorphometric parameters and BMD
30	See Table 2	Cross-sectional	25% reduction in 1–25(OH)2vitD and 35% reduction in PTH in patients compared to controls 37.5% increase in urinary pyridinium cross-links in patients compared to controls No difference in serum and urinary calcium, 25OHvitD, and serum BALP

Abbreviation: PTH, parathyroid hormone.
Bone formation markers: BALP, bone-specific alkaline phosphatase; osteocalcin; PICP, carboxyterminal procollagen of type 1 collagen.
Bone resorption markers: ICTP, carboxyterminal telopeptide region of type 1 collagen; D-PYR, deoxypyridinoline; CTx, C-telopeptide.

fracture risk (2,4). BMD, as measured by dual-photon absorptiometry is a well-known predictor of fracture risk in the general population (2–6). However, the observation of decreased BMD is not sufficient to state that the prevalence of osteoporosis is increased in the particular AS population, until an increase in fractures is demonstrated. In particular, new bone formation, such as syndesmophytes, observed in AS, might change the biomechanical parameters and the strength of the bone and thus might change the relationship between BMD and fractures.

Several studies have evaluated the prevalence of osteoporotic fractures in AS (8,9,14,18–23,34). As shown in Table 4, various results have been obtained, with both low and high levels of vertebral fractures, the observed prevalence ranging from 0% to 40.9%. These studies differed in the design, the studied population, and especially the definition of vertebral fracture. The studies in which the highest fracture prevalences were demonstrated used morphometric methods, which are more reproducible than subjective assessment but may overestimate the prevalence of fractures (9,19,22,34).

The studies comparing the prevalence of vertebral fractures in AS patients and in the general population resulted in more homogeneous results. Two cross-sectional studies demonstrated an increased vertebral fracture prevalence in AS women (8.3% vs. 1.9%) and men (16.7% vs. 2.6%; odds ratio = 5.92; 95% confidence interval = 1.4–23.8), compared to older control patients (9,19). It is noteworthy that, in the second work, the patients suffered mild AS (defined as a mobile lumbar spine, radiographically normal hips, and absent or incipient syndesmophytes). A population-based cohort study evaluated the fracture incidence in an inception cohort of 158 AS patients, in comparison with the expected rates from the same community (35). In 2398 person-years of observation, there was no difference in the risk of limb fractures, and an increased risk of vertebral compression fractures, in AS patients compared to controls (standardized morbidity ratio = 7.6, 95% confidence interval = 4.3–12.6). The increase in risk tended to be greater in men than in women (standardized morbidity ratio of 10.7 and 4.2, respectively), but without reaching statistical significance. After 30 years of follow-up, the estimated cumulative incidence of limb fractures was 26%, the same as that expected in the general population, while it was 14% for vertebral compression fractures (3.4% expected).

Thus, although some bias cannot be excluded (selection bias in cross-sectional studies and ascertainment bias in the population-based study), it seems likely that at least the risk of vertebral compression fractures is increased in AS compared to the general population. On the contrary, no increased risk in the main complication of osteoporosis, i.e., the femoral fracture, was demonstrated. However, it is difficult to conclude on this point. The femoral fracture risk is difficult to assess because such events are less frequent, and usually occur at an older age than vertebral fractures, so the above-mentioned study might have suffered from lack of statistical power (4).

Determinants of Fracture Risk

Since BMD is related to fractures in the general population, and is reduced in AS, one could suppose that the increase in the vertebral fracture risk in AS is correlated with the decrease in BMD. However, this does not appear clearly in the studies that evaluated both BMD and fractures (Table 4).

Several hypotheses can be proposed for explanation. First is the overestimation of lumbar BMD due to redistribution of bone. However, no difference in BMD between fractured and nonfractured patients was demonstrated in patients with no or incipient syndesmophytes (19). Second, in AS, an increase in other risk factors for fractures, such as decreased mobility and muscle weakness, might reduce the proportion of BMD-related risk in the total fracture risk. Third, as stated above, morphometric methods may overestimate the prevalence of vertebral fractures, and may have rated some other spinal deformities as fractures. Finally, the absence of correlation might be due to a lack of statistical power, and it must be reminded that the relationship between BMD and fractures in the general population was established on much larger population than those studied in AS.

The relationship between fractures and other parameters have been evaluated in some studies (9,19,22,34). Although heterogeneous results were obtained, the fracture risk appears to be positively related to the disease duration and negatively to reduced spine mobility, the last correlation being difficult to interpret since the reduced spine mobility might be due, in part, to the fractures themselves.

Clinical Manifestations

Osteoporotic vertebral fractures are usually associated with an acute back pain, which ranges from mild to intolerable (4). Chronic pain can persist for years, frequently leading to difficulties in day-to-day activities (4). In addition, height loss and kyphosis can occur, particularly in the most advanced stages. Numerous vertebral fractures do not come to medical attention, but they can, however, lead to functional loss (4,36). Hip fractures are associated with increased death and disability. In the year following the hip fracture mortality is increased by 12% to 20% compared to the general population, and one-half of the survivors present a loss of physical function at one year (4,5).

The clinical consequences of osteoporotic fractures in AS patients have not been extensively evaluated. In one study, none of the eight patients with vertebral fractures had symptoms clearly attributable to fracture nor had previous X rays requested to rule out a fracture (9). However, numerous symptomatic vertebral fractures in AS are probably misdiagnosed, being wrongly attributed to the disease. The long-term consequences of AS osteoporotic fractures are not well known. They might be involved in the kyphosis and vertebral restriction observed in some patients (37).

Insufficiency fractures have been described in AS (38). Insufficiency fractures often involve the pelvis, the legs, and the feet, and usually present as a sudden pain and, if involving the legs or the feet, localized swelling. Radiological signs being frequently delayed, the diagnosis can be difficult, particularly in AS, if the clinical manifestations are wrongly attributed to the disease.

Finally, it seems likely that the transpinal fractures, which are a well-known complication of advanced AS, are mostly due to the loss of the shock-absorbing properties of the ankylosed spine, since the cervical spine, which is not involved in classical osteoporosis, is the most susceptible site (39–41). However, osteoporosis may act as a cofactor.

PATHOPHYSIOLOGY OF LOW BMD IN AS

The etiology of bone loss in AS remains uncertain. Numerous potential factors, such as immobility, decreased intestinal absorption of calcium and vitamin D, hormonal status, treatment with nonsteroidal anti-inflammatory drugs (NSAIDs), and local or systemic inflammatory cytokine release, have been proposed.

Table 4 Compression Vertebral Fractures in AS Patients

Reference	Patients	Design	Evaluation	Results: fractures
8	See Table 1	See Table 1	Fractures noted qualitatively on x-rays	1 AS patient with a thoracic vertebral fracture (5.3%)
9	See Table 1	See Table 1	Thoracic and lumbar spine radiographs. Measure of anterior, central, and posterior vertebral heights. Algorithm based on normal female ranges of vertebral heights used to define fractures	8 patients with fractures (X rays available in 75 patients) BMD not related to fractures Fracture rate = 13.7% in male and 8.3% in female (1.9% in a 1035 reference woman population) Fractures related to disease duration, age, and spine mobility
14	See Table 1	See Table 1	Thoracolumbar spine radiographs. Fracture defined as 20% reduction in body vertebral height at any hedge	1 transdiscal fracture
18	See Table 1	See Table 1	Pelvic and lumbar spine radiographs. Method for assessing fractures not stated	No patient with fracture
19	See Table 1	See Table 1	Thoracolumbar spine radiographs Measurement of vertebral anterior, middle and posterior heights. Definition of fracture based on normal ranges of vertebral heights	Vertebral fracture in 11 patients (16.7%) and 1 control (2.6%) Longer disease duration in patients with compared to without fractures (mean = 12.4 vs. 9.3 yr) No BMD differences in fractured, compared to nonfractured patients
20	See Table 1	See Table 1	Thoracolumbar spine radiographs at the end of the follow-up. Fractures assessed using Genant semiquantitative method	2 patients (3.7%) with vertebral fracture
21	See Table 1	See Table 1	Thoracolumbar spine X rays read by two readers who assessed the presence or not of vertebral fractures	Vertebral fractures in 3 patients (4.3%)

22	See Table 1	See Table 1	Thoracolumbar spine radiographs. Fracture defined as a ratio anterior/posterior vertebral height <0.85. Biconcave vertebra defined as a ratio midvertebra/posterior vertebral height <0.8	Vertebral fractures in 9 patients (40.9%). Prevalence of fractures higher in grade 2 AS
23	See Table 2	Longitudinal	Pelvic and lumbar spine radiographs. Method for assessing fractures not stated	No patient with fracture
23	See Table 1	See Table 1	Thoracic and lumbar spine radiographs. Fracture defined as a ratio anterior/posterior vertebral height <0.8 (thoracic vertebrae) or 0.85 (lumbar vertebrae)	1 patient (5.6%) with vertebral fracture
34	98 men, 13 women, median age and disease duration = 41 and 17 yr	Cross-sectional	Cervicothoracolumbar spine radiographs. Fracture defined as a ratio anterior/posterior vertebral height <0.8 (thoracic vertebrae) or 0.85 (lumbar vertebrae) Biconcave vertebra defined as a ratio midvertebra/posterior vertebral height <0.8	Compression fracture in 18 cases (16%) and biconcave fractures in 5 others. No correlation between fractures and age, disease duration, ESR, CRP. Fractures associated with a greater syndesmophyte X-ray score, and with decrease spine mobility
35	158 AS patients (121 men, 38 women)	Retrospective population based cohort study, follow-up: 2398 person-years	Diagnosis of fracture on the basis of medical and radiologists' reports. Fractures through posterior elements or transverse processes of vertebrae, and cervical fractures were recorded separately	15% of patients had fractures before diagnosis (most frequently hands and forearms), and 26% had fracture during the follow-up (most frequently spine). No increased risk of limb fracture compared to general population. Increased risk of vertebral fracture compared to general population (standardized morbidity ratio = 10.7 in men, 4.2 in women, gender difference non significant)

*Abbreviation:*BMD, bone mineral density.

Pain and stiffness reduce activity and mobility in some AS patients, and inactivity, being a well-known risk factor for osteoporosis, has been suggested as an etiologic factor for AS bone loss (4,5). However, some authors found low bone mass in AS patients with regular exercise therapy or similar levels of exercise and sport participation as controls, both in patients with normal or reduced spine mobility (12,13,15). In a longitudinal study, the two-year changes in BMD were not related to baseline spine mobility or to parameters of clinical activity (20). These results suggest that impaired mobility and reduced activity do not play a major role in AS bone loss. It probably acts, however, as a cofactor.

Some authors have postulated the role of decreased intestinal absorption of calcium and vitamin D. In favor of this hypothesis, the mineralization defects observed on bone biopsy in one study, and the demonstration of high prevalence of inflammatory gut lesions in AS patients, which might be related to disease activity (33,42). However, as stated earlier, neither serum and urinary calcium, nor serum 25OHvitD is decreased in AS patients compared to controls. Moreover, one could expect that a decrease in intestinal calcium and vitamin D absorption should induce an increase in serum PTH level, whereas PTH was found normal in most studies, and decreased in one. In addition, in this last study, PTH was negatively correlated with inflammatory parameters, a finding that is not consistent with a primary decrease in intestinal calcium and vitamin D absorption during a flare-up of the disease. Moreover, the serum PTH and 25OHvitD were not found to be correlated with BMD and bone loss (24,26).

The role of hormonal status in AS bone loss has been discussed since numerous hormones interfere with bone metabolism, and hence a decrease in some hormones, such as testosterone, has been described in other inflammatory disorders. However, hormone levels, including gonadotrophins, testosterone, progesterone, dehydroepiandrosterone, cortisol, growth hormone, prolactin, and thyroid stimulating hormone, were found normal in AS, except in one study in which 17β-estradiol was decreased in 10 AS menstruating women, in comparison with controls (8,10,18,43–46). Thus, hormonal status is probably not involved in bone loss in AS patients, although additional studies on estrogen levels in women, particularly nonmenopausal women, are needed.

The use of NSAIDs has been suggested, since these drugs, widely used in AS, inhibit prostaglandin synthesis, which has an anabolic effect on bone. Long-term treatment of indomethacin has been shown to reduce vertebral bone mass and strength in ovariectomized rats (47). On the other hand, it has been suggested that diclofenac sodium inhibits bone resorption, at least in postmenopausal women (48). There are only few data from clinical studies in AS. In a cross-sectional study, there was no difference in urinary crosslink excretion between patients treated or not treated with NSAIDs (27). In a two year longitudinal study evaluating bone loss in AS patients, the duration of past treatment with NSAIDs was not related to the two-year percentage changes in BMD (20). Corticosteroids can decrease bone mass and increase the fracture risk (49). These drugs are not frequently used in AS. Moreover, the patients included in the studies evaluating bone mass and fractures in AS were not treated, or were rarely treated with corticosteroids. Thus, corticosteroids might increase bone loss in treated patients, but are not the main determinant of low BMD in the whole AS population.

Numerous authors have suggested that systemic inflammatory cytokines might be implicated in bone loss. This hypothesis is based on several data: (i) bone loss is related to persistent systemic inflammation in other inflammatory rheumatic disorders, particularly rheumatoid arthritis (50); (ii) bone loss and turnover are increased in active AS; (iii) molecules associated with systemic inflammation, such as interleukin 1, and particularly tumor necrosis factor α (TNFα), stimulate bone resorption, mostly through the induction of receptor activator of NF-κB ligand (RANKL) and, in TNF-transgenic mice, osteoprotegerin, an inhibitor of RANKL, blocks TNF-mediated bone loss (51,52); (iv) increased soluble TNFα and TNFα messenger RNA (mRNA) expression (53,54) have been documented in serum and sacroiliac joints of AS patients; and (v) an increase in BMD was demonstrated six months after initiation of infliximab, a TNFα inhibitor, in AS patients (55). Consequently, although the relationship between circulating serum concentrations of inflammatory cytokines and bone loss has to be evaluated in longitudinal studies for confirmation, inflammation and circulating pro-inflammatory cytokines probably act as important contributors to generalized bone loss in AS.

Finally, the diffuse bone loss might be increased in some structures, particularly vertebral bodies, by focal inflammation and release of pro-inflammatory cytokines. The rate of bone loss might be higher at the lumbar spine than at the femoral neck and, although possibly explained by lack of statistical power, an increase in femoral fracture risk has not been demonstrated at this time. Spondylitis and spondylodiscitis are well-known features of AS, and can lead to focal erosions or to destructive lesions (56). These inflammatory processes can be detected by magnetic resonance imaging (MRI) even in early stages of the disease and in asymptomatic patients, and regress after treatment with TNFα blockers (57,58). In addition, a correlation between the gadolinium enhancement and the sacroiliac histologic scores of inflammation in AS has been demonstrated, and an increased TNFα mRNA expression has been documented in the sacroiliac joints of AS patients (54,59).

Taken together, several factors are probably involved in AS bone loss, including impaired mobility, and particularly systemic and possibly local inflammation and pro-inflammatory cytokines. Large longitudinal studies are needed to increase our knowledge of AS bone loss pathophysiology, and thus improve prevention and treatment in clinical practice.

LOW BMD AND OSTEOPOROSIS IN AS IN CLINICAL PRACTICE

At present, there are no guidelines or consensus regarding the detection and prevention of bone loss and osteoporosis in AS. Moreover, as stated above, data are lacking on some important points, such as the relationship between BMD and fracture in AS, or the prevalence of hip fractures. In addition, no long-term study aiming at preventing or treating bone loss and osteoporosis has been conducted in AS. Thus, the purpose stated in this chapter should be regarded as reflecting the authors' opinion. In this opinion, until evaluated correctly, the unknown data in AS should be completed by the knowledge on primary osteoporosis for the clinical management in AS (e.g., the decreased hip BMD in AS should be regarded as predicting an increased hip fracture risk).

Should AS Patients Be Screened for Bone Loss and Osteoporosis

In our opinion, AS patients should be screened for osteoporosis. The question of whether such screening should be proposed in the whole population or in selected patients is not solved. Since there are evidences that bone loss is increased in patients with persistent inflammation, screening should be proposed at least in these patients. However, as no model predicting bone loss with maximal sensibility and specificity has been established, and as AS course can fluctuate, the screening could be proposed in all patients. Subsequent monitoring could be realized in patients at high risk for osteoporosis, such as those with persistent systemic inflammation, and/or low bone mass, and/or additional predisposing factors for osteoporosis, e.g., low dietary calcium intake, excess of alcohol intake, menopause, and other conditions associated with osteoporosis (3–5). Although conflicting results have been published on the spondyloarthropathies disease subtype, inflammatory bowel disease associated with AS must be regarded as an indication for BMD assessment (60).

Which Screening Technique Should Be Used?

At present, DXA is the standard and most widely used technique to evaluate bone mass and fracture risk. In AS, there are some potential limitations to the use of DXA:

1. Lumbar BMD is overestimated in patients with lumbar syndesmophytes or interapophyseal joint and interpedicular ankylosis. However, if physicians are aware of that, they can only take into account the BMD measured at the hip (BMD at any site is of value in making the diagnosis of osteoporosis) (4). They can also consider alternative techniques, such as lumbar DXA in lateral projection, or quantitative computer tomography, but these techniques have limited access, and have a low precision (1,61).
2. The relationship between DXA-measured BMD and fracture risk, and the WHO definition of osteoporosis have been established in postmenopausal women, whereas most AS patients are male. However, although data are limited, it has been suggested that the same BMD criteria used to diagnose osteoporosis in women can be applied in men (62).
3. There is no clear relationship between DXA-measured BMD and fractures in AS.

In spite of these limitations, waiting for large prospective studies evaluating the relationship between DXA-measured BMD and fractures in AS, it is likely that DXA should be used as a screening and monitoring technique in AS.

Prevention and Treatment of Bone Loss and Osteoporosis in AS

Even though there are currently no scientific data regarding this point, some measures appear as reasonable:

1. Preventive measures, such as dietary advice, exercise regimens, and treatment of underlying conditions increasing the fracture risk;
2. Prevention of bone loss and osteoporosis in patients treated with corticosteroids, according to the current recommendations (49); and
3. In patients with fractures, prescription of drugs that have been proved to reduce the incidence of fractures in osteoporosis (63).

In patients with low bone mass and no prevalent fracture, it is not possible to suggest any systematic measure. In these patients, the prevention of osteoporotic fractures must be discussed case by case, taking into account strong additional risk factors, such as inflammatory bowel diseases and persistent inflammation.

Finally, physicians should take into account that some drugs used for anti-inflammatory treatments in patients with refractory AS, i.e., those with the maximal risk of bone loss, might have an additional positive effect on bone mass, and possibly on fracture risk:

1. Pamidronate has been proposed for the treatment of refractory AS (64,65). Apart from the anti-inflammatory effects, this drug is a potent antiresorptive agent, which belongs to the molecular class of bisphosphonates. It has been shown to reduce the incidence of fractures in children with osteogenesis imperfecta and in osteoporotic men and women, and to increase bone mass in rheumatoid arthritis patients (66–68). To our knowledge, the effects of pamidronate on BMD have not been evaluated in AS.

2. TNFα-blockers have been shown to induce a rapid and significant improvement in numerous patients with active AS (69,70). In addition to the anti-inflammatory effect, a significant 2.2–3.6% increase in spine, total hip, and trochanter BMD was demonstrated six months after initiation of infliximab, a TNFα inhibitor (55).

Conclusion: Main Points Regarding BMD and Osteoporosis in AS Patients for Clinical Practice

1. In AS, BMD is decreased, and the prevalence of osteoporosis is increased.
2. The prevalence of osteoporotic fractures is increased in AS patients, compared to the general population, and might be an important determinant of invalidity, and particularly of kyphosis.
3. Some fractures are probably misdiagnosed. Physicians should be aware that an acute back pain in AS is not necessarily due to a flare-up of the disease, and could sometimes be related to an osteoporotic vertebral fracture.
4. DXA-screening and monitoring for low BMD and osteoporosis should be performed at least in patients at high risk for osteoporosis, particularly those with persistent systemic inflammation. The results of screening should be interpreted with the knowledge that lumbar BMD can be overestimated in some patients, particularly those with long-standing disease.
5. Preventive measures for bone loss must be proposed to AS patients.
6. Antiosteoporotic drug therapy must be prescribed in patients with fractures.

REFERENCES

1. Bessant R, Harris C, Keat A. Audit of the diagnosis, assessment, and treatment of osteoporosis in patients with ankylosing spondylitis. J Rheumatol 2003; 30:779–782.
2. Consensus development conference: diagnosis, prophylaxis, and treatment of osteoporosis. Am J Med 1993; 94:646–650.
3. Consensus development conference. Who are candidates for prevention and treatment of osteoporosis? Osteoporosis Int 1997; 7:1–6.
4. Meunier PJ, Delmas PD, Eastell R, et al. Diagnosis and management of osteoporosis in postmenopausal women: clinical guidelines. Clin Ther 1999; 21:1025–1044.
5. Newitt MC. Epidemiology of osteoporosis. Rheum Clin North Am 1994; 3:535–559.
6. Riggs BL, Melton LJ. The worldwide problem of osteoporosis: insights afforded by epidemiology. Bone 1995; 17(suppl):505S–511S.
7. Assessment of fracture risk and its application to screening for postmenopausal osteoporosis; report of a WHO Study group. WHO technical report series 843. Geneva: World Health Organization, 1994.

8. Bronson WD, Walker SA, Hillman LS, Keisler D, Hoyt T, Allen SH. Bone mineral density and biochemical markers of bone metabolism in ankylosing spondylitis. J Rheumatol 1998; 25:929–935.

9. Donnelly S, Doyle DV, Denton A, Rolfe I, McCloskey EV, Spector TD. Bone mineral density and vertebral compression fracture rates in ankylosing spondylitis. Ann Rheum Dis 1994; 53:117–121.

10. Grisar J, Bernecker PM, Aringer M, et al. Ankylosing spondylitis, psoriatic arthritis, and reactive arthritis show increased bone resorption, but differ with regard to bone formation. J Rheumatol 2002; 29:1430–1436.

11. Meirelles ES, Borelli A, Camargo OP. Influence of disease activity and chronicity on ankylosing spondylitis bone mass loss. Clin Rheumatol 1999; 18:364–368.

12. Mullaji AB, Upadhyay SS, Ho EKW. Bone mineral density in ankylosing spondylitis. DEXA comparison of control subjects with mild and advanced cases. J Bone Joint Surg 1994; 76-B:660–665.

13. Pimentel Dos Santos F, Constantin A, Laroche M, et al. Whole body and regional bone mineral density in ankylosing spondylitis. J Rheumatol 2001; 28:547–549.

14. Toussirot E, Michel F, Wendling D. Bone density, ultrasound measurements and body composition in early ankylosing spondylitis. Rheumatology 2001; 40:882–888.

15. Will R, Palmer R, Bhalla AK, Ring F, Calin A. Osteoporosis in early ankylosing spondylitis: a primary pathological event? Lancet 1989; 2:1483–1485.

16. El Maghraoui A, Borderie D, Cherruau B, Edouard R, Dougados M, Roux C. Osteoporosis, body composition, and bone turnover in ankylosing spondylitis. J Rheumatol 1999; 26:2205–2209.

17. Speden DJ, Calin AI, Ring FJ, Bhalla AK. Bone mineral density, calcaneal ultrasound, and bone turnover markers in women with ankylosing spondylitis. J Rheumatol 2002; 29:516–521.

18. Lee YSL, Schlotzhauer T, Ott SM, et al. Skeletal status of men with early and late ankylosing spondylitis. Am J Med 1997; 103:233–241.

19. Mitra D, Elvins DM, Speden DJ, Collins AJ. The prevalence of vertebral fractures in mild ankylosing spondylitis and their relationship to bone mineral density. Rheumatology 2000; 39:85–89.

20. Maillefert JF, Aho LS, El Maghraoui A, Dougados M, Roux C. Changes in bone density in patients with ankylosing spondylitis: a 2-year follow-up prospective study. Osteoporos Int 2001; 12:605–609.

21. Devogelaer JP, Maldague B, Malghem J, Nagant de Deuxchaines C. Appendicular and vertebral bone mass in ankylosing spondylitis. A comparison of plain radiographs with single- and dual-photon absorptiometry and with quantitative computed tomography. Arthritis Rheum 1992; 35:1062–1067.

22. Sivri A, Kilinç S, Gökçe-Kutsal Y, Ariyürek M. Bone mineral density in ankylosing spondylitis. Clin Rheumatol 1996; 15:51–54.

23. Juanola X, Mateo L, Nolla JM, Roig-Vilaseca D, Campoy E, Roig-Escofet D. Bone mineral density in women with ankylosing spondylitis. J Rheumatol 2000; 27:1028–1031.

24. Gratacos J, Collado A, Pons F, et al. Significant bone mass in patients with early, active ankylosing spondylitis. Arthritis Rheum 1999; 42:2319–2324.

25. Franck H, Keck E. Serum osteocalcin and vitamin D metabolites in patients with ankylosing spondylitis. Ann Rheum Dis 1993; 52:343–346.

26. Mitra D, Elvins DM, Collins AJ. Biochemical markers of bone metabolism in mild ankylosing spondylitis and their relationship with bone mineral density and vertebral fractures. J Rheumatol 1999; 26:2201–2204.

27. Marhoffer W, Stracke H, Masoud I, et al. Evidence of impaired cartilage/bone turnover in patients with active ankylosing spondylitis. Ann Rheum Dis 1995; 54:556–559.

28. Toussirot E, Ricard-Blum S, Dumoulin G, Cedoz JP, Wendling D. Relationship between urinary pyridinium cross-links, disease activity, and disease subsets of ankylosing spondylitis. Rheumatology 1999; 38:21–27.

29. MacDonald AG, Birkinshaw G, Durham B, Bucknall RC, Fraser WD. Biochemical markers of bone turnover in seronegative spondylarthropathy: relationship to disease activity. Br J Rheumatol 1997; 36:50–53.

30. Lange U, Jung O, Teichmann J, Neeck G. Relationship between disease activity and serum levels of vitamin D metabolites and parathyroid hormone in ankylosing spondylitis. Osteoporos Int 2001; 12:1031–1035.

31. Wendling D, Dumoulin G. Spondylarthrite ankylosante et paramètres phosphocalciques. Rev Rhum 1991; 58:279–281.

32. Lange U, Teichmann J, Stracke H. Correlation between plasma TNF-alpha, IGF-1, biochemical markers of bone metabolism, markers of inflammation/disease activity, and clinical manifestations in ankylosing spondylitis. Eur J Med Res 2000; 5:507–511.

33. Szejnfeld VL, Monier-Faugere MC, Bognar BJ, Bosi Ferraz M, Malluche HH. Systemic osteopenia and mineralization defect in patients with ankylosing spondylitis. J Rheumatol 1997; 24:683–688.

34. Ralston SH, Urquhart GDK, Brzeski M, Sturrock RD. Prevalence of vertebral compression fractures due to osteoporosis in ankylosing spondylitis. Br J Rheumatol 1990; 300:563–565.

35. Cooper C, Carbone L, Michet CJ, Atkinson EJ, O'Fallon WM, Melton LJ. Fracture risk in patients with ankylosing spondylitis: a population-based study. J Rheumatol 1994; 21:1877–1882.

36. Nevitt MC, Ettinger B, Black DM, et al. The association of radiographically detected vertebral fractures with back pain and function: a prospective study. Ann Intern Med 1998; 128:793–800.

37. Geusens P, Vosse D, van der Heijde D, et al. High prevalence of thoracic vertebral deformities and discal wedging in ankylosing spondylitis patients with hyperkyphosis. J Rheumatol 2001; 28:1856–1861.

38. Mäenpää HM, Soini I, Lehto MUK, Belt EA. Insufficiency fractures in patients with chronic inflammatory joint diseases. Clin Exp Rheumatol 2002; 20:77–79.

39. Braun J, Pincus T. Mortality, course of disease and prognosis of patients with ankylosing spondylitis. Clin Exp Rheumatol 2002; 20(suppl 28):S16–S22.

40. Hunter T, Dubo HJC. Spinal fractures complicating ankylosing spondylitis. A long-term follow-up study. Arthritis Rheum 1983; 26:751–759.

41. Sieper J, Braun J, Rudwaleit M, Boonen A, Zink A. Ankylosing spondylitis: an overview. Ann Rheum Dis 2002; 61(suppl III):iii8–iii18.

42. Baeten D, De Keyser F, van Damme N, Veys EM, Mielants H. Influence of the gut and cytokine patterns in spondylarthropathy. Clin Exp Rheumatol 2002; 20(suppl 28): S38–S42.

43. Jimenez-Balderas FJ, Tapia-Serrano R, Madero-Cervera JI, Murrieta S, Mintz G. Ovarian function studies in active ankylosing spondylitis in women. Clinical response to estrogen therapy. J Rheumatol 1990; 17:497–502.

44. Mitra D, Elvins DM, Collins AJ. Testosterone and testosterone free index in mild ankylosing spondylitis: relationship with bone mineral density and vertebral fractures. J Rheumatol 1999; 26:2414–2417.

45. Straub RH, Struharova S, Schölmerich J, Härle P. No alteration of serum levels of adrenal and gonadal hormones in patients with ankylosing spondylitis. Clin Exp Rheumatol 2002; 20(suppl 28):S52–S59.

46. Toussirot E, Nguyen NU, Dumoulin G, Regnard J, Wendling D. Insulin-like growth factor-I and insulin-like growth factor binding protein-3 serum levels in ankylosing spondylitis. Br J Rheumatol 1998; 37:1172–1176.

47. Saino H, Matsuyama T, Takada J, Kaka T, Ishii S. Long-term treatment of indomethacin reduces vertebral bone mass and strength in ovariectomized rats. J Bone Miner Res 1997; 12:1844–1850.

48. Bell NH, Hollis BW, Shary JR, et al. Diclofenac sodium inhibits bone resorption in post menopausal women. Am J Med 1994; 96:349–353.

49. American College of Rheumatology Ad Hoc Committee on Glucocorticoid-Induced Osteoporosis. Recommendations for the prevention and treatment of glucocorticoid-induced osteoporosis. 2001 update. Arthritis Rheum 2001; 44:1496–1503.
50. Gough AKS, Lilley J, Eyre S, Holder RL, Emery P. Generalised bone loss in patients with early rheumatoid arthritis. Lancet 1994; 344:23–27.
51. Goldring SR. Bone and joint destruction in rheumatoid arthritis. What is really happening? J Rheumatol 2002; 29(suppl 65):44–48.
52. Schett G, Redlich K, Hayer S, et al. Osteoprotegerin protects against generalized bone loss in tumor necrosis factor-transgenic mice. Arthritis Rheum 2003; 48:2042–2051.
53. Gratacos J, Collado A, Fidella X, et al. Serum cytokines (IL-6, TNF-alpha, IL-1 beta and IFN-gamma) in ankylosing spondylitis: a close relation between serum IL-6 and disease activity and severity. Br J Rheumatol 1994; 33:927–931.
54. Braun J, Bollow M, Neure L, et al. Use of immunohistologic and in situ hybridization techniques in the examination of sacroiliac joint biopsy specimens from patients with ankylosing spondylitis. Arthritis Rheum 1995; 38:499–505.
55. Allali F, Breban M, Porcher R, Maillefert JF, Dougados M, Roux C. Increase in bone mineral density of spondyloarthropathy patients treated with anti-TNF alpha therapy. Ann Rheum Dis 2003; 62:347–349.
56. Resnick D, Niwayama G. Ankylosing spondylitis. In: Resnick D, Niwayama G, eds. Diagnosis of Bone and Joints Disorders. 2nd ed. Philadelphia: WB Saunders, 1988: 1103–1170.
57. Bollow M, Enzweiler C, Taupitz M, et al. Use of contrast enhanced magnetic resonance imaging to detect spinal inflammation in patients with spondyloarthritides. Clin Exp Rheumatol 2002; 20(suppl 28):S167–S174.
58. Bollow M, Fischer T, Reisshauer H, et al. Quantitative analyses of sacroiliac biopsies in spondylarthropathies: T cells and macrophages predominate in early and active sacroiliitis-cellularity correlates with the degree of enhancement detected by magnetic resonance imaging. Ann Rheum Dis 2000; 59:135–140.
59. Braun J, Baraliakos X, Golder W, et al. Magnetic resonance imaging examinations of the spine in patients with ankylosing spondylitis, before and after successful therapy with infliximab. Evaluation of a new scoring system. Arthritis Rheum 2003; 48:1126–1136.
60. Roux C, Abitbol V, Chaussade S, et al. Bone loss in patients with inflammatory bowel disease: a prospective study. Osteoporos Int 1995; 5:156–160.
61. Bessant R, Keat A. How should clinicians manage osteoporosis in ankylosing spondylitis?. J Rheumatol 2002; 29:1511–1519.
62. Kanis JA, Johnell O, Oden A, De Laet C, Mellstrom D. Diagnosis of osteoporosis and fracture threshold in men. Calcif Tissue Int 2001; 69:218–221.
63. DeSanti A, Buchman A. Current and emerging therapies in osteoporosis. Expert Opin Pharmacother 2002; 3:835–843.
64. Maksymowych WP, Jhangri GS, Fitzgerald AA, et al. A six-month randomized, controlled, double-blind dose–response comparison of intravenous pamidronate (60 mg versus 10 mg) in the treatment of nonsteroidal antiinflammatory drug-refractory ankylosing spondylitis. Arthritis Rheum 2002; 46:766–773.
65. Haibel H, Braun J, Maksymowych WP. Bisphosphonates—targeting bone in the treatment of spondyloarthritis. Clin Exp Rheumatol 2002; 20(suppl 28):S162–S166.
66. Glorieux FH. Bisphosphonate therapy for severe osteogenesis imperfecta. J Pediatr Endocrinol Metab 2000; 13(suppl 2):989–992.
67. Brumsen C, Papapoulos SE, Lips P, et al. Daily oral pamidronate in women and men with osteoporosis: a 3-year randomized placebo-controlled trial with a 2-year open extension. J Bone Miner Res 2002; 17:1057–1064.
68. Eggelmeijer F, Papapoulos SE, van Paassen HC, et al. Increased bone mass with pamidronate treatment in rheumatoid arthritis. Results of a three-year randomized, double-blind trial. Arthritis Rheum 1996; 39:396–402.

69. Braun J, Brandt J, Listing J, et al. Treatment of active ankylosing spondylitis with inflix-imab: a randomised controlled multicentre trial. Lancet 2002; 359:1187–1193.
70. Gorman JD, Sack KE, Davis C. Treatment of ankylosing spondylitis by inhibition of tumor necrosis factor α. N Engl J Med 2002; 346:1349–1356.

8

Analysis of Posture in Patients with Ankylosing Spondylitis

Sandra D. M. Bot
Institute for Research in Extramural Medicine, VU University Medical Center, Amsterdam, The Netherlands

Margo Caspers
BGZ Wegvervoer, Gouda, The Netherlands

Idsart Kingma
Department of Human Movement Sciences, VU University Amsterdam, Amsterdam, The Netherlands

INTRODUCTION

The chronic inflammation associated with ankylosing spondylitis (AS) affects the sacroiliac joints and the synovial joints of the spine. Bony fusion of these joints and ossification of the longitudinal ligaments leads to total immobility of the spine. The fusion of joints and the adoption of a less painful posture may lead to an increasing kyphosis at later stages of the disease (1). As a consequence of the spinal kyphosis, patients are not able to sit, stand, or lie comfortably. In severe cases, patients may be unable to look above the level of the horizon, causing problems in daily activities, like talking to another person, participating in traffic, and getting something above their head.

From a biomechanical point of view, the spinal kyphosis causes a forward and downward shift of the center of mass (COM) of the trunk in the sagittal plane. The forward displacement is especially problematic because it threatens the whole body balance. Murray et al. (2) showed that a significant proportion of AS patients had poor balance compared to asymptomatic subjects. In order to maintain the whole body balance, patients have to compensate for the forward displacement of the trunk COM. In asymptomatic subjects the normal sagittal plane curves of the spine tend to balance each other in such a way that the head, trunk, and pelvis are lined up vertically (3–6). However, in patients with AS the spine is immobile, and hence only the mobile joints of the lower extremities can compensate for the sagittal displacement of the trunk COM. A patient may compensate by extension of the hips, flexion of the knees, and plantar flexion of the ankles. Compensation by the ankles is very efficient in that it demands little plantar flexion of the ankle joints to maintain whole body

123

balance. However, it hardly influences the horizontal view. When the hips are used for compensation a larger change in joint angle is needed to reach the same result concerning the COM displacement compared to compensation by the ankle joints. With respect to the field of vision, this is beneficial, as the more the trunk is rotated posteriorly, the more the field of vision increases, which will enhance the performance of daily activities. Due to the progress of the disease, the compensation by the hips may become insufficient because of the limited range of motion (ROM) in extension direction. Consequently, a permanent displacement of the trunk COM may result in later stages of AS, potentially leading to the need to flex the knees or plantar flex the ankles to prevent falling or to see the horizon. The former compensation would, as already mentioned, be inefficient with respect to the field of vision, whereas the latter compensation would cause rapid fatigue of the quadriceps muscles during standing.

Knowledge of the way patients counterbalance the shift of the body COM could be instrumental in designing more optimal conservative and invasive treatment procedures. Up to now, no biomechanical approach has been used to evaluate the posture of patients with AS. We therefore analyzed the possible mechanisms used to compensate for the sagittal displacement of the trunk COM.

BIOMECHANICS

Biomechanics can be defined as the application of mechanical principles to biological systems. It is differentiated from more classical mechanical engineering primarily by the materials of interest, that is, tissue rather than metals, and it requires a detailed knowledge of the relevant anatomy and physiology of the structures involved. Its focus on the mechanics of a biological system, rather than a clinical focus on the diagnosis and treatment of an injury, differentiates biomechanics from medicine. Examples of biomechanics in health care include the design of artificial joints, the analysis of flow patterns in vascular grafts, gait analysis, and the design of work environments to reduce physical stresses on workers.

The mechanical aspects of human movement are often studied with the help of linked segments models. In such an approach the human body is modeled as a chain of rigid body segments, interconnected by joints. By applying the mechanical principles to each individual body segment, starting at one end of the chain, intersegmental reaction forces and moments can be calculated. In addition, locations of the COM of individual body segments can be "summed up" to obtain the location (under static conditions) or the trajectory (under dynamic conditions) of the COM of the whole body. Besides the application of mechanical principles, human anthropometry is needed to be able to describe the biomechanics of human motion. Included in these measurements are the lengths and weight of specific body parts.

HYPOTHETICAL COMPENSATION MECHANISM

In patients with AS, the spinal kyphosis causes a forward and downward shift of the COM of the trunk. When the other segments do not change position, it will induce a forward and downward shift of the body COM with respect to the base of support (i.e., the feet). In order to keep balance, patients have to compensate for the displacement of the body COM. In Figure 1 this mechanism is explained. Extension of the hip joints, flexion of the knees, and plantar flexion of the ankles, all can be of support

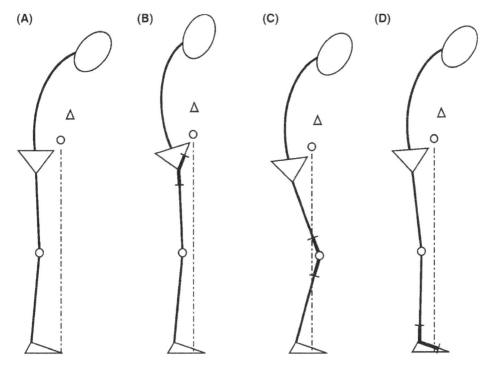

Figure 1 The spinal kyphosis causes a forward and downward shift of the COM of the trunk (Δ), which induces a forward and downward shift of the body COM (O) with respect of the base of support (**A**). The patient has to correct for this shift by extension of the hips (**B**), flexion of the knees (**C**), or plantar flexion of the ankles (**D**). *Abbreviation*: COM, center of mass.

in rotating the body COM over the base of support. We presumed that patients with AS would use hip extension to compensate for the forward displacement of the trunk COM, preserving equilibrium when standing straight. Extension of the hips induces a posterior rotation of the pelvis, inducing a large posterior rotation of the trunk, in contrast to compensation by the knees or ankles. When the deformity progresses and the hip joints are fully extended, this compensation may become insufficient and additional flexion of the knees or plantar flexion of the ankle joints may be needed to compensate for the increased forward inclination of the trunk.

RESEARCH METHODS

To enable evaluation of the mechanisms used to compensate for the shift of the trunk COM we asked four male patients with progressive spinal kyphosis because of severe AS to participate voluntarily in this study. Clinical examination showed that there was no movement possible in the lumbar and thoracal spine. Standard radiographs of the whole spine showed a classic bamboo spine with complete calcification of the disks and bridging syndesmophytes in all patients. One of the patients had a total hip replacement (left side). The other patients had full ROM of the hip joint and none of the patients had problems in the knees or ankles. For all subjects, standing height, total body mass, and length of all segments were measured. Demographic data of the patients are shown in Table 1.

Table 1 Demographic Characteristics of the Patients Participating in the Study

Patient	Age (yrs)	Body mass (kg)	Stature (m)
1	43	68	1.58
2	42	68	1.70
3	77	79	1.68
4	28	75	1.75

The patients stood barefoot on a force platform and were asked to adopt seven different predefined postures, standing as motionlessly and symmetrically as possible for a few seconds. The following postures were recorded: (i) standing relaxed (i.e., the individual habitual standing posture), (ii) standing straight, (iii) standing with maximally extended hips and straight knees, (iv) in between straight standing and maximal hip flexion, (v) standing in maximal hip flexion, (vi) standing with flexed knees with horizontal view, and (vii) standing with maximally extended knees. The postures were recorded by a video camera while simultaneously the forces at the foot–floor interface were registered by a forceplate. The forceplate recordings enabled us to assess the whole body balance by relating the point of application of the ground reaction force [i.e., the center of pressure (COP), which equals the horizontal position of the body COM under static conditions] to the base of support formed by the feet. The COP was expressed as a percentage of distance from heel to toe.

White markers with contrasting black circles were placed on the skin to indicate the location of anatomical landmarks, enabling precise recording of those landmarks from the video images (Fig. 2A). The coordinates of these landmarks were determined by digitizing the video images with a personal computer. From those landmarks, COM locations of the body segments were calculated according to Plagenhoef (7). A two-dimensional linked segment model of the subjects was constructed from these data to calculate the biomechanical parameters (Fig. 2B).

Using the recordings of postures ii, iv and v, the center of gravity of the trunk was calculated from the recordings of the COM locations of the other segments and from the COP with the aid of an optimization method according to Kingma et al. (8). The joint angles of the hip, knee, and ankle joints were defined as the front angle between the distal and proximal segment (Fig. 3). The inclination of a segment was defined as the angle between a horizontal tariff and a line indicating the longitudinal axis of the segment.

We compared joint angles and COP over the various postures. Furthermore, the patients' joint angles of hip, knee, and ankle were compared to data of 18 healthy, asymptomatic male subjects (age 21–27 years) standing relaxed.

ACTUAL COMPENSATION MECHANISM

The COP and trunk angle in the first posture (standing relaxed), the third posture (standing with maximal extension of the hips and straight knees), and seventh posture (standing with maximally extended knees) were compared to examine whether hip and ankle joints could prevent the forward displacement of the trunk COM, without compensation by flexing the knees (Table 2). Only patient 2 was able to fully extend his legs in postures iii and vii, the other patients still had some knee flexion. The results are inconsistent: in patients 1 and 2 the COP moved toward the toes when they stood with maximal extended hips; however in patient 4 the COP moved slightly toward the center of the base of support. When the patients stood with maximal

(A)   (B)

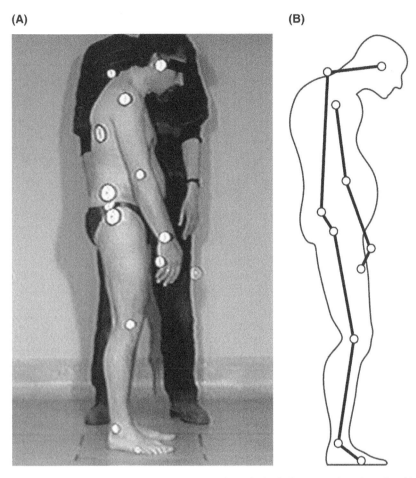

Figure 2 (A) White markers with contrasting black circles were placed on the skin to indicate the location of predefined anatomical landmarks. (B) The coordinates of the anatomical landmarks were determined by digitizing the video images and a two-dimensional linked segment model was constructed.

extended knees, the COP moved slightly toward the toes compared to standing relaxed. The trunk bend forward in three patients when asked to maximally extend their knees (posture vii) compared to standing relaxed (Table 2). The changes of the COP were small relative to the joint movements, which means the patients were compensating for the displacement of the COM. In contrast to our expectations the patients did not extend their hips to induce a large increase in trunk angle as a compensation for the displacement of the trunk COM. Moreover, as will be outlined in more detail subsequently, our results indicate that the patients were hardly able to extend their hips any further when standing relaxed.

Hip

The hip angles in postures i (standing relaxed), ii (standing straight), and iii (standing with maximally extended hips and knees) were compared to examine the potential compensation of forward trunk COM displacement by the hip joint (Table 3). Maximal

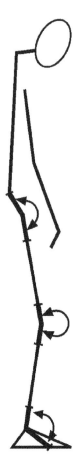

Figure 3 Joint angles were defined as the front angle between the distal and proximal segment.

extension of the hip was obtained by asking the subjects to extend the hips maximally with straight knees. Surprisingly, the patients did not show an increased hip extension to compensate for the forward trunk COM displacements when standing relaxed. In fact, the patients showed on average 16° less hip extension compared to

Table 2 COP and Trunk Angle in Standing Relaxed (Posture i), Standing with Maximal Hip Extension (Posture iii) and Standing with Extended Knees (Posture vii)

Patient	COP (%)[a]			Trunk angle (°)		
	Posture i	Posture iii	Posture vii	Posture i	Posture iii	Posture vii
1	28	37	33	90	96	79
2	34	44	35	91	93	86
3[b]	–	–	–	73	80	76
4	29	26	32	94	97	81

[a]Expressed as a percentage of the distance from heel to toe.
[b]Forceplate data of subject 3 was not available because of an error in the forceplate registration.
Abbreviation: COP, center of pressure.

Table 3 Angle of the Hip Joints (Degrees) in Standing Relaxed (Posture i), Standing Straight (Posture ii), and Standing with Maximal Extension of the Hips (Posture iii)

Patient	Posture i	Posture ii	Posture iii
1	187	185	191
2	209	208	209
3	190	196	193
4	192	191	190

healthy subjects. Moreover, when comparing posture i to posture ii or posture iii, a difference of only one to six degrees was found between these postures. In addition, there was no difference in knee and ankle angles between these postures. This means that the patients were hardly able to extend their hips any further when standing relaxed. The hips appeared to be almost in maximal extension in all three postures. This indicates that these patients had flexed hips when standing straight, which enlarges rather than compensates for the problem of forward trunk COM displacement as it induces an anterior rotation of the trunk. Apparently, the expected compensation by the hip joints is not possible.

Knees

The knees of three patients were more flexed (196° to 209°) compared to asymptomatic subjects (mean 185° ± 6°), and when the patients were asked to adopt a posture that enabled them to see above the horizon, knee flexion further increased (Table 4). The ability to see above the level of the horizon depends on the deformity of the spine, which differed among the patients. One patient was able to see above the horizon without compensation by flexing the knees. Standing with flexed knees will take more effort and will result in earlier fatigue than standing with straight legs. As a consequence the knees may become overloaded.

Ankles

Flexion of the ankles is a third way to compensate for the displacement of the trunk COM. A small change of the ankle joints induces a large shift of the upper body. However, compensating by the ankle joints induces almost no posterior rotation of the trunk. Therefore, the horizontal view hardly increases, which is a disadvantage of this compensation. The angle of the ankles of two patients (118° and 111°) was

Table 4 Knee Flexion (Degrees) in Standing Relaxed (Posture i) and with Horizontal View (Poster vi)

Subject	Posture i	Posture vi
1	199	232
2[a]	190	–
3	209	220
4	195	220

[a]Subject 2 was able to see the horizon without the need of compensation.

larger compared to the mean ankle angle of healthy subjects (mean $104° \pm 4°$) in posture i. One of the patients (patient 2) had straight legs when standing relaxed and thus it can be concluded that he only used his ankles to compensate for the forward displacement of the trunk COM.

DISCUSSION

The results above indicate that patients with spinal kyphosis compensate for the displacement of the trunk COM by flexion of the knees and/or plantar flexion of the ankles. Hip extension becomes limited and therefore it is not possible to compensate by a posterior rotation of the pelvis. The lumbar spine is immobile in patients with AS and it is assumable that pelvic tilt is limited as a result of the fused sacroiliac joints, which may result in a reduced ROM of the hip joint. Therefore, it is plausible that maximal hip extension cannot be reached. However this does not explain why the patients could hardly perform hip extension at all, when standing erect.

Decreased Hip Extension

Several explanations for a decreased hip extension can be found. First, morning stiffness and pain are common in patients with AS (9). It is possible that pain prevents further hip extension. Simkin et al. (10) suggested the patient adopts a flexed posture in an attempt to alleviate pain. Secondly, besides a direct consequence of pain in the hip joints, pain may also have a long-term effect as it can lead to a deliberate immobilization and in turn to muscle atrophy after a period of time. The ability to extend the hips may thus become insufficient because of muscle weakness. Another explanation for the limited extension is osteoarthritis of the hips. Progressively destructive hip arthritis is a common complication in patients with AS. Loss of joint space caused by osteoarthritis leads to a reduced ROM (11,12).

Therapy

Symptoms of AS are worse with inactivity and are relieved with exercise. As a result, a proper exercise program is a crucial element of treatment. Therapeutic goals are to preserve as much mobility as possible and to encourage good body posture so that fusion can occur in a less disabling posture. The emphasis in treatment usually focuses on spinal mobility. Only little attention has been paid to the ROM of the hips. Our results showed that where spinal kyphosis cannot completely be prevented, preservation of hip joint extension is essential. This is because only hip extension restores balance as well as a functionally acceptable field of vision, without inducing rapid development of fatigue in patients with AS. Bulstrode et al. (13) investigated the effects of daily passive stretching of the hip joints during a three week inpatient physiotherapy course. Their results showed that passive stretching resulted in a significant increase in the range of all movements of hip joints except for flexion. Conservative therapy might prevent or delay the limitation of the hip extension and thus should focus not only on spinal mobility, but also on prevention of hip joint mobility restrictions.

Limitations of the Present Investigation

Although we have attempted to accurately define all variables presented in this chapter, a few aspects merit discussion. In calculating the joint angles, we used the front angle between the distal and proximal segment instead of the zero-measurement, which is generally used in clinical practice (14). As a consequence the joint angles should not be interpreted as such, yet should be viewed relative to each other.

The joint angles of the hip and knee, as well as the knee and the ankle, are dependent on each other. Flexion of the knees results in a decrease in hip angle and ankle angle, which complicates reviewing the components of the compensation mechanism separately. However, comparing the hip angle during standing relaxed, straight, or with maximally extended hips, showed that the patients were hardly able to extend their hips. Thus, it may be concluded that the hip joints are no longer involved in balance control and patients compensate by flexion of the knees and/or plantar flexion of the ankles.

ADVICE

The four patients of this study, all with a spinal deformity caused by AS, could not use their hip joints to counterbalance the displacement of the trunk COM. Conservative therapy should not only focus on pain reduction, anti-inflammation, and spinal mobility, but also on the mobility of the hip joints. If further immobilization of the hip joints can be prevented the patient will have a larger ROM to compensate for the forward shift of the COP together with restoring the field of vision, which might diminish the posture problems.

REFERENCES

1. Carette S, Graham D, Little H, Rubenstein J, Rosen P. The natural disease course of ankylosing spondylitis. Arthritis Rheum 1983; 26(2):186–190.
2. Murray HC, Elliott C, Barton SE, Murray A. Do patients with ankylosing spondylitis have poorer balance than normal subjects? Rheumatology (Oxford) 2000; 39(5):497–500.
3. Bernhardt M, Bridwell KH. Segmental analysis of the sagittal plane alignment of the normal thoracic and lumbar spines and thoracolumbar junction. Spine 1989; 14(7):717–721.
4. Voutsinas SA, MacEwen GD. Sagittal profiles of the spine. Clin Orthop 1986; 210: 235–242.
5. Jackson RP, McManus AC. Radiographic analysis of sagittal plane alignment and balance in standing volunteers and patients with low back pain matched for age, sex, and size. A prospective controlled clinical study. Spine 1994; 19(14):1611–1618.
6. Gelb DE, Lenke LG, Bridwell KH, Blanke K, McEnery KW. An analysis of sagittal spinal alignment in 100 asymptomatic middle and older aged volunteers. Spine 1995; 20(12):1351–1358.
7. Plagenhoef S. Anatomical data for analyzing human motion. Res Q Exerc Sport 1983; 54:169–178.
8. Kingma I, Toussaint HM, Commissaris DA, Hoozemans MJ, Ober MJ. Optimizing the determination of the body center of mass. J Biomech 1995; 28(9):1137–1142.
9. Sigler JW, Bluhm GB, Duncan H, Ensign DC. Clinical features of ankylosing spondylitis. Clin Orthop 1971; 74:14–19.
10. Simkin PA, Downey DJ, Kilcoyne RF. Apophyseal arthritis limits lumbar motion in patients with ankylosing spondylitis. Arthritis Rheum 1988; 31(6):798–802.

11. Resnick D, Dwosh IL, Goergen TG, Shapiro RF, D'Ambrosia R. Clinical and radiographic "reankylosis" following hip surgery in ankylosing spondylitis. AJR Am J Roentgenol 1976; 126(6):1181–1188.
12. Bisla RS, Ranawat CS, Inglis AE. Total hip replacement in patients with ankylosing spondylitis with involvement of the hip. J Bone Joint Surg Am 1976; 58(2):233–238.
13. Bulstrode SJ, Barefoot J, Harrison RA, Clarke AK. The role of passive stretching in the treatment of ankylosing spondylitis. Br J Rheumatol 1987; 26(1):40–42.
14. Greene WB, Heckman JD, eds. Clinical Measurement of Joint Motion. Rosemont, Illinois: American Academy of Orthopedic Surgeons, 1994.

9

Sagittal Balance of the Spine in Ankylosing Spondylitis

Pierre Roussouly, Sohrab Gollogly, and Frederic Sailhan
Department of Orthopaedic Surgery, Centre Des Massues, Lyon, France

INTRODUCTION

Ankylosing spondylitis (AS) is an inflammatory arthritis that primarily affects the spine and sacroiliac joints (1–4). Advanced stages of the disease are characterized by a progressive stiffening of the spine and thorax as reactive syndesmophytes bridge the intervertebral disks and the entire spine becomes a fixed lever arm. The sagittal balance of the patient often deteriorates during the course of the disease, producing a rigid thoracolumbar kyphosis that can be a significant source of pain and disability. The surgical management of this deformity is complicated, with controversies regarding different treatment approaches (5–14). In this chapter, the clinical and radiographic evaluation of the thoracolumbar kyphosis and the secondary compensatory changes in sagittal alignment are reviewed. The preoperative planning of a corrective osteotomy is then discussed.

The changes in sagittal alignment that are induced by ankylosing spondylitis can be divided into two different categories: the primary deformity of thoracolumbar kyphosis, and the compensatory changes in the position of the pelvis and lower extremities. A severe thoracolumbar kyphosis results in a downward tilt of the head and face (4). The ability of the patient to see above the level of the horizon progressively worsens. The center of gravity moves anteriorly, resulting in the stooped, downward looking posture that is characteristic of advanced ankylosing spondylitis (Fig. 1B). In an attempt to rectify this situation, the patient flexes the ankles and knees, extends the hips, retroverts the pelvis, and tilts the entire rigid segment of the spine backwards (Fig. 1A). This posture is usually unable to completely compensate for the thoracolumbar kyphosis. Therefore, the standing position of the patient represents the maximal posterior tilt of the pelvis, and the maximal extension of the hips and flexion of the knees and ankles that the patient is physiologically capable of. This position is biomechanically inefficient, and painful, and the patient fatigues easily while walking or standing (4,5,8,11,13,15,16).

A complete assessment of the sagittal balance of the patient with ankylosing spondylitis includes anterior/posterior and lateral radiographs of the spine from the occiput to the proximal femurs. In some cases, the kyphosis is so severe that

(A)   **(B)**

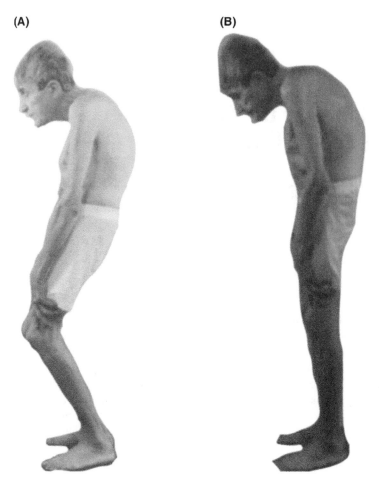

Figure 1 Clinical photographs of a patient with ankylosing spondylitis and a severe thoracolumbar kyphosis. (**A**) The patient is standing in the compensated position with the knees flexed. (**B**) When the knees are extended, the effect of the deformity on the direction of the gaze worsens.

the occiput and the pelvis cannot be captured on the same vertically oriented long cassette. Several exposures may be required, and clinical photographs may also be necessary in order to document the severity of the deformity.

RADIOGRAPHIC DESCRIPTION OF SAGITTAL DEFORMITY

Previous authors have described many techniques for measuring the changes in the sagittal balance of the patient with AS (11,15,17–20). The location and orientation of physical and radiographic points are used to document the position of the head, the orientation of the gaze, the characteristics of the thoracic and lumbar kyphosis, and the orientation of the pelvis. These parameters are reviewed in order, beginning proximally with the position of the head and the direction of the gaze.

The *sagittal vertical axis from the external auditory canal* is used to document the location of the head with respect to the normal center of gravity (Fig. 2). In a normal

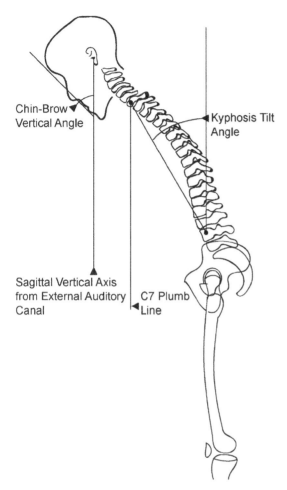

Chin-Brow
Vertical Angle

Kyphosis Tilt
Angle

Sagittal Vertical Axis
from External Auditory   C7 Plumb
Canal   Line

Figure 2 The measurement of the physical and radiographic severity of the kyphotic deformity includes a description of the chin-brow to vertical angle; the position of the sagittal vertical axis from the external auditory canal; the C7 plumb line; and the kyphosis tilt angle. In this example, the inferior limit of kyphosis is found at the L4 vertebral body.

patient, this line is considered to be very close to the center of gravity, and always intersects the supporting area of the feet. In a patient with a severe deformity, this line will pass anterior to the feet if the knees and ankles are extended. Compensatory changes in the position of the lower extremities will usually bring the projection of this line back to a more normal location. The *chin-brow to vertical angle* is defined by the angle subtended between a line drawn from the chin to the brow and the vertical axis. It is considered to be perpendicular to the direction of gaze. With increasing kyphosis, the chin-brow axis tilts downward, resulting in a gaze that has a limited ability to see above the horizon. Extension of the hips, and flexion of the knees and ankles attempts to compensate for the deformity and return the angle to zero.

A description of the characteristics of the sagittal profile of the spine begins proximally with a measurement of the *C7 plumb line*. This is a vertical line drawn from the middle of the vertebral body of C7. In a normal patient, it intersects the posterior edge of the superior endplate of S1. The C7 plumb line moves anteriorly with increasing amounts of uncompensated kyphosis. However, the position of the C7 plumb line with respect to the pelvis varies according to the relative degree of extension and flexion of the lower extremities.

Kyphosis is measured with the Cobb method. The proximal and distal limits of the segment of the spine where the vertebral bodies are in a position of flexion with respect to each other are identified. In the normal patient, the spine is considered to be kyphotic between T1 and the thoracolumbar junction. In the patient with ankylosing spondylitis, the entire cervical, thoracic, and lumbar spine can become kyphotic. The angle between the superior endplate of the proximal vertebral body of the kyphotic curve and the inferior endplate of the distal vertebral body defines the global kyphosis. In order to further characterize the sagittal shape of the spine, the *inflection point* where the kyphosis transitions to lordosis and the *apex* of the curve can also be identified. In severe kyphosis, the inflection point generally moves inferiorly, into the lumbar spine. The position of the apex is variable, and can occur in the cervicothoracic, thoracic, thoracolumbar, or lumbar areas of the spine. The relationship between the location of the apex of the deformity and the site of the corrective osteotomy has a significant effect on postoperative sagittal balance.

The amount of *lordosis* in the spine is assessed with the same technique of measurement as the Cobb method. In the normal patient, the spine is considered to be lordotic between L1 and the sacrum, where the vertebral bodies are in a position of extension with respect to each other. In severe kyphotic deformities, both the inflection point between kyphosis and lordosis and the apex of the lordotic curve move distally. This reduces the global amount of lordosis and the number of vertebral bodies in a lordotic orientation. Often, the apex of the remaining lumbar lordosis is located close to the lumbosacral junction. Postoperatively, the position of the corrective osteotomy will become the location of the new apex of lordosis.

The *kyphosis tilt angle* is a positional parameter that is defined as the angle between the vertical axis and a line drawn from the center of T1 to the center of the inferior kyphotic vertebral body. This angle describes the tilt induced by the global kyphosis. When the entire spine is kyphotic and L5 is the inferior vertebral body in kyphosis, the kyphosis tilt angle is equivalent to the *spinal tilt angle*. Both the kyphosis and spinal tilt angles are dependent upon positional changes in the lower extremities. With extension of the knees, the kyphosis tilt angle increases. With extension of the hips, retroversion of the pelvis, and flexion of the knees and ankles, the kyphosis tilt angle is reduced.

The relationship between the alignment of the pelvis and the lumbar spine is a very important determinant of sagittal balance. The radiographically identifiable points of the pelvis that are used to describe lumbopelvic anatomy include the superior endplate of S1 and the center of the femoral heads. Legaye et al. (19) have described three angles between these radiographic landmarks that regulate spinal sagittal curves (Fig. 3). These angles are called *pelvic incidence* (PI), *pelvic tilt* (PT), and *sacral slope* (SS). Pelvic incidence is defined as the angle between the perpendicular to the sacral plate at its midpoint and a line connecting the same point to the center of the bicoxofemoral axis. In normal subjects, this angle measures approximately 52°, with a range from 34° to 84°. The measurement of this angle does not change with the position of the patient, and it is considered an anatomic constant after the cessation of growth. Pelvic tilt is defined as the angle between a vertical line originating at the center of the bicoxofemoral axis and a line drawn between the same point and the middle of the superior endplate of S1. The angle of pelvic tilt describes the amount of rotation of the pelvis around the femoral heads. In normal

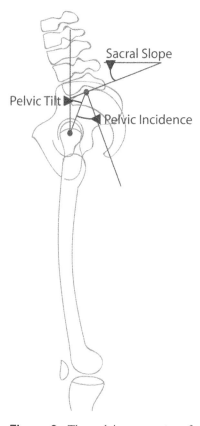

Figure 3 The pelvic parameters for defining the sagittal alignment of the lumbopelvic junction are shown. The sacral slope (SS) is defined as the angle between the superior endplate of S1 and the horizontal axis. Pelvic tilt (PT) is defined as the angle between a line drawn from center of the hip axis to the center of the superior endplate of S1 and the vertical axis. Pelvic incidence (PI) is defined as the angle between a line drawn from center of the hip axis to the center of the superior endplate of S1 and perpendicular to the endplate. These three angles are linked by the geometric equation of PI = SS + PT.

subjects, this angle measures 12°, with a range from −5° to 30°. Sacral slope is defined as the angle between the superior endplate of S1 and the horizontal axis. In normal subjects, this angle is approximately 40°, with a range from 20° to 65°. Sacral slope and pelvic tilt are positional parameters that can be affected by changes in the alignment of the lower extremities. Pelvic incidence is a shape parameter that is not affected by changes in the alignment of the lower extremities. These angles are geometrically related such that pelvic incidence is equal to the sum of the angles of sacral slope and pelvic tilt: PI = SS + PT.

The *sacral end offset* is an additional positional parameter that can be used to define the position of the pelvis and lower extremities with respect to the base of the spine and the hip axis. This parameter is defined as the horizontal distance between the projection of the center of the superior endplate of S1 and the center of the femoral heads. In normal subjects, the center of the sacral endplate is normally located over the center of the femoral heads. With the knees in extension, the center of the knee joint is also located along the same vertical axis. With increasing amounts of kyphosis, compensatory changes in the alignment of the pelvis places the center of the sacral endplate posterior to the center of the femoral heads. In order to compensate for a posterior shift in the base of the spine, the patient bends the knees so that they are located anterior to the center of the femoral heads. An estimate of the amount of compensation that is required in order to assume a balanced standing position can be determined by measuring the offset between the center of the sacral endplate and the center of the knee joint.

The alignment of the lower limbs influences the appearance, description, and measurement of sagittal alignment (11,13,14). In a normal population, a comfortable standing position is found when the femoral shafts are vertical, defining the neutral position of the hip joint. With severe kyphosis, the alignment of the lower limbs changes in an attempt to compensate for the anterior position of the center of gravity and the downward direction of the gaze. The knees and ankles are flexed, the hips are extended, and the pelvis is tilted posteriorly in order to bring the entire spine backwards (Fig. 4) (5,8,11,13,15,16). Measuring these adaptive changes with radiography is difficult. Mangione and Senegas have described the *pelvic femoral shaft angle* (PFA) between the long axis of the femoral shafts and a vertical axis originating at the center of the femoral heads (1). When the knees are in extension, the PFA is equal to zero, and when the knees are flexed, the angle increases. Adaptive extension of the hips can be measured with this angle because there is a relationship between pelvic tilt and the pelvic femoral shaft angle, such that PT = extension of the hips + PFA. This angle is often difficult to use clinically, because only the very proximal portion of the femoral shafts are visible on a plain lateral radiograph of the entire spine and pelvis. Due to the anatomy of the proximal femur and the natural anterior bow of the shaft, it is often difficult to accurately determine the long axis of the femur from just the proximal portion of the bone. If an additional long lateral radiograph of the pelvis and lower extremities is made, then the extension of the hips, flexion of knees and ankles, and retroversion of the pelvis with respect to the lower limbs can be measured and documented. However, this is rarely a part of the radiographic evaluation of the patient with kyphosis.

Several authors have demonstrated that the radiographic appearance of kyphosis is dependent upon the position of the lower extremities (11,13). It is not possible to measure the position of the lower extremities on the same lateral radiograph as the spine and pelvis. Therefore, it is important to describe the relationship between the pelvis and the spine in a way that is independent of the position of the hips, knees, and ankles. The *spino-pelvic angle* (SPA) is defined as the angle between a line from the center of T1 to the center of the sacral endplate and a line from the center of the sacral endplate to the center of the hip axis (Fig. 5). In the presence of a kyphotic deformity, the angle increases significantly. The *spino-sacral angle* (SSA) is defined as the angle between a line from the center of T1 to the center of the sacral endplate and the sacral endplate itself. In a healthy population, this angle is strongly correlated with the sacral slope (Pearson correlation coefficient = 0.92) with the geometric equation of SSA = 99 + 0.9 (SS). In addition, there is a geometric relationship between the spino-pelvic angle and the spino-sacral angle and the pelvic incidence: SPA = SSA + 90 – PI.

In a healthy population, the spine is flexible. Therefore, the parameters that are used to describe sagittal balance provide information about both the shape and position of the spine. For example, the measurement of kyphosis and lordosis on a single radiograph describes a shape, since the radiograph captures the spine in a specific position. However, the shape can change, altering the position of radiographic landmarks with respect to each other. In the measurement of sagittal alignment, the only

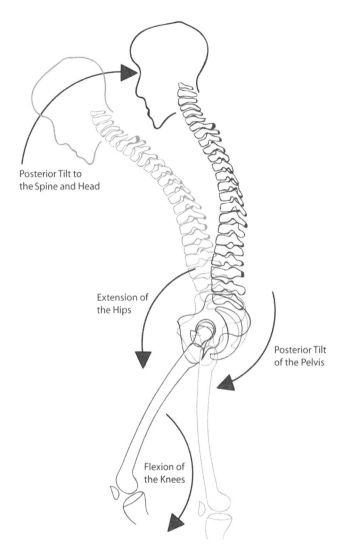

Posterior Tilt to
the Spine and Head

Extension of
the Hips

Posterior Tilt
of the Pelvis

Flexion of
the Knees

Figure 4 In the case of a severe thoracolumbar kyphotic deformity, the trunk is displaced anterior to the pelvis. In an effort to compensate for this deformity and to bring the center of mass back over the feet and the direction of the gaze closer to the horizontal axis, the entire spine must be tilted backwards. With the adaptive changes that occur in severe ankylosing spondylitis and kyphosis, the posterior tilt is maximal and the sacral slope is nearly zero.

parameter that does not change with the position of the patient is pelvic incidence. In a normal population there is a large range of variability in pelvic incidence from 34° to 84°. The geometric relationship between pelvic incidence, sacral slope, and pelvic tilt ($PI = SS + PT$) links this anatomic constant to parameters that are dependent upon the position of the patient. When a kyphotic deformity occurs, the inflection point between kyphosis and lordosis usually moves inferiorly, and the global amount of lordosis decreases. To compensate for the loss of lumbar lordosis, the patient tilts the pelvis posteriorly, increasing the sacral end offset. As the sum of the sacral slope and the pelvic tilt is equal to pelvic incidence, the ability of the spine to compensate for the deformity is limited by the patient's native anatomic alignment. A patient

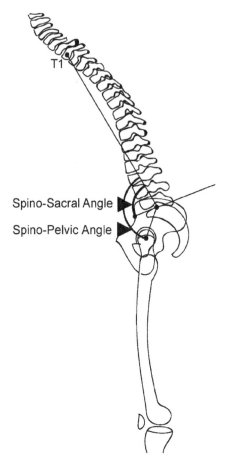

Spino-Sacral Angle

Spino-Pelvic Angle

Figure 5 The spino-pelvic angle (SPA) is defined as the angle between a line from the center of T1 to the center of the sacral endplate and a line from the center of sacral endplate to the center of the hip axis. The spino-sacral angle (SSA) is defined as the angle between a line from the center of T1 to the center of the sacral endplate and the sacral endplate itself.

with a large pelvic incidence is able to compensate for a kyphotic deformity by inducing a large posterior tilt to the pelvis, which increases the sacral end offset and flattens the sacral slope. However, a patient with a very low pelvic incidence does not have the same capacity to accommodate the deformity as their ability to induce a large posterior tilt to the pelvis is diminished and the maximum sacral end offset is less. Geometrically, a pelvic incidence of 35 (the lower limit of normal) theoretically limits the pelvic tilt to a range from –5 to 35, and the sacral slope to a range from 0 to 40. A pelvic incidence of 80 (the upper limit of normal) theoretically limits the pelvic tilt to a range from –5 to 75, and the sacral slope to a range from 0 to 85.

In summary, the stages of adaptation to a significant kyphosis with anterior displacement of the center of gravity proceeds as follows: (i) in order to maintain C7/T1 over the endplate of the sacrum, pelvic tilt is first increased by extension of the hips; and (ii) once the amount of pelvic tilt reaches the maximum, the knees are flexed in order to tilt the rigid spine and pelvis posteriorly. These compensatory mechanisms are related by the fact that pelvic tilt is equal to the sum of hip extension (HE) and the pelvic femoral angle ($PT = HE + PFA$). Therefore, when the pelvic incidence is small, the amount of pelvic tilt is limited and large increases in the sacral end offset are not possible. In contrast, with a large pelvic incidence, it is possible to accommodate the deformity through a significant pelvic tilt with a large increase in the sacral end offset.

PREOPERATIVE PLANNING FOR KYPHOSIS CORRECTION

The goals of surgical correction of sagittal malalignment in ankylosing spondylitis are to decrease the cosmetic and functional effects of the deformity, reduce the patient's pain, and increase their ability to stand and walk comfortably without fatigue (1,6,8,15,21). A number of techniques for inducing a posterior tilt to the spine and returning the gaze to the horizontal have been described (2,5–10,12,15,17,18,21,22). These techniques include an opening wedge anterior osteotomy, vertebral body corpectomy and realignment, multiple posterior wedge osteotomies of the posterior elements only, and osteotomy of the anterior and posterior column with either an "eggshell" or pedicle subtraction technique. The techniques, complications, and clinical results of these procedures have been extensively reviewed elsewhere. Briefly, opening wedge anterior osteotomies are associated with the risk of severe and irreversible vascular and neurologic complications (2,23–25). Multiple posterior osteotomies do not have the ability to correct large deformities, and there are concerns about the risk of multiple pseudoarthroses and loss of correction over time with this technique (10,12). Selecting the location for the osteotomy and the degree of desired correction is a subject of considerable controversy. The unpredictable nature of the vascular supply to the spinal cord in the thoracic spine and the decreased ratio between the size of the neural elements and the space available for the cord makes correction of the deformity in the thoracic spine very challenging. There is an increased margin of safety in performing realignment surgery in the lumbar spine, and currently, there is a trend toward performing the correction inferior to the level of the *conus medullaris*. A posteriorly based osteotomy of the posterior and anterior columns of the spine with a pedicle subtraction technique appears to be associated with the best published clinical results in terms of degree of correction, number of complications, and patient satisfaction (6,8,10). It should be emphasized that purely thoracic or cervicothoracic kyphosis is not well corrected with a lumbar osteotomy distal to the deformity and the clinical results are likely to be inferior. However, published reports have diminished the enthusiasm for performing a corrective osteotomy in the thoracic spine and the theoretical advantages are often outweighed by the technical difficulty of the procedure and the unpredictability of vascular and neurologic complications (2,21,23).

In the process of preoperative planning, it is important to determine both how much correction is desirable, and how much correction is achievable. The amount of correction in the sagittal plane that can be achieved with a posteriorly based osteotomy is limited by the size of the closing wedge that can be safely created in the lumbar spine and then closed with modern pedicle fixation devices. In the published results with pedicle subtraction and eggshell osteotomies, single level corrections of more than 40° are rare (6,8,10). If more than 40° or 45° of correction is desirable, then multiple closing wedges of the spine are likely to be necessary.

As the desired standing position for the patient after the operation is with the knees in extension, it can be beneficial to proceed with preoperative planning with a radiograph taken in this position. This represents the uncompensated position of standing and the radiographic appearance of the deformity is affected by the extension of the knees. In many patients, the degree of deformity does not allow the spine to be captured on a vertically oriented cassette. Therefore, clinical photographs may be necessary in order to document the preoperative standing position. As some compensation is likely to occur postoperatively, it is necessary to determine which measurements of spinal and pelvic alignment should be used to plan the osteotomy. Van Royen et al. (11) have described a method based upon a trigonometric relationship between sagittal balance of the spine and the sacral endplate angle. Their method utilizes nomograms to show a relationship between the level and degree of correction on the horizontal position of the C7 plumb line. Van Royen et al. (11) and Suk et al. (16) have also described the use of chin-brow vertical angle to determine the amount of correction of kyphosis that is desired. This clinical measurement has also been described as a means of evaluating the technical success of the operation (16). However, these techniques do not take into account the influence of the shape of the pelvis on the deformity and the position of the inferior limbs is not controlled. In our experience, we have found that a preoperative plan that places the T1 vertebral body directly above the superior endplate of S1 provides a reasonable guide for the amount of correction that should be achieved with surgery.

The amount of correction that is needed to place the center of the T1 vertebral body directly above the sacral endplate with the patient's knees in extension is determined by the amount of kyphosis and the alignment of the spine and pelvis. Patients who have a large pelvic incidence have an increased ability to compensate for a large thoracoabdominal kyphosis. A patient with a low value for pelvic incidence is more likely to require a corrective osteotomy earlier than a patient with a high value for pelvic incidence. In our experience, we have found that patients with a low-grade pelvic incidence become symptomatic much earlier than patients with a high-grade pelvic incidence and an equivalent amount of kyphosis. This appears to be the result of the fact that when kyphosis is associated with a low-grade pelvic incidence the patient's spinal balance deteriorates. A patient with poor spinal balance must choose between two inefficient and fatiguing positions: with the knees in extension the center of gravity is well forward and the erector spine and hamstrings are under tension; with the knees flexed, the center of gravity is restored to a more normal position, but the quadriceps musculature tires in this position. Therefore, it is not necessary to wait until a large kyphotic deformity is present before performing a surgical correction in a patient with a low-grade pelvic incidence.

Currently, our indications for surgical correction of the sagittal alignment of the spine in the presence of a kyphotic deformity are as follows: with a low-grade pelvic incidence of $<40°$, we will offer the patient sagittal realignment surgery when they have sufficient symptoms and evidence of sagittal imbalance. Clinically, we find that this often occurs with relatively small amounts of kyphosis, but with evidence of a large anterior shift in the center of gravity (Fig. 6A). In contrast, we find that patients with a high-grade pelvic incidence of more than 50° tolerate much larger amounts of kyphosis. In this situation, we are able to counsel the patient that they are likely to enjoy a longer duration without disabling symptoms before they require realignment surgery (Fig. 6B), but they are likely to require a larger osteotomy in order to restore optimal spinal balance.

In our research on asymptomatic individuals without evidence of sagittal imbalance, we have found that the center of T1 is always positioned directly above S1, independent of the value for the sacral slope. In planning sagittal realignment surgery, the optimal strategy for correction of the profile of the rigid spine and pelvis is to restore the center of T1 directly above S1. However, in many instances, the amount

(A)   (B)

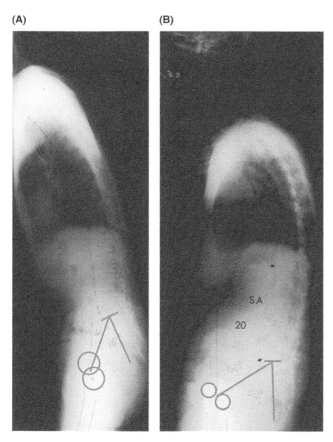

Figure 6 An illustration of the effect of kyphosis on sagittal balance in a patient with kyphosis associated with (**A**) a low-grade pelvic incidence of 46° and (**B**) a high-grade pelvic incidence of 60°. In the presence of a low-grade pelvic incidence, there is evidence of a large anterior shift in the center of gravity, even with small amounts of kyphosis. In contrast, a patient with a high-grade pelvic incidence is able to compensate for larger amounts of kyphosis.

of kyphotic deformity makes this correction impossible. We base our preoperative plan upon a radiograph of the entire spine between the occiput and the proximal femurs. It is not necessary to calculate the osteotomy based upon a radiograph taken with the patient's knees in full extension because the *rigid* fused spine and pelvis provides sufficient information. Using the spino-sacral angle, we calculate the amount of correction required to place the center of T1 directly over the sacral endplate (Fig. 7). If the desired amount of correction is <45°, we feel that this can be achieved with a single-level posteriorly based pedicle subtraction osteotomy in the lumbar spine. The goal of this osteotomy is to restore the center of gravity to a position where the patient can stand with the knees in extension, as this is a biomechanically advantageous position. Knee flexion is a compensatory change in the alignment of the spine, pelvis, and lower limbs that can accommodate the anterior displacement of the center of gravity, but at a significant cost to the patient because it is fatiguing.

In some instances, we have noticed that the patient will adopt a standing position with the knees in slight flexion because the amount of correction is insufficient to return the center of T1 directly over the center of S1. The ability of the spine and

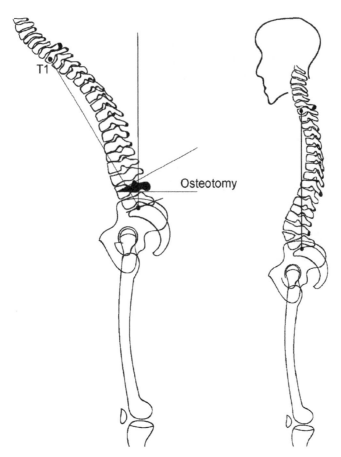

Figure 7 Using a preoperative radiograph taken with the patient's knees in extension, the amount of correction required to place the center of T1 directly above the sacral endplate is calculated. This correction is accomplished with a posteriorly based pedicle subtraction osteotomy.

pelvis to attain a balanced position after an osteotomy can depend upon the relative extension of the hips and posterior tilt of the pelvis. If the patient is able to hyper-extend their hips and retrovert the pelvis until T1 is centered over S1, they will be able to compensate for the residual anterior displacement of the center of gravity and stand with the knees in extension (Fig. 8). However, if their hip extension is limited, by coexisting degenerative arthritis of the hip, for example, then they will continue to stand with a slight amount of knee flexion in order to obtain a balanced profile. The theoretical limit to compensatory changes in the alignment of the spine, pelvis, and hips occurs when the sacral slope becomes horizontal. If T1 is not centered over S1 and this limit has been reached, the patient will not be able to obtain a balanced standing position and will continue to stand with flexed knees.

If it is also considered desirable to increase the sacral slope (and thereby decrease the pelvic tilt), the value for the desired increase in the sacral slope must be added to the amount of correction that will bring T1 over the center of S1 with zero sacral slope. For example, if 30° of correction is necessary to return T1 over S1 with zero sacral slope, but an increase of 10° of pelvic tilt is desirable, then the osteotomy must accomplish 40° of sagittal correction.

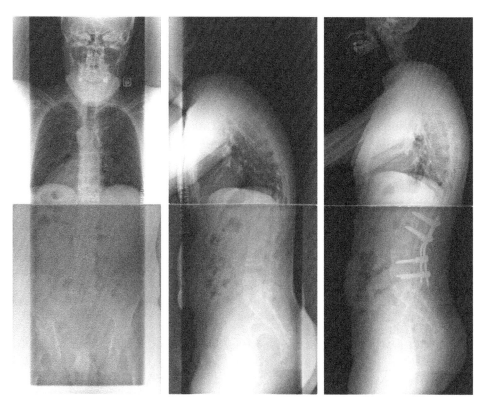

Figure 8 A clinical case of a corrective osteotomy in the setting of a low-grade pelvic incidence. The A/P and lateral preoperative radiographs of a 52-year-old male with ankylosing spondylitis are shown. After a 40° corrective osteotomy, the patient's sagittal balance has been restored.

The level of the osteotomy will determine the new position of the apex of lumbar lordosis. Therefore, we plan the osteotomy so that the superior endplate of the vertebral body at the proximal end of the osteotomy is as horizontal as possible. In some situations, we are able to achieve a posterior tilt to the superior endplate. We make every attempt to avoid segmental kyphosis at the superior end of the fusion as we speculate that this creates a situation that places the patient at risk of fracture of the fused segments of the spine or the development of a pseudoarthrosis in a location that is under tension.

In conclusion, the surgical management of the sagittal profile of the patient with a kyphotic deformity in the context of ankylosing spondylitis is complicated. Appropriate clinical and radiographic evaluation of the compensatory changes in sagittal alignment requires full length standing A/P and lateral radiographs of the spine. Several techniques exist for the preoperative planning of a corrective osteotomy. We favor a plan that places the center of T1 directly over the sacral endplate, restoring the center of gravity to a more balanced position. We have discussed a number of compensatory changes in the alignment of the spine, pelvis, and hips that have an effect on the final standing position of the patient after the osteotomy has been performed. Knowledge of these compensatory changes helps the operating surgeon to predict the effect of the osteotomy on the final sagittal balance of the patient.

REFERENCES

1. Mangione P, Senegas J. Sagittal balance of the spine. Rev Chir Orthop Reparatrice Appar Mot 1997; 83(1):22–32.
2. McMaster MJ, Coventry MB. Spinal osteotomy in akylosing spondylitis. Technique, complications, and long-term results. Mayo Clin Proc 1973; 48(7):476–486.
3. Smith-Petersen MN, Larson CB, Aufranc OE. Osteotomy of the spine for correction of flexion deformity in rheumatoid arthritis. Clin Orthop 1969; 66:6–9.
4. White AA III, Panjabi MM, Thomas CL. The clinical biomechanics of kyphotic deformities. Clin Orthop 1977; 128:8–17.
5. Berven SH, Deviren V, Smith JA, Emami A, Hu SS, Bradford DS. Management of fixed sagittal plane deformity: results of the transpedicular wedge resection osteotomy. Spine 2001; 26(18):2036–2043.
6. Bridwell KH, Lewis SJ, Edwards C, Lenke LG, Iffrig TM, Berra A, Baldus C, Blanke K. Complications and outcomes of pedicle subtraction osteotomies for fixed sagittal imbalance. Spine 2003; 28(18):2093–2101.
7. Hehne HJ, Zielke K, Bohm H. Polysegmental lumbar osteotomies and transpedicled fixation for correction of long-curved kyphotic deformities in ankylosing spondylitis. Report on 177 cases. Clin Orthop 1990; 258:49–55.
8. Kim KT, Suk KS, Cho YJ, Hong GP, Park BJ. Clinical outcome results of pedicle subtraction osteotomy in ankylosing spondylitis with kyphotic deformity. Spine 2002; 27(6):612–618.
9. McMaster MJ. A technique for lumbar spinal osteotomy in ankylosing spondylitis. J Bone Joint Surg Br 1985; 67(2):204–210.
10. Van Royen BJ, De Gast A. Lumbar osteotomy for correction of thoracolumbar kyphotic deformity in ankylosing spondylitis. A structured review of three methods of treatment. Ann Rheum Dis 1999; 58(7):399–406.
11. Van Royen BJ, De Gast A, Smit TH. Deformity planning for sagittal plane corrective osteotomies of the spine in ankylosing spondylitis. Eur Spine J 2000; 9(6):492–498.
12. Van Royen BJ, Slot GH. Closing-wedge posterior osteotomy for ankylosing spondylitis. Partial corporectomy and transpedicular fixation in 22 cases. J Bone Joint Surg Br 1995; 77(1):117–121.
13. Van Royen BJ, Toussaint HM, Kingma I, Bot SD, Caspers M, Harlaar J, Wuisman PI. Accuracy of the sagittal vertical axis in a standing lateral radiograph as a measurement of balance in spinal deformities. Eur Spine J 1998; 7(5):408–412.
14. Vaz G, Roussouly P, Berthonnaud E, Dimnet J. Sagittal morphology and equilibrium of pelvis and spine. Eur Spine J 2002; 11:80–87.
15. Camargo FP, Cordeiro EN, Napoli MM. Corrective osteotomy of the spine in ankylosing spondylitis. Experience with 66 cases. Clin Orthop 1986; 208:157–167.
16. Suk KS, Kim KT, Lee SH, Kim JM. Significance of chin-brow vertical angle in correction of kyphotic deformity of ankylosing spondylitis patients. Spine 2003; 28(17): 2001–2005.
17. Boachie-Adjei O, Bradford DS. Vertebral column resection and arthrodesis for complex spinal deformities. J Spinal Disord 1991; 4(2):193–202.
18. Danisa OA, Turner D, Richardson WJ. Surgical correction of lumbar kyphotic deformity: posterior reduction "eggshell" osteotomy. J Neurosurg 2000; 92(suppl 1):50–56.
19. Legaye J, Duval-Beaupere G, Hecquet J, Marty C. Pelvic incidence: a fundamental pelvic parameter for three-dimensional regulation of spinal sagittal curves. Eur Spine J 1998; 7(2):99–103.
20. Pile KD, Laurent MR, Salmond CE, Best MJ, Pyle EA, Moloney RO. Clinical assessment of ankylosing spondylitis: a study of observer variation in spinal measurements. Br J Rheumatol 1991; 30(1):29–34.

21. Chen PQ. Correction of kyphotic deformity in ankylosing spondylitis using multiple spinal osteotomy and Zielke's VDS instruments. Taiwan Yi Xue Hui Za Zhi 1988; 87(7):692–699.
22. Noun Z, Lapresle P, Missenard G. Posterior lumbar osteotomy for flat back in adults. J Spinal Disord 2001; 14:311–316.
23. Fox MW, Onofrio BM, Kilgore JE. Neurological complications of ankylosing spondylitis. J Neurosurg 1993; 78(6):871–878.
24. Lichtblau PO, Wilson PD. Possible mechanism of aortic rupture in orthopaedic correction of rheumatoid spondylitis. J Bone Joint Surg Am 1956; 38A(1):123–127.
25. Weatherley C, Jaffray D, Terry A. Vascular complications associated with osteotomy in ankylosing spondylitis: a report of two cases. Spine 1988; 13(1):43–6.

10

Planning the Restoration of View and Balance in Ankylosing Spondylitis

Theo H. Smit

Department of Physics and Medical Technology, VU University Medical Center, Amsterdam, The Netherlands

ABSTRACT

Patients with ankylosing spondylitis (AS; Bechterew's disease) may develop severe kyphotic deformities of the spine with strong medical, psychological, and social impairments. Due to the rigidity of the spine, surgical correction is the only option to effectively restore horizontal view and spinal balance. It is not trivial, though, to select the level and amount of correction and to predict the outcome of the surgery. This is partly due to the large variety of sagittal deformations and compensation strategies exposed by AS patients, partly also to a lacking definition of good spinal balance and view angle. In the following, it is argued that a well-balanced spine has a fundament in a sacral endplate angle of 40° with respect to the horizon. Further, it is suggested to use the so-called Frankfort horizontal to define the natural cranium position and view angle. Given the circumstance that the spine is a rigid rod, deformities resulting from AS can precisely be quantified. Also, elementary goniometry can be used to plan optimal view angle and spinal balance. However, the question is: what is a good spinal balance? This has to be established in a broad clinical follow-up study; the analytical tools presented here will be helpful in finding the relevant parameters in an accurate way.

INTRODUCTION

In AS, also referred to as Bechterew's disease, the anterior and posterior longitudinal ligaments ossify and fuse the vertebral bodies from the occiput down to the sacrum. The resulting rigid beam of bone may show severe kyphotic deformities in the cervical and thoracolumbar regions, with curvatures up to more than 100° (1,2). As a consequence, the patient is no longer able to see the horizon, which leads to social isolation and psychological stress. Additionally, serious medical complications may occur, depending on the level and severity of the kyphosis. At the cervical level, problems arise with chewing and swallowing (i.e., eating and drinking), and skin care

149

under the chin. Patients with deformities at the thoracolumbar level may show respirational, pulmonal, cardiac, and intestinal problems of various degrees. Moreover, the severe kyphotic deformation induces an anterior displacement of the center of mass (COM) of the trunk, which makes the patient continuously feel as if falling forward. In order to compensate for the downward view angle and the sagittal unbalance, the patient's only option is a backward rotation of the pelvis, which is generally realized by extension of the hips, eventually accompanied by flexion of the knees and the ankles (Fig. 1A) (3,4). This is a fatiguing standing position with high muscular stresses, leading to increased loading of hips and knees and an increased risk of osteoarthrosis.

As the spine has become a rigid beam in AS patients, surgical correction is the only option to restore large deviations from horizontal view and sagittal balance. Such a correction is performed by one or more wedge osteotomies, which are stabilized in extension by internal fixation (5). There is no consensus in literature on the best level of an osteotomy. One concept holds that the major correction should be performed in the area of the main deformation, i.e., at the apex of kyphosis (6,7). This eliminates the strongest curvatures of the ankylosed spine, and it optimally releases the spinal cord tension, as well as the pressure on the abdomen, thorax, and/or throat. In another concept, the osteotomy is preferably applied in the lower lumbar region, because more balance correction is achieved for the same correction angle (8,9). This approach does not necessarily conflict with the first concept, but a kyphotic deformity seldom has its apex in the lumbar spine. There are other arguments,

(A)   **(B)**   **(C)**

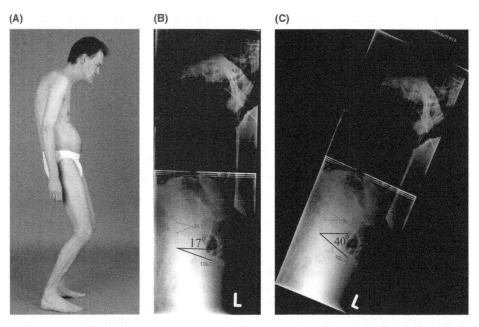

Figure 1 Defining the foundation of the balanced spine in AS. (**A**) AS patient showing the typical compensation mechanisms: a tilted pelvis and flexed knees and ankles. (**B**) X-ray of the same patient, showing an SEA of approximately 17°. (**C**) The ideal SEA of 40° is achieved by turning the X-ray over 23° clockwise. This is a well-defined position excluding the patient's compensation mechanisms in the lower extremities, which allows for comparisons between pre- and postoperative X-rays, and between individuals. *Abbreviations*: AS, ankylosing spondylitis; SEA, sacral endplate angle.

though, to select a certain level of osteotomy. For example, in the thoracic region, correction is often difficult because of the rib cage, which requires an anterior release of the thoracic spine followed by a posterior correction with compression instrumentation (10). In the cervical spine, an extending osteotomy requires complete exposure of the spinal cord (11), and there is a considerable risk of rupture of the vertebral artery. Postoperatively, the patient is obliged to wear a halo-thoracic brace for several months. Also in the lumbar region there are potential complications. Kim et al. (12), for example, report that their Asian patients who had an osteotomy at L4 complained of more difficulty in sitting on the floor, which is a serious complication in Eastern societies. Generally, reducing operation risk and postoperative complications is often (and appropriately) of overriding importance in the choice of the level of osteotomy, even if this results in a suboptimal restoration of view and balance.

Despite all surgical considerations, restoration of horizontal view and spinal balance are the main objectives of an intervention in AS, because social isolation and muscular pain are the biggest problems for AS patients (13,14). However, to predict the effect of a wedge osteotomy on view angle and sagittal balance is not trivial, as evidenced among others by reports on iatrogenic extension deformities due to overcorrecting the ankylosed spine (15). Also under correction has been reported (9). While the view angle after the intervention is mainly determined by the angle of the osteotomic wedge, the resulting spinal balance strongly depends on the level of osteotomy and the form of the curvature. Both view angle and sagittal balance corrections, however, are affected by the compensation strategies of the AS patient: pelvic tilt and flexion of knees and ankles effectively veil the full consequence of kyphotic deformation. So not only view angle and sagittal balance, but also the compensation strategies exploited by the AS patient should be considered in the preoperative planning.

In the following, considerations for the best position of the pelvis are discussed, and the parameters for view angle and sagittal balance are introduced. Mathematical rules for preoperative planning are derived, based on the circumstance that the ankylosed spine essentially is a rigid rod. The possibilities and limitations of the planning procedure will be discussed.

THE FUNDAMENT OF A BALANCED SPINE

A major goal of surgical intervention in patients with AS is to restore spinal balance in the sagittal plane. However, a complicating factor is that spinal balance is not well defined, especially for AS patients. From the biomechanical point of view, a plumb line from the collective COM of trunk, arms, and head, should intersect the hip axis and the supporting area of the feet; this minimizes both muscular effort and joint loading. It is very difficult, though, to exactly locate the COM in an individual, let alone in an AS patient (16). Length, thoracic and abdominal girth, posture, position of head and arms, and many more parameters are of influence. A mechanical approach thus is not of practical use. Alternatively, radiographic landmarks can be used. The difficulty again is that they may be well described for healthy individuals, but they are of limited use in individual AS patients. Nevertheless, this seems to be the only option for preoperative planning aiming at the restoration of spinal balance.

Spinal balance does not only refer to the shape of the spine, but also to its position in the field of gravity. Spatial orientation of the basis of the spine (i.e., the pelvis, or more particular, the sacrum) has been a subject of many studies (17–21). In standing healthy individuals, the sacral endplate (i.e., the superior surface of the sacrum) makes an angle of approximately 40° with the horizon (18,20,21). With the sacral endplate in this position, the hip joints are not in full extension, thus allowing for compensatory movements. These are not only necessary during activities like walking, bending, or carrying weights, but also in cases of muscular unbalance and sagittal spine deformities. In fact, this mechanism is fully exploited by AS patients, leaving no possibility for additional correction and increasing the risk for falling and fracturing of the spine (Fig. 1A) (22–24). Another advantage of a natural position of the pelvis is that it allows the lower extremities to be stretched, thereby minimizing the muscular effort to maintain balance and thus minimizing the joint loads and the risk of osteoarthrosis. Therefore, it is postulated that also in AS patients, sacral endplate angle (SEA) should be 40° with respect to the horizon (Fig. 1). Apart from achieving a more physiological and comfortable SEA, defining SEA at 40° provides a reliable and reproducible reference for quantifying the view angle, balance, and spinal deformity in AS patients. After all, the compensation mechanisms in the pelvis and legs exploited by the AS patient no longer interferes with the view angle and sagittal balance as currently determined by lateral X-rays and photographs. As a result, the severity and progress of the kyphosis can unambiguously be quantified with respect to a well-defined reference.

PARAMETERS FOR SPINAL BALANCE

Quantifying spinal balance has been a subject of extensive research in the last two decades and various describing parameters have been introduced (19,21,25–38). Generally, these parameters can be classified as angulations, curvatures, and plumb lines.

Angulations basically refer to the position of the pelvis, or more particularly, the sacrum, which serves as fundament for the spine. The position of the pelvis or spine in the gravitational field is expressed in terms of pelvic tilt, sacral slope, pelvic angle, or pelvic incidence, all of which are mutually related and show strong correlations with the sagittal curvatures of the spine (27,36,37,39). In healthy subjects, the sacral plate angle is in the order of 40°, but in AS patients this angle is strongly decreased (18,20,21). Kim et al. (12), for example, measured an average sacro-horizontal angle of $8 \pm 13°$ in 45 patients. This pelvic tilt is accomplished by extension of the hips and flexion of the knees and ankles, and is a direct indication of an unbalanced spine. Pelvic angulation in a relaxed standing position thus has some value as a measure for spinal unbalance. It must be recognized, however, that compensation strategies may change due to, e.g., muscle fatigue, and that pelvic tilt changes with posture. Pelvic tilt is also related to the amount of deformation of the ankylosed spine itself: stronger and more distal curvatures require more compensation for balance and view. For planning an osteotomy, therefore, it is most practical to start from a well-balanced position of the fundament, i.e., with an SEA of some 40° (Fig. 1).

Sagittal curvatures also have been studied extensively in healthy patients (19,21,26,29–34,36,37,39–41). Generally, spinal curvatures can be adapted in order to compensate for deviating pelvic angulations or shifts in the COM. It is well known, for example, that there is a strong correlation between the inclination of the sacral endplate and lumbar lordosis and, to a lesser extent, between lumbar lordosis and thoracic kyphosis (21,37). Also, changing the position of the arms substantially influences spinal balance and thus the sagittal curvatures (19,33,38). In AS patients, the compensatory mechanism of the spine is obviously lost, because the spine has become a rigid rod as a result of the disease. For the same reason, sagittal curvatures are hardly of interest for the planning of a corrective osteotomy, although the total curvature of the spine could be a direct measure for the amount of angular correction required to restore the view angle. It is interesting to note that in AS patients, increased thoracic kyphosis is generally accompanied by a decreased lumbar lordosis: in healthy persons, increased thoracic kyphosis usually goes with an increased lumbar lordosis in order to maintain balance (21,37). This suggests that the compensatory mechanism of the spine itself is already eliminated as the characteristic kyphosing process proceeds. This has important implications for understanding the biological process of progressing kyphosis in AS.

While view angle is related to the total sagittal curvature, spinal balance is related to the relative position of plumb lines. Sagittal plumb lines for spinal balance have been measured in various ways and shown to have wide cross-sectional variations in different volunteer and patient populations (21,30,31,33,42–46). Plumb lines thus are not very accurate, but have the advantage of their simplicity in practical use. In order to evaluate balance in the whole thoracolumbar spine, the plumb line from C7 is most commonly used. Advantages of this plumb line are that it roughly intersects the posterior edge of the sacral endplate, and that is does not depend on the inclination of the sacral endplate in healthy volunteers (21,26,30,31,47). The primary difficulty of using this plumb line is in determining the location of C7. The vertebral body of C7 is often eclipsed by the projection of the shoulders in lateral radiographs. This reduces reliability and reproducibility of spinal balance measurements by different observers (35). Alternatively, T4 can be used, which is easier and more reliably visualized; also radiographical landmarks of the skull are useful (34,48). In AS patients eligible for surgical correction, the plumb line from C7 runs far anteriorly from the sacrum due to the strong kyphotic deformation of the spine (9). The horizontal distance between the plumb line and some pelvic landmark thus can be used as a practical measure for spinal balance in the pre- and postoperational evaluation (9).

ESTABLISHING THE ANGULAR CORRECTION

Restoration of the view angle is the most important reason for intervention in AS patients (9,13,14). Establishing the required amount of angular correction thus should be the first step in preoperative planning. The most direct and reliable procedure would be to take a lateral radiograph of sacrum, spine, and cranium; to position the sacral endplate in the optimum position of 40° to the horizon (Fig. 1); and to determine the angular position of an anatomic reference plane as a measure for view angle. A useful parameter for this purpose could be the so-called Frankfort plane, which is considered in the field of cephalometry as a true horizontal for a person standing upright (49–51). The Frankfort plane is radiographically defined by the lower edge of the eye sockets and the most upper point of the bony external auditory meatuses (Fig. 2), and is directly related to the field of view (52). In the ideal case, the SEA and the Frankfort plane thus should make an angle of 40°. Important advantages of this approach are that only one lateral radiograph is needed to determine all parameters, and that the measurement does not depend on the incidental posture of the patient.

Although this method is reliable and straightforward, it has not been used in clinical practice, or at least has not been described in the clinical literature. As a rule, longitudinal radiographs of the spine do not include the cranium, which in fact could be quite difficult for AS patients with severe kyphoses, as the projection of head and spine would not fit on one radiograph. So, practically, other methods and measures

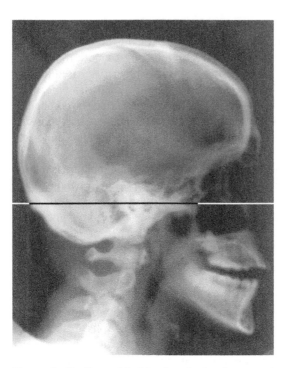

Figure 2 Radiographical landmarks for the natural position of the head. A well-established measure in the field of cephalometry is the Frankfort plane, which can be used as a true-horizontal plane equivalent. The Frankfort plane is defined by the lower edge of the eye sockets and the most upper point of the bony external auditory meatuses.

are sought to estimate the required angular correction. One way to approximate the radiographic assessment of the Frankfort plane would be to take a longitudinal radiograph of the spine and a photograph of the patient standing in the same position. Methods have been developed to determine the soft Frankfort plane (the Frankfort plane determined on a photograph by external soft tissue landmarks), and that could be related to the SEA as determined by the radiograph in order to calculate the required correction angle (Fig. 3) (53,54). Drawbacks of this approach are that measurements have to be made on two separate recordings, and the assumption has to be made that the patient has maintained the same posture.

Currently, the most common way to estimate the required correction makes use of the chin-brow to vertical angle (CBVA) (9,55,56). The angular correction is assessed by measuring CBVA in two positions: first, the patient is asked to stand in a position with hips and knees extended; then, the patients is asked to restore his view angle as close to normal as possible. The difference in CBVA is the required correction. However, this method fully neglects the compensation mechanisms explored by the AS patient and thereby underestimates the required correction angle. Therefore, Van Royen et al. (9) defined the required correction angle as the CBVA correction, added with the deviation of the SEA from 40°. Still, this method has some drawbacks. First, three recordings are needed to determine the required correction angle. Second, it is assumed that the patient is actually able to restore a normal CBVA; considering his physical impairments, this is in fact highly questionable. Finally, it assumes that pelvic tilt is the same in the radiograph and the photograph in which the patient stretches his knees and ankles; this, in fact, could differ considerably in successive

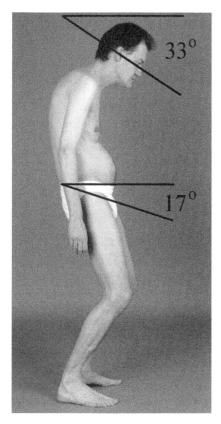

Figure 3 Estimation of the required correction angle using the soft Frankfort plane. Assuming that the radiograph (Fig. 1B) and the photograph have been taken with the patient in the same position, the SEA is 17°. The deviation from the ideal position is 40° – 17° = 23°. The Frankfort plane—considered to be the true-horizon equivalent—makes an angle of 33° with the horizon. The total required correction thus is 23° + 33° = 56°. For discussion see text. *Abbreviation*: SEA, sacral endplate angle.

lateral recordings (3). Despite these drawbacks, the CBVA correction, added with the SEA deviation from 40°, seems to result in an acceptable practical guideline for angular correction (9).

PREDICTING POSTOPERATIVE SPINAL BALANCE

Having defined the optimal position of the sacrum and the cranium (Figs. 1 and 2), the required angular correction for an AS patient can easily be calculated (Fig. 3). What remains to be determined is the level of osteotomy that gives an optimal sagittal balance. As pointed out earlier, there is no exact definition for sagittal balance, and this is more so a problem in AS patients. In the following, the C7 plumb line will be used as an alternative measure.

Consider an ankylosed spine, the posture of which is defined by the angulation of the sacral endplate and the position of the center of the vertebral body C7. The SEA is optimally placed at 40° with respect to the horizon, and the origin of the coordinate system is chosen at its posterior edge (Fig. 4). The position of

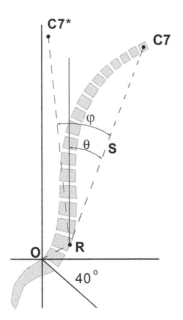

Figure 4 Calculation of sagittal balance after surgery. C7 denotes the position of the center of the vertebral body of C7 preoperatively. After correction over an angle φ around rotation point R, C7 moves to C7*. The x-coordinate of C7* (x_{C7^*}) defines the position of the plumb line of C7.

(the center of) vertebra C7 is defined as (x_{C7}, y_{C7}). The wedge osteotomy effectively introduces a rotation φ of the upper spine and cranium around a point R (x_R, y_R), defined by the type and level of surgery. In case of a closing wedge procedure, R lies at the middle of the anterior edge of the vertebral body involved; in case of an open-wedge procedure, R lies at the posterior edge of the intervertebral disc involved; in case of a multi-segmental wedge osteotomy, R is located centrally to the osteotomies at the anterior rim of the spine. With S the distance between C7 and R, the coordinates of C7 after the operation, $C7^* = (x_{C7^*}, y_{C7^*})$, are:

$$x_{C7^*} = x_R + S \sin(\theta - \varphi) \tag{1}$$

$$y_{C7^*} = y_R + S \cos(\theta - \varphi) \tag{2}$$

with θ defined as shown in Figure 4, or mathematically:

$$S \cos(\theta) = y_{C7} - y_R \tag{3}$$

$$S \sin(\theta) = x_{C7} - x_R \tag{4}$$

Using Equations (3) and (4), and the goniometric equation:

$$\sin(\theta - \varphi) = \sin(\theta) \cos(\varphi) - \cos(\theta) \sin(\varphi) \tag{5}$$

the position of the plumb line C7 after the operation (x_{C7^*}) can be expressed in terms of the required correction angle φ and the positions of R and C7:

$$x_{C7^*} = x_R + (x_{C7} - x_R) \cos(\varphi) - (y_{C7} - y_R) \sin(\varphi) \tag{6}$$

Knowing the required correction angle φ and the position of C7, and choosing the type and level of osteotomy (i.e., the position of R), the surgeon can thus precisely determine the postoperative position of plumb line C7. Reversibly, the surgeon may wish to aim at a certain position of plumb line C7 (i.e., x_{C7^*}), and derive the best level of osteotomy. To that end, Equation (6) can be rewritten into

$$y_R = y_{C7} - [x_R - x_{C7^*} + (x_{C7} - x_R)\cos(\varphi)]/\sin(\varphi) \qquad (7)$$

which describes a line of mathematical solutions for R (x_R, y_R). The optimal position of R is found at the intersection of this line with the spine (Fig. 5).

As a result of the stiffened spine in AS patients, the postoperative sagittal balance can be calculated with mathematical precision. However, unlike optimal SEA and required view angle correction, optimal postoperative sagittal balance is difficult to define. Plumb line C7 likely has to run several centimeters in front of the posterior edge of the sacral endplate, but a real number is hard to give. Van Royen et al. (9) showed a case of under correction, in which the position of the plumb line C7 postoperatively was more than 20 cm anterior; the correction had been limited to only 23° for surgical reasons, instead of the intended 35°. At six years follow-up, the C7 plumb line shifted anteriorly to 26 cm. A relation between this kyphotic progression and insufficient surgical correction is suggestive, but as yet speculative. Nonetheless, the other case described in that paper had a postoperative plumb line at 7.5 cm anterior, and showed no progression of the kyphosis after four years follow-up. Obviously, data of many more patients are required in order to see if there actually exists a relationship between the postoperative C7 plumb line position and progression of the kyphotic deformation. This could also shed some light on the role of mechanical balance in the development and progression of thoracolumbar

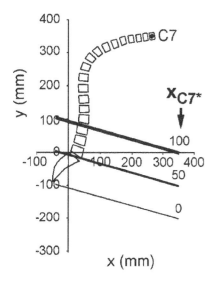

Figure 5 Determination of the optimal level of osteotomy (i.e., the position of point R) for three values of aimed postoperative plumb line position (x_{C7^*} = 0, 50, and 100). In the case of this particular patient, the required correction angle was determined at 30° (9). The graph shows that the postoperative plumb line will run at 100 mm in front of the posterior edge of the sacral endplate if an open-wedge osteotomy is performed at the discus L3–L4. Choosing

kyphosis in AS patients. Such a study also could help to define an optimum postoperative sagittal balance, based on the C7 plumb line or any other radiographic landmark.

SUMMARY AND DISCUSSION

AS may lead to severe rigid kyphotic deformities in the spine, resulting in a loss of horizontal view and sagittal balance. AS patients with a hyperkyphosis may partially compensate for their discomfort by tilting the pelvis, but they ultimately require a surgical intervention, mainly because of muscular pain and social isolation. A rigid kyphosis cannot be straightened up, but a well-planned wedge osteotomy can restore a natural view angle and sagittal balance. How to accomplish this, is the question at hand.

The first step in planning an osteotomy is to acknowledge the fact that AS patients must compensate for their loss of horizontal view and sagittal balance by extending their hips and bending their knees and ankles. This reduces the effects of hyperkyphosis at the cost of muscular fatigue and pain. Therefore, it is suggested that the pelvic alignment should be restored to its natural position, which is with the SEA at some 40°. The pelvis in this position forms a good fundament for the balanced spine, reduces the muscular effort to maintain balance, reduces the risk of developing osteoarthrosis, and restores the compensation possibilities of the lower extremities.

The second parameter of interest is the view angle, which also should be as natural as possible. It is suggested here to use the so-called Frankfort plane, which is known to be a true horizon equivalent in healthy persons and closely connected to the field of view. One whole-body radiograph allows clinicians to determine both the SEA and the Frankfort plane, independent of the posture of the patient while recording. The required correction angle for the wedge osteotomy thus now becomes the sum of the deviation of the SEA from 40° and the deviation of the Frankfort plane from the true horizontal.

Finally, sagittal balance has to be considered. As the COM cannot be determined from radiographs, related parameters must be used, like radiographic landmarks. The plumb line from C7 has some drawbacks, but is commonly used to quantify spinal balance. In healthy persons, it more or less runs through the posterior edge of the sacral endplate; in AS patients with hyperkyphosis, it is shifted anteriorly by 20–50 cm. Restoration probably should aim at a position <10 cm for acceptable spinal balance, but optimal values are unknown and only can be established in a clinical study.

The proposed procedure for planning the restoration of view and balance in AS patients is based on anatomical and biomechanical considerations, and can be performed with mathematical precision. The surgical procedure, however, cannot always meet the prescriptions resulting from the planning. Apart from the clinical considerations mentioned in the introduction (complication risk, postoperative handicaps, etc.), it should be recognized that the surgical procedure is less accurate than the planning procedure. For example, it is most difficult to determine the exact angle of the osteotomic wedge, and part of the correction can be lost postoperatively. Computer-assisted surgery could be of much help in this respect. A problem of a different nature is formed by off-sagittal deformations; in order to see the horizon, some patients turn their head, thereby introducing a scoliotic deformation in their stiffening spine. This requires a true three-dimensional planning procedure, instead of the two-dimensional approach discussed here. Nonetheless, the basic assumptions for preoperative planning—the position of sacrum and cranium—remain valid also in the three-dimensional case.

Discussing accuracy, it also should be recognized that accuracy is not imperative for clinical success. For AS patients with severe kyphosis, a correction of more than 20° is a dramatic improvement of their situation (13,14). Not surprisingly, close to 100% of the patients are satisfied with the outcome of a corrective osteotomy. However, some follow-up studies do suggest that insufficient correction may be related to a progressive kyphosis after the operation. This needs to be confirmed in a broader clinical study, and the planning procedure presented here provides an excellent analytical tool for that purpose. This future clinical study also should address the problem of defining optimal sagittal balance.

REFERENCES

1. Duff SE, Grundy PL, Gill SS. New approach to cervical flexion deformity in ankylosing spondylitis. Case report. J Neurosurg 2000; 93(suppl 2):283–286.
2. Thiranont N, Netrawichien P. Transpedicular decancellation closed wedge vertebral osteotomy for treatment of fixed flexion deformity of spine in ankylosing spondylitis. Spine 1993; 18(16):2517–2522.
3. Bot SD, Caspers M, Van Royen BJ, Toussaint HM, Kingma I. Biomechanical analysis of posture in patients with spinal kyphosis due to ankylosing spondylitis: a pilot study. Rheumatology (Oxford) 1999; 38(5):441–443.
4. Van Royen BJ, Toussaint HM, Kingma I, et al. Accuracy of the sagittal vertical axis in a standing lateral radiograph as a measurement of balance in spinal deformities. Eur Spine J 1998; 7(5):408–412.
5. Van Royen BJ, De Gast A. Lumbar osteotomy for correction of thoracolumbar kyphotic deformity in ankylosing spondylitis. A structured review of three methods of treatment. Ann Rheum Dis 1999; 58(7):399–406.
6. Simmons EH. Kyphotic deformity of the spine in ankylosing spondylitis. Clin Orthop 1977; 128:65–77.
7. Niemeyer T, Hackenberg L, Bullmann V, Liljenqvist U, Halm H. Technik und ergebnisse der monosegmentalen transpedikulären wirbelkörpersubtraktionsosteotomie bei patienten mit spondylitis ankylosans und fixierter kyphotischer deformität. Z Orthop Ihre Grenzgeb 2002; 140(2):176–181.
8. Van Royen BJ, Slot GH. Closing-wedge posterior osteotomy for ankylosing spondylitis. Partial corporectomy and transpedicular fixation in 22 cases. J Bone Joint Surg Br 1995; 77(1):117–121.
9. Van Royen BJ, De Gast A, Smit TH. Deformity planning for sagittal plane corrective osteotomies of the spine in ankylosing spondylitis. Eur Spine J 2000; 9(6):492–498.
10. Bradford DS, Schumacher WL, Lonstein JE, Winter RB. Ankylosing spondylitis: experience in surgical management of 21 patients. Spine 1987; 12:238–243 (Erratum: Spine 1987; 12:590–592).
11. Urist MR. Osteotomy of the cervical spine; report of a case of ankylosing rheumatoid spondylitis. J Bone Joint Surg Am 1958; 41-A:833–843.
12. Kim KT, Suk KS, Cho YJ, Hong GP, Park BJ. Clinical outcome results of pedicle subtraction osteotomy in ankylosing spondylitis with kyphotic deformity. Spine 2002; 27:612–618.
13. Halm H, Metz-Stevenhagen P, Zielke K. Results of surgical correction of kyphotic deformities of the spine in ankylosing spondylitis on the basis of the modified arthritis impact measurement scales. Spine 1995; 20:1612–1619.
14. Metz-Stevenhagen P, Krebs S, Volpel HJ. Operationsmethoden zur behandlung der totalkyphose bei der spondylitis ankylosans. Orthopäde 2001; 30:988–995.

15. Sengupta DK, Khazim R, Grevitt MP, Webb JK. Flexion osteotomy of the cervical spine: a new technique for correction of iatrogenic extension deformity in ankylosing spondylitis. Spine 2001; 26(9):1068–1072.

16. Kingma I, Toussaint HM, Commissaris DA, Hoozemans MJ, Ober MJ. Optimizing the determination of the body centre of mass. J Biomech 1995; 28:1137–1142.

17. Ferguson AB. Clinical and roentgenographic interpretation of lumbosacral anomalies. Radiology 1934; 22:548–558.

18. Hellems HK, Keats TE. Measurement of the normal lumbosacral angle. Am J Roentgenol 1971; 113:642–645.

19. Stagnara P, de Mauroy JC, Dran G, Gonon GP, Costano G, Dimnet J, Pasquet A. Reciprocal angulation of vertebral bodies in a sagittal plane: approaches to references for the evaluation of kyphosis and lordosis. Spine 1982; 7:335–342.

20. Mangione P, Gomez D, Senegas J. Study of the course of the incidence angle during growth. Eur Spine J 1997; 6:163–167.

21. Jackson RP, Peterson MD, McManus AC, Hales C. Compensatory spinopelvic balance over the hip axis and better reliability in measuring lordosis to the pelvic radius on standing lateral radiographs of adult volunteers and patients. Spine 1998; 23:1750–1767.

22. Murray GC, Persellin RH. Cervical fracture complicating ankylosing spondylitis: a report on eight cases and review of the literature. Am J Med 1982; 70:1033–1041.

23. Hitchon PW, From AM, Brenton MD, Glaser JA, Torner JC. Fractures of the thoracolumbar spine complicating ankylosing spondylitis. J Neurosurg 2002; 97(suppl 2): 218–222.

24. Bessant R, Keat A. How should clinicians manage osteoporosis in ankylosing spondylitis? J Rheumatol 2002; 29:1511–1519.

25. During J, Goudfrooij H, Keessen W, Beeker TW, Crowe A. Toward standards for posture. Postural characteristics of the lower back system in normal and pathologic conditions. Spine 1985; 10(1):83–87.

26. Voutsinas SA, MacEwen GD. Sagittal profiles of the spine. Clin Orthop 1986; 210: 235–242.

27. Duval-Beaupere G, Robain G. Visualization on full spine radiographs of the anatomical connections of the centres of the segmental body mass supported by each vertebra and measured in vivo. Int Orthop 1987; 11:261–269.

28. Abitbol MM. Sacral curvature and supine posture. Am J Phys Anthropol 1989; 80: 379–389.

29. Bernhardt M, Bridwell KH. Segmental analysis of the sagittal plane alignment of the normal thoracic and lumbar spines and thoracolumbar junction. Spine 1989; 14:717–721.

30. Jackson RP, McManus AC. Radiographic analysis of sagittal plane alignment and balance in standing volunteers and patients with low back pain matched for age, sex, and size. A prospective controlled clinical study. Spine 1994; 19:1611–1618.

31. Gelb DE, Lenke LG, Bridwell KH, Blanke K, McEnery KW. An analysis of sagittal spinal alignment in 100 asymptomatic middle and older aged volunteers. Spine 1995; 20:1351–1358.

32. Korovessis PG, Stamatakis MV, Baikousis AG. Reciprocal angulation of vertebral bodies in the sagittal plane in an asymptomatic Greek population. Spine 1998; 23: 700–704.

33. Vedantam R, Lenke LG, Keeney JA, Bridwell KH. Comparison of standing sagittal spinal alignment in asymptomatic adolescents and adults. Spine 1998; 23:211–215.

34. Korovessis P, Stamatakis M, Baikousis A. Segmental roentgenographic analysis of vertebral inclination on sagittal plane in asymptomatic versus chronic low back pain patients. J Spinal Disord 1999; 12:131–137.

35. Jackson RP, Kanemura T, Kawakami N, Hales C. Lumbopelvic lordosis and pelvic balance on repeated standing lateral radiographs of adult volunteers and untreated patients with constant low back pain. Spine 2000; 25:575–586.

36. Jackson RP, Hales C. Congruent spinopelvic alignment on standing lateral radiographs of adult volunteers. Spine 2000; 25(21):2808–2815.

37. Vaz G, Roussouly P, Berthonnaud E, Dimnet J. Sagittal morphology and equilibrium of pelvis and spine. Eur Spine J 2002; 11:80–87.

38. Marks MC, Stanford CF, Mahar AT, Newton PO. Standing lateral radiographic positioning does not represent customary standing balance. Spine 2003; 28:1176–1182.

39. Marty C, Boisaubert B, Descamps H, et al. The sagittal anatomy of the sacrum among young adults, infants, and spondylolisthesis patients. Eur Spine J 2002; 11:119–125.

40. Gracovetsky S, Farfan H. The optimum spine. Spine 1986; 11:543–573.

41. Troyanovivich SJ, Cailliet R, Janik TJ, Harrison DD, Harisson DE. Radiographic mensuration characteristics of the sagittal lumbar spine from a normal population with a method to synthesize prior studies of lordosis. J Spinal Disord 1997; 10:380–386.

42. LaGrone MO. Loss of spinal lordosis: a complication of spinal fusion for scoliosis. Orthop Clin North Am 1988; 19:383–393.

43. LaGrone MO, Bradford DS, Moe JH, Lonstein JE, Winter RB, Ogilvie JW. Treatment of symptomatic flatback after spinal fusion. J Bone Joint Surg Am 1988; 70:569–580.

44. Swank SM, Mauri TM, Brown JC. The lumbar lordosis below Harrington instrumentation for scoliosis. Spine 1990; 15:181–186.

45. DeWald RL. Revision surgery for spinal deformity. Am Acad Orthop Surg Instr Course Lect 1992; 41:235–250.

46. Shufflebarger HL, Clark CD. Thoracolumbar osteotomy for postsurgical sagittal imbalance. Spine 1992; 17(suppl):S287–S290.

47. Schulz AB, Ashton-Miller JA. Biomechanics of the spine. In: Mow VC, Hayes WC, eds. Basic Orthopaedic Biomechanics. New York: Rave Press, 1991:336–374.

48. Jackson RP. Letter to the editor. Spine 2002; 27:1950–1951.

49. Ricketts RM. New perspectives on orientation and their benefits to clinical orthodontics—part I. Angle Orthod 1975; 45:238–248.

50. Strait DS, Ross CF. Kinematic data on primate head and neck posture: implications for the evolution of basicranial flexion and an evaluation of registration planes used in paleoanthropology. Am J Phys Anthropol 1999; 108:205–222.

51. Leitao P, Nanda RS. Relationship of natural head position to craniofacial morphology. Am J Orthod Dentofacial Orthop 2000; 117:406–417.

52. Ricketts RM, Schullof RJ, Bahga L. Orientation-Sella-nasion or Frankfort horizontal. Am J Orthod 1976; 69:648–654.

53. Ferrario VF, Sforza C, Miani A, Tartaglia G. Craniofacial morphometry by photographic evaluations. Am J Orthod Dentofacial Orthop 1993; 103:327–337.

54. Ferrario VF, Sforza C, Germano D, Dalloca LL, Miani A Jr. Head posture and cephalometric analyses: an integrated photographic/radiographic technique. Am J Orthod Dentofacial Orthop 1994; 106:257–264.

55. Simmons EH. Ankylosing spondylitis: surgical considerations. In: Roltman RH, Simeone FA, eds. The Spine. 2. 3rd ed. Philadelphia: WB Saunders, 1992; 1447–1511.

56. Van Royen BJ, De Kleuver M, Slot GH. Polysegmentallumbar posterior wedge osteotomies for correction of kyphosis in ankylosing spondylitis. Eur Spine J 1998; 7:104–110.

11

Medical Treatment for Ankylosing Spondylitis: An Overview

Corinne Miceli-Richard and Maxime Dougados
Department of Rheumatology, Cochin Hospital, AP-HP, René Descartes University, Paris, Cedex, France

Medical treatment for ankylosing spondylitis (AS), as well as for the different clinical forms of spondyloarthropathies (SpA), comprises a broad range of pharmacologic treatments: nonsteroidal anti-inflammatory drugs (NSAIDs), corticosteroids, disease-modifying antirheumatic drugs (DMARDs), and the more recent biological drugs. The management of patients with AS also includes procedures such as rest, programs of physical exercises, and physiotherapy (see chap. 13). Patient's education is another important point to consider. An overview of the medical treatments proposed in AS is proposed herein.

NONSTEROIDAL ANTI-INFLAMMATORY DRUGS

Until the development of noninflammatory drugs, the therapeutic management of SpA was extremely limited. The past 60 years have been marked by a considerable development of NSAIDs, maintaining the same efficacy while diminishing adverse events. This development provided rheumatologists with the first line treatment for SpA. Overall, NSAIDs are effective in every painful manifestation of SpA. However, graduation of efficacy is often noted according to the location of the disease, axial involvement and/or enthesitis being classically more sensitive to NSAIDs in comparison to peripheral arthritis. NSAID treatments induce improvement of pain and function and help maintain normal mobility. Bedtime intake of a long-acting NSAID is recommended in order to cover the inflammatory and painful phases of the disease that occur at night. Nevertheless, an additional morning dose of a short-acting NSAID is often necessary.

Response to NSAIDs often differs markedly among patients, and several NSAIDs may have to be tried in order to identify which is the most effective for a particular patient (1). NSAIDs should also be used at the appropriate dosage before being considered as inefficient. High doses are sometimes required in severe cases.

NSAIDs have a quick-acting symptomatic effect but the question remaining in a patient well controlled by NSAIDs is whether such treatment has to be taken systematically and continuously on a daily basis or only "at request." A continuous administration of these drugs may facilitate the concomitant required physical therapy and may have a beneficial structural effect (2). On the contrary, a continuous daily intake may increase the risk of NSAIDs toxicity. Further studies in this field, in particular evaluating the coxibs, are required.

In daily practice, the current view is to restrict NSAIDs to the active phase of the disease. If NSAID treatment leads to a remission, a therapeutic discontinuation can distinguish between an NSAID-related improvement and the onset of a non-active phase of the disease that does not justify continuation of treatment. If a flare-up occurs at discontinuation of NSAIDs, the treatment should be reintroduced.

CORTICOSTEROIDS

Corticosteroids can provide a therapeutic option in case of patients who are refractory or intolerant to the NSAID treatment. Nevertheless, in daily practice, oral cortico-steroids appear less effective in AS than in other rheumatic inflammatory conditions such as rheumatoid arthritis. Unfortunately, no controlled trial has addressed that particular point. Moreover, oral administration of corticosteroids over a long period is often associated with side effects. Therefore, their use in AS is quite limited.

Intravenous methylprednisolone pulse therapy in AS can be useful in acute phases of the disease but short-term relapses are often observed in daily practice, justi-fying the concomitant use of other therapeutic options (3). Conversely, intra-articular corticosteroids (including sacroiliac joints and facets joints) are widely used in AS with a very effective response in most cases (4).

SECOND LINE AGENT IN MEDICAL TREATMENT OF AS

Many SpA patients have a mild disease with a good clinical response to NSAIDs. Nevertheless, some patients have clinical, biological, and/or radiological elements of poor prognosis or are refractory to NSAIDs with persistent signs of active disease (5). In this particular set of patients, the initiation of second line agents or DMARDs may be necessary. Nevertheless, such slow acting drugs [i.e., sulfasalazine (SLZ) or methotrexate (MTX)] may at best induce a symptomatic improvement. Few placebo-controlled studies have been performed in order to evaluate the efficacy of these drugs leading to the conclusion that none of them can be considered as DMARDs in AS as their efficacy has not been established in this disorder.

Sulfasalazine

This drug is one of the most investigated for the treatment of AS. Since 1986, different placebo-controlled trials of relatively small sample size have been reported (6,7). A statistically significant improvement was observed among patients receiving SLZ, either in terms of functional index or in most of the clinical and laboratory variables [morning stiffness, chest expansion, erythrocyte sedimentation rate (ESR), C-reactive protein (CRP)], suggesting the efficacy of this drug in AS (6,7). A potential effect of SLZ in axial symptoms was suggested in the subgroup of patients with shorter disease duration (<6 years) (7). Such a trend has never been confirmed to date.

In the 1990s, two large placebo-controlled trials have been conducted (8,9). SLZ was effective when the analysis was restricted to the subgroup of SpA patients with peripheral arthritis. No significant difference was evidenced by analyzing the whole group of patients, irrespective of the axial or peripheral manifestations. No clear improvement of axial symptoms was observed in both trials, perhaps due to the inclusion of a high proportion of patients with a long-standing disease. Efficacy of SLZ has also been reported for peripheral arthritis in psoriatic and reactive arthritis or proposed in the prevention of recurrent anterior uveitis associated with AS (10–12).

Overall, the main conclusions regarding SLZ in SpA are:

- SLZ is effective in SpA with peripheral arthritis.
- SLZ is probably effective in the prevention of anterior uveitis associated with AS.
- The efficacy of SLZ in axial manifestations is more debatable.

Methotrexate

Three open prospective trials have studied MTX in AS, suggesting a potential efficacy in this indication (13–15). An improvement of the biological parameters of inflammation—ESR and/or CRP—was observed (13,15). Efficacy was reported among patients with peripheral arthritis or axial disease (13,15). Marshall and Kirwan (16) have reported a poor clinical response to MTX in AS in a more recent prospective trial, but a better efficacy was noted in the subgroup of patients with peripheral arthritis. Nevertheless, the relevance of such studies is limited (small sample size, not placebo-controlled). Therefore, further long-term placebo-controlled studies are necessary to address the role of MTX in AS, specifically in axial forms of the disease. Unfortunately, large placebo-controlled trials testing the efficacy of MTX in AS are unlikely to be performed in the future because MTX is already widely used in daily practice in AS by the rheumatologist community, even in the absence of proven benefits in the axial disease.

ᴅ-Penicillamine

A double-blind placebo-controlled trial did not demonstrate any significant improvement of clinical or biological parameters in AS patients receiving ᴅ-penicillamine compared with placebo (17).

Gold Salt, Antimalarial, Cyclosporin A, Leflunomide, Azathioprine

No placebo-controlled trials are available to evaluate the efficacy of these treatments in AS as only few case reports have been reported (18–20).

Thalidomide

A potential efficacy of thalidomide for the treatment of AS has been first reported by Breban et al. (21) in a case report of two patients with a severe and disabling AS, resistant to the medical treatment proposed until the introduction of thalidomide. An obvious clinical improvement of both patients was observed within three to six months, correlated with a decrease in CRP and ESR. Three years after this first publication, a one-year open-label trial of thalidomide in AS was reported by a Chinese group (22). Thirty male patients were included in this trial. Treatment was given at a daily dosage of 200 mg and followed during 12 months. A 20% improvement in four out of seven items from a composite index was considered as the primary endpoint: Bath AS Disease Activity Index (BASDAI), Bath AS Functional Index (BASFI), duration of the morning stiffness, total body pain and spinal pain on a four-point Likert scale, and patient and physician global assessment on a four-point scale. According to that definition, 80% of patients were responders to the treatment. Biological parameters of inflammation normalized in more than 50% of patients within 12 months or less.

Side effects were reported with variable frequencies and were roughly correlated to the therapeutic schemes proposed in the different studies: a higher rate of dropout was observed in the French study where the initial dosage of thalidomide was 300 mg; no dropout due to side effects was reported in the Chinese study where the initial dosage was 50 mg with a progressive increment until 200 mg/day. The most frequent side effects were drowsiness, constipation, dizziness, and dry mouth. Paresthesias and peripheral neuropathies were also reported, but to a lesser extent. Nevertheless, a close monitoring of the patients is necessary as well as an accurate contraception. In the reported studies, no birth abnormalities were observed under that last condition.

This drug has an anti-tumor necrosis factor (TNF) α activity by enhancing messenger RNA (mRNA) degradation (23). An inhibition of interleukin-12 has also been reported (24). More recent studies have evidenced that thalidomide increases natural killer cell cytotoxicity and augments T-cell proliferation (25,26). The clinical efficacy of thalidomide might be related to those biological effects. The main goal of the pharmacological industry is now to develop more potent and less toxic drugs, notably without teratogenic effects. Two classes of second generation analogs have been synthesized: immunomodulatory drugs (IMIDs) and selective cytokines inhibitory drugs (SelCIDs). These drugs are much more potent than thalidomide at inhibiting TNFα production in vitro and are currently being assessed in the treatment of cancer patients (27–29). Nevertheless, further applications in chronic inflammatory diseases are expected.

Pamidronate and Biotherapies in AS

Bisphosphonates also possess anti-inflammatory properties. Therefore, besides their wide use in bone disorders, bisphosphonate therapy has been proposed in AS. Open studies performed in that indication have shown hopeful results leading to controlled evaluation of pamidronate in AS. Biotherapies as TNFα blockers have also demonstrated convincing results in AS. Details about these treatments are provided elsewhere (see chap. 12).

Finally, the management of patients with AS includes some other procedures such as patient education, rest, physical exercises, and physiotherapy (see chap. 13). In fact, stiffness and spinal deformities are unlikely to be prevented by drugs alone. In parallel with pharmacotherapy, these procedures are of great importance in reducing stiffness and spinal ankylosis, and thus improving the patient's quality of life.

REFERENCES

1. Dougados M, Revel M, Khan MA. Spondyloarthropathy treatment: progress in medical therapy. Baillieres Clin Rheumatol 1998; 12:717–736.

2. Wanders A, van der Heijde D, Landewé R, et al. Inhibition of radiographic progression in ankylosing spondylitis by continuous use of NSAIDs. Arthritis Rheum 2003; 48(suppl):S532.

3. Peters ND, Ejstrup L. Intravenous methylprednisolone pulse therapy in ankylosing spondylitis. Scand J Rheumatol 1992; 21:134–138.

4. Maugars Y, Mathis C, Berthelot JM, Charlier C, Prost A. Assessment of the efficacy of sacroiliac corticosteroid injections in spondylarthropathies: a double-blind study. Br J Rheumatol 1996; 35:767–770.

5. Amor B, Santos RS, Nahal R, Listrat V, Dougados M. Predictive factors of the long term outcome of spondylarthropathies. J Rheumatol 1994; 21:1883–1887.

6. Dougados M, Boumier P, Amor B. Sulphasalazine in ankylosing spondylitis: a double blind controlled study in 60 patients. Br Med J (Clin Res Ed) 1986; 293:911–914.

7. Nissila M, Lehtinen K, Leirisalo-Repo M, Luukkainen R, Mutru O, Yli-Kerttula U. Sulfasalazine in the treatment of ankylosing spondylitis. A twenty-six-week, placebo-controlled clinical trial. Arthritis Rheum 1988; 31:1111–1116.

8. Clegg DO, Reda DJ, Abdellatif M. Comparison of sulfasalazine and placebo for the treatment of axial and peripheral articular manifestations of the seronegative spondylarthropathies. A Department of Veterans Affairs Cooperative Study. Arthritis Rheum 1999; 42:2325–2329.

9. Dougados M, van der Linden S, Leirisalo-Repo M, et al. Sulfasalazine in the treatment of spondylarthropathy. A randomized, multicenter, double-blind, placebo-controlled study. Arthritis Rheum 1995; 38:618–627.

10. Clegg DO, Reda DJ, Mejias E, et al. Comparison of sulfasalazine and placebo in the treatment of psoriatic arthritis. A Department of Veterans Affairs Cooperative Study. Arthritis Rheum 1996; 39(12):2013–2020.

11. Clegg DO, Reda DJ, Weisman MH, et al. Comparison of sulfasalazine and placebo in the treatment of reactive arthritis (Reiter's syndrome). A Department of Veterans Affairs Cooperative Study. Arthritis Rheum 1996; 39:2021–2027.

12. Benitez-Del-Castillo JM, Garcia-Sanchez J, Iradier T, Banares A. Sulfasalazine in the prevention of anterior uveitis associated with ankylosing spondylitis. Eye 2000; 14: 340–343.

13. Biasi D, Carletto A, Caramaschi P, Pacor ML, Maleknia T, Bambara LM. Efficacy of methotrexate in the treatment of ankylosing spondylitis: a three-year open study. Clin Rheumatol 2000; 19:114–117.

14. Creemers MC, Franssen MJ, van de Putte LB, Gribnau FW, van Riel PL. Methotrexate in severe ankylosing spondylitis: an open study. J Rheumatol 1995; 22:1104–1107.

15. Sampaio-Barros PD, Costallat LT, Bertolo MB, Neto JF, Samara AM. Methotrexate in the treatment of ankylosing spondylitis. Scand J Rheumatol 2000; 29:160–162.

16. Marshall RW, Kirwan JR. Methotrexate in the treatment of ankylosing spondylitis. Scand J Rheumatol 2001; 30(6):313–314.

17. Steven MM, Morrison M, Sturrock RD. Penicillamine in ankylosing spondylitis: a double blind placebo controlled trial. J Rheumatol 1985; 12(4):735–737.

18. Durez P, Horsmans Y. Dramatic response after an intravenous loading dose of azathioprine in one case of severe and refractory ankylosing spondylitis. Rheumatology (Oxford). 2000; 39:182–184.

19. Grasedyck K, Schattenkirchner M, Bandilla K. The treatment of ankylosing spondylitis with auranofin. Z Rheumatol 1990; 49:98–99.

20. Geher P, Gomor B. Repeated cyclosporine therapy of peripheral arthritis associated with ankylosing spondylitis. Med Sci Monit 2001; 7:105–107.

21. Breban M, Gombert B, Amor B, Dougados M. Efficacy of thalidomide in the treatment of refractory ankylosing spondylitis. Arthritis Rheum 1999; 42:580–581.

22. Huang F, Gu J, Zhao W, Zhu J, Zhang J, Yu DT. One-year open-label trial of thalidomide in ankylosing spondylitis. Arthritis Rheum 2002; 47:249–254.

23. Moreira AL, Sampaio EP, Zmuidzinas A, Frindt P, Smith KA, Kaplan G. Thalidomide exerts its inhibitory action on tumor necrosis factor alpha by enhancing mRNA degradation. J Exp Med 1993; 177:1675–1680.

24. Moller DR, Wysocka M, Greenlee BM, et al. Inhibition of IL-12 production by thalidomide. J Immunol 1997; 159:5157–5161.

25. Davies FE, Raje N, Hideshima T, et al.Thalidomide and immunomodulatory derivatives augment natural killer cell cytotoxicity in multiple myeloma. Blood 2001; 98:210–216.

26. Haslett PA, Corral LG, Albert M, Kaplan G. Thalidomide costimulates primary human T lymphocytes, preferentially inducing proliferation, cytokine production, and cytotoxic responses in the CD8+ subset. J Exp Med 1998; 187:1885–1892.

27. Corral LG, Haslett PA, Muller GW, et al. Differential cytokine modulation and T cell activation by two distinct classes of thalidomide analogues that are potent inhibitors of TNF-alpha. J Immunol 1999; 163:380–386.

28. Muller GW, Chen R, Huang SY, et al. Amino-substituted thalidomide analogs: potent inhibitors of TNF-alpha production. Bioorg Med Chem Lett 1999; 9(11):1625–1630.

29. Marriott JB, Westby M, Cookson S, et al. CC-3052: a water-soluble analog of thalidomide and potent inhibitor of activation-induced TNF-alpha production. J Immunol 1998; 161: 4236–4243.

12

Biologic Therapies in Spondyloarthritides—The Current State

Joachim Sieper
Department of Medicine and Rheumatology, University Medicine Charité,
Freie Universität Berlin, Universitatsklinikum Benjamin Franklin, Berlin, Germany

Juergen Braun
Rheumazentrum Ruhrgebiet, Herne and Ruhr-University, Bochum, Germany

INTRODUCTION

Ankylosing spondylitis (AS), together with reactive arthritis (ReA), arthritis/ spondylitis spectrum associated with psoriasis (Pso) and inflammatory bowel disease (IBD) and undifferentiated spondyloarthritides (uSpA) are part of the spondyloarthritides (SpA). AS is the most frequent subtype of SpA followed by uSpA and psoriatic arthritis (PsA). The prevalence of the whole group of SpA has been recently estimated between 0.6% and 1.9% with an implicated AS prevalence between 0.1% and 1.1% (1–4). AS and PsA are regarded as the SpA subsets with the most severe course of disease.

Nonsteroidal anti-inflammatory drugs (NSAID) were until recently the only agents with proven efficacy and, based on their good anti-inflammatory properties, should perform the basis of any treatment for AS (5,6). This should always be supplemented by intensive physiotherapy, which has recently been shown to be effective using modern tools for measuring outcome (7). However, beyond this, therapeutic options for patients suffering from AS have been limited during the last decades. Especially and in contrast to rheumatoid arthritis (RA), no disease modifying antirheumatic drug (DMARD) has been available. It is even more surprising that glucocorticoids do not work well, although good studies on this subject are missing (5). We could recently show that leflunomide does not improve axial symptoms at all, while there was some improvement in peripheral arthritis in those AS patients with arthritis (8). Taken together, there was a clear need for more effective therapies for AS patients (9).

TNFα-BLOCKING AGENTS IN RHEUMATIC DISEASES

Today there are three main biologic agents targeting tumor necrosis factor alpha (TNFα): the chimeric monoclonal Immunoglobin G1 (IgG1) antibody infliximab, the recombinant 75 kDa TNF receptor IgG1 fusion protein etanercept, and the fully humanized monoclonal antibody adalimumab. All three anti-TNF agents clearly work in RA. Infliximab has been approved in RA in combination with methotrexate (MTX) because less human antichimeric antibodies and somewhat less adverse events did occur with this regimen in RA, while etanercept and adalimumab have been approved as monotherapy (10). However, all agents work better when MTX is added. For PsA, etanercept and infliximab can be prescribed both inside the European Community (EC) and the United States. Furthermore, both infliximab and etanercept have received approval for AS both for the EC and the United States. Treatment trials with adalimumab in AS patients are ongoing.

THE ROLE OF TNFα IN AS

The sacroiliac joint (SIJ), the vertebral bodies, and the entheses are the most characteristic and almost pathognomonic sites involved in SpA (11,12). Inflammation at the interphase of cartilage and bone has been convincingly demonstrated by magnetic resonance imaging (MRI) and by immunohistological investigations of SIJ biopsies (12–17). Dense mononuclear infiltrates invading the cartilage have been described in the SIJ, especially in early cases, and TNFα messenger RNA has been described in inflamed SIJ (15). These results clearly demonstrated that AS is an inflammatory disorder, a statement which was sometimes doubted in the past, mostly because of the lack of response to DMARDs and glucocorticoids and because of the predominance of ankylosis in later stages. Thus, although RA is pathogenetically clearly different from AS, there is evidence for a pathogenetic role for TNFα in both diseases. Furthermore, TNFα is expressed in the gut of patients with IBD and anti-TNFα therapy with infliximab is effective for induction and maintenance therapy of Crohn's disease (CD) (18–20). This is of relevance because AS and the whole group of the SpA are associated with IBD, as such patients may develop AS and many patients with primary AS show histological gut lesions similar to CD (21). In addition, the gut and joint symptoms of patients with CD treated with infliximab have been reported to improve in a small number of patients (22). The efficacy of infliximab seems to be less convincing in ulcerative colitis but further study is needed (23,24). In contrast, etanercept, the 75 kDa TNF receptor fusion protein seems not to work in CD, while there are no data on adalimumab yet (25,26).

EFFECT OF ANTI-TNF THERAPY IN AS

Infliximab

In the first open pilot study on anti-TNF therapy in AS that was performed in Berlin, infliximab in a dosage of 5 mg/kg improved the disease activity of severe AS patients with a mean disease duration of five years when given at week zero, two, and six. Nine of 10 patients showed an improvement of >50% in disease activity at week 12, as measured by the Bath AS Disease Activity Index (BASDAI) (27,28). After the first three infusions, treatment was stopped and restarted once a relapse occurred, defined as 80% of the initial activity (29). As the first symptoms returned after a mean of six weeks and a relapse occurred after a mean of 12 weeks, a six-week treatment interval was chosen in the following randomized controlled trial (RCT) (30).

Several open label studies on infliximab in AS have all, very interestingly, shown a similar efficacy (31–40). In a Belgian study, 21 SpA patients including 11 with AS were treated with infliximab with a similar dose regimen as in the Berlin study, but the patients had a longer disease duration (15 years) and a longer time interval of 14 weeks was chosen between the infusions. The spinal and peripheral symptoms of all SpA patients improved significantly (31). In the one year follow-up, relapses occurred in 16% at week 20, in 68% at week 34, and in 79% at week 48 after last treatment and before retreatment (32). Week six and eight after the last infusion was not evaluated, thus, a direct comparison with the Berlin study regarding time at relapse is not possible. However, these data indicate that, similar to our pilot study, patients will relapse once treatment is stopped (27).

In Canada there were two studies, one with 24 and one with 21 AS patients; in France there were 50 AS patients, and in Spain 42 SpA patients (33–36). In the Canadian and the Spanish studies, there was a tendency that patients with long disease duration and advanced radiographic disease/ankylosis had less benefit from therapy (33,36). In the French study, even around 80% of the patients showed a 50% improvement, probably because only C-reactive protein (CRP)-positive and human leukocyte antigen (HLA)-B27 positive patients were included (see also the following about prediction of response) (35). In the second Canadian study, a relatively small dose of 3 mg/kg every eight weeks was sufficient to cause improvement in a substantial proportion of patients (see also the following for discussion on doses/interval) (34).

In a Greek study, 25 mostly HLA-B27+ AS patients with a mean disease duration of 14 years and active axial disease were treated with infliximab 5 mg/kg given every eight weeks for one year (38). The primary end point [reduction of pain by >20% on a 100-mm visual analog scale (VAS)] was reached by 92% of patients, improvement of 50% was obtained in 84% of patients, and of 70% in 52%. These data indicate that in open studies, more similar to daily clinical practice, a response rate for 50% improvement can even be expected in a percentage of up to 80% of patients.

Infliximab can even increase the bone mineral density (BMD) which can be reduced in AS due to local and systemic inflammation and immobility of the spine. After six months of infliximab therapy, the BMD, as measured by dual energy X-ray absorptiometry (DXA), was found to be significantly increased in 31 patients with a mean age of 40 years and a mean disease duration of 18 years by about 3% at the lumbar spine and by about 2% at the femoral neck (39).

The efficacy of infliximab in AS in a dosage of 5 mg/kg every six to eight weeks, which was so convincingly demonstrated in the open label trials, could subsequently be confirmed in three placebo-controled studies (evidence class A) (30,40,41). In the first multicenter study, 70 AS patients with a BASDAI ≥4 and spinal pain on a VAS ≥4 were included (30). The primary outcome parameter, a 50% improvement of BASDAI, was achieved in 53% of the patients treated with infliximab compared with 8% on placebo. Other parameters such as Bath AS Functional Index (BASFI), Bath AS Metrology Index (BASMI), short form (SF)-36 (a parameter for quality of life), peripheral arthritis, and enthesitis showed a similar clear-cut improvement. There was some evidence that patients with elevated CRP levels had a greater benefit than those with low or normal levels (see also the following for discussion of prediction of response) (38). In a similar study design, 40 patients with active SpA (including a majority of patients with AS) were treated with infliximab 5 mg/kg every eight weeks, the same results were obtained (40). In the so far largest international multicenter placebo-controlled trial very similar response rates were observed in the infliximab-treated group versus the placebo-treated group (41). Taken together, both peripheral and spinal manifestations of AS clearly improve on anti-TNF therapy. This includes severe enthesitis which also improves, as assessed both clinically and by ultrasound (42). Recent results from imaging follow-up studies, performed in patients from the German placebo-controlled double-blind study, with spinal MRI assessing both acute and chronic spinal changes, showed also a significant effect of infliximab on disease progression (30,43). Thus, both subjective parameters, such as the patient-based BASDAI and objective parameters improve significantly.

After the three-month placebo phase, the 70 patients from the German RCT are now being treated with infliximab at the same dose for another four years. After 54 weeks, 78% of the patients were still being treated with infliximab, and after two years still 70% (37,44). The intent-to-treat primary efficacy analysis at week 54 showed that almost 50% of the patients still achieved 50% improvement in BASDAI score. In the completer analysis, the mean BASDAI scores showed continuous improvement over 54 weeks down to a low disease activity level of 2.5. This further decrease of the BASDAI was significant when the 12-week value was compared with the 54-week value. Furthermore, the dosage of NSAID could be reduced in about 70% of patients. This continuous efficacy is of special interest because no concomitant treatment with DMARDs or glucocorticoids was permitted. Thus, in this study with the drug given in the indicated dosage and interval, the inhibition of infliximab by the possible production of anti-infliximab antibodies does not seem to be of clinical significance. This ongoing study will provide more information about the long-term efficacy and safety of infliximab in AS.

Regarding the optimal dosage of infliximab in SpA only limited data are available. In a small study of six patients with undifferentiated spondyloarthritis we found the dose of 3 mg/kg to be effective; however, 5 mg/kg was slightly superior (45). Some published and unpublished observations from different groups suggest that up to 50% of patients are doing well with a lower dose and/or a longer interval (34). However, more studies are needed on this subject.

Etanercept

Treatment of AS with the soluble TNFα receptor, etanercept, has also been studied in several studies. After initial positive results from an open study, three double-blind placebo-controlled trials have now been published which prove the efficacy of etanercept in AS (evidence class A) (46–49). In the first study, 40 patients were treated either with etanercept 2×25 mg (20 patients) or placebo (20 patients) subcutaneous (47). In contrast to our infliximab and etanercept studies, DMARDs and steroids were allowed to be continued during the study in 40% and 25% of patients, respectively (30,48). The main outcome parameters—morning stiffness and nocturnal spinal pain—improved significantly in the etanercept but not in the placebo group after four months of treatment. In the multicenter trial performed in Berlin, 30 AS patients with active disease (BASDAI ≥ 4) were randomized for the initial placebo-controlled period of six weeks duration which was followed by an observational phase lasting 24 weeks (48). The placebo group was switched to etanercept after six weeks and both groups were treated with etanercept for three months. NSAID treatment could be continued but DMARDs and steroids were withdrawn. Treatment with etanercept was significantly better than placebo with an at least 50% regression of disease activity in 57% of these patients at week six, versus only 6% in the placebo group. Disease relapses occurred at a mean of 6.2 ± 3 weeks after cessation of etanercept treatment. No severe adverse events, including major infections, were observed during this trial.

In the very recently published international trial, 277 patients were treated with either etanercept 25 mg ($n = 138$) or placebo ($n = 139$) s.c. twice weekly for 24 weeks (49). In this study, the Assessment in Ankylosing Spondylitis (ASAS) working group criteria for improvement were used as the primary outcome measure (50). The ASAS 20% improvement was achieved by 59% of patients in the etanercept group versus 28% of the patients in the placebo group at week 12, and by 57% versus 22% of patients, respectively, at week 24. The ASAS 50% and 70% response at week 24 was 45% in the etanercept group versus 10% in the placebo group and 28% in the etanercept group versus 5% in the placebo group, respectively. All differences were highly significant.

The group from Leeds has reported in a small study with 10 SpA patients, including seven patients with AS, that etanercept, obviously similar to infliximab, had a positive influence on the BMD of patients treated with this therapy, in contrast to a control group treated in a nonblinded way with conventional treatment (51).

TNF-BLOCKING AGENTS IN UNDIFFERENTIATED SPONDYLOARTHRITIS

There are many patients who have symptoms suggestive of SpA but do not fulfill the diagnostic criteria for any of the defined SpA subtypes. These patients have often been classified as uSpA by use of the European Spondyloarthropathy Study Group (ESSG) criteria (52). According to these criteria, patients with uSpA have either inflammatory back pain or asymmetrical peripheral arthritis predominantly of the lower limbs plus one additional manifestation characteristic of SpA such as enthesitis. Given the fact that especially patients with axial uSpA (preradiograph AS) have the same disease as patients with established radiographic AS (only at a different time point and stage) there is an urgent need to classify these patients in one set of criteria, and also to give the possibility to extend the indication for the treatment of AS with TNF-blockers to these early forms. We have most recently suggested an approach of how to diagnose these early forms (preradiographic) of AS reliably (53).

Preliminary data indeed suggest that both infliximab and etanercept are effective in the treatment of severe active uSpA patients (31,45). Peripheral arthritis, enthesitis, and spinal symptoms improved equally in six uSpA patients treated with infliximab (45). In a similar study 10 uSpA patients, treated with 2×25 mg etanercept twice a week s.c., responded similarly well (54). Taken together, anti-TNF therapy is a promising therapy for patients with severe uSpA.

TNF-BLOCKING AGENTS IN UVEITIS

Anterior uveitis (AU) occurs in 20–30% of patients with AS. Although it normally runs a benign course, in a few patients it can be refractory to conventional therapy. There is some evidence from controlled trials that sulfasalazine does prevent attacks (55,56). The response of patients with all kinds of inflammatory eye disease to anti-TNF has been recently looked at in a limited number of patients (57,58). At the moment the role of TNF-blockers for this indication is not clear: improvement and worsening of inflammatory eye disease have been reported during anti-TNF treatment. In one study, 16 patients, most of whom received etanercept for either inflammatory eye disease or associated joint disease, were studied retrospectively (57).

Although all 12 patients with active arthritis experienced improvement in joint disease, only six (38%) improved with their eye disease. Five patients even developed inflammatory eye disease for the first time while taking etanercept. In another study, there was some improvement of ocular inflammation in patients with chronic uveitis associated with partly antinuclear antibody-positive (ANA$^+$) juvenile chronic arthritis upon treatment with etanercept (58). However, because uveitis in HLA-B27 positive patients has a different course and a different pathogenesis compared with ANA-positive patients with juvenile arthritis these two groups should be studied separately in the future.

Beneficial effects of infliximab in a dosage of 10 mg/kg in seven patients with acute onset of HLA-B27-associated AU were reported from Austria (59). These patients were followed up for a mean period of 17 months. Total resolution of AU was achieved with infliximab as the only anti-inflammatory drug in all but one patient. A relapse was seen in four patients after a median of five months. The authors concluded that infliximab appears to be an efficacious therapeutic agent in acute HLA-B27-associated uveitis and might be an alternative or supplement to steroid treatment. Recently other reports about a successful treatment of uveitis with infliximab have been reported (60,61). The experience with infliximab in our study was also positive as only one versus three patients in the placebo group developed AU over three months (30). However, the natural course of AU in SpA is rather benign in the majority of patients. Thus, anti-TNF therapy should only be considered in severe refractory cases. Controlled studies in homogenous patient populations and a systematic comparison to local and systemic steroid therapy are needed. Severe uveitis in patients with Behcet's disease has also been successfully treated with infliximab (62).

SIDE EFFECTS OF ANTI-TNF THERAPY

Given the outstanding efficacy of the TNF-blockers in the treatment of AS the question of potential side effects is of greatest importance. There are clearly side effects which have to be considered in patients treated with anti-TNF agents. After the first years of experience with anti-TNF therapy the following types of adverse events seem to be of special concern for patients treated with anti-TNF therapy: (*i*) infections including tuberculosis (TB), (*ii*) lymphoma, (*iii*) demyelinating disorders/neuropathy, (*iv*) congestive heart failure, (*v*) occurrence of autoantibodies, lupus-like syndromes and other autoimmunities, (*vi*) infusion/injection and hypersensitivity reactions, (*vii*) occurrence of psoriatic skin lesions and CD, and (*viii*) other side effects.

Infections

In a recent report from Spain, mainly on RA patients, 71 participating centers sent data on 1578 treatments with infliximab (86%) or etanercept (14%) of 1540 patients (63). The estimated incidence of TB associated with infliximab in RA patients was 1893 per 100,000 in the year 2000 and 1113 per 100,000 in the year 2001. However, in the first five months of 2002, after official guidelines were established for TB prevention in patients treated with biologics, only one new TB case was registered, suggesting that the screening program is effective. Although the percentage of patients treated with etanercept was much smaller, no TB case occurred during treatment with etanercept. In a previous study a higher rate of TB cases during treatment with infliximab in comparison with etanercept has also been reported (64). In a recent report from Belgium 107 patients with SpA were treated with infliximab (65). Eight severe infections occurred, including two reactivations of TB and three retropharyngeal abscesses. Infliximab had to be stopped in five patients with severe infections. In our own placebo-controlled infliximab study in AS we observed one patient with lymph node TB; however, this study was started before patients were regularly screened for previous exposure to TB. In this study, there was no other severe infection (37).

Lymphoma

Under the U.S. Food and Drug Administration (FDA) MedWatch program, lymphoproliferative disorders were identified following treatment with etanercept or infliximab (66). The majority of cases (81%) were non-Hodgkin's lymphomas. The interval between initiation of therapy with etanercept or infliximab and the development of lymphoma was very short (median eight weeks). In two cases lymphoma regression was observed following discontinuation of anti-TNF treatment without specific cytotoxic therapy against lymphoma. However, on the background of the known predisposition of patients with RA and CD to lymphoma and the known excess of lymphoma in patients treated with other immunosuppressive drugs, a clear increase cannot be demonstrated at the moment for the development of lymphoma during treatment with TNF-blockers, although longer observation and a higher number of patients are necessary. No lymphoma has been reported in AS patients treated with TNF-blockers, although the small numbers of patients with AS or other SpA treated so far does not presently allow any conclusions about this side effect (37,45).

Neurologic Events

The U.S. FDA MedWatch program identified 19 patients with neurologic events during anti-TNF therapy, 17 following etanercept and two following infliximab administration (67). All neurologic events were temporally related to anti-TNFα therapy, with partial or complete resolution on discontinuation. Until more long-term safety data are available, anti-TNFα therapy should be avoided in patients with preexisting multiple sclerosis and discontinued when new neurologic signs and symptoms occur. No new neurologic events have so far been reported in AS patients treated with TNF-blockers (37,49,65).

Heart Failure

TNF-blockers have been tested as a treatment for patients with severe chronic heart failure. There was no difference in the outcome between patients treated with etanercept or placebo (68). In a trial treating patients with infliximab for this indication more patients died in the infliximab group compared with the placebo group, however only when treated with the high dose of 10 mg/kg but not in the 5 mg/kg group (69). At the lower doses there was no safety issue with regard to the use of infliximab. Indeed, a large postapproval report from the United States for the treatment of RA with TNF-blockers did not find higher heart-related safety issues compared with RA patients not treated with TNF-blockers (70). Again, no data on this are available for AS patients. However, because of the younger age of this group of patients an even lower risk can be expected compared with RA.

Induction of Autoantibodies and Autoimmunity

Anti-TNF therapy may lead to formation of ANAs. In patients with RA, anti-double-stranded (ds) deoxyribonucleic acid (DNA) antibodies of Immunoglobin M (IgM) class may be induced by infliximab; the frequency is dependent on the method used (71). Only one of the 156 patients treated with infliximab developed a self-limiting clinical lupus-like syndrome; this patient developed high titers of anti-dsDNA antibodies of IgG, IgM, and Immunoglobin A (IgA) class.

In another recent study, sera from 62 RA and 35 SpA patients treated with inflix-imab were tested at baseline and during therapy (72). Initially, 32 of 62 RA patients (51.6%) and six of 35 SpA (17.1%) patients tested positive for ANAs. After infliximab treatment, these numbers shifted to 82.3% and 88.6%, respectively. At baseline, none of the RA or SpA patients had anti-dsDNA antibodies. After infliximab treatment, seven RA and six SpA patients became positive for anti-dsDNA antibodies. All seven anti-dsDNA-positive RA patients had IgM and IgA anti-dsDNA antibodies. During the observation period, no IgG anti-dsDNA antibodies or lupus-like symptoms were observed. The development of anti-nucleosome, anti-histone, or anti extractable nuclear antigen (ENA) antibodies following infliximab treatment was observed in some patients, but the numbers were not statistically significant. Taken together, development of ANA is a rather frequent event in patients on infliximab therapy, while anti-DNA antibodies occur infrequently and is only rarely associated with lupus-related symptoms. In the one year follow-up study of AS patients treated with infliximab we also observed an increase in the percentage of patients becoming ANA-positive while there was no increase in our one year follow-up study in AS patients treated with etanercept (29,48,73).

Allergic Reactions to Infliximab or Etanercept

Side effects due to infusion or injection reactions occur with both infliximab and etanercept. In a large study with a total of 165 consecutive patients who received 479 infliximab infusions, the overall incidence of infusion reactions to infliximab was 6.1% (29 of 479) of infusions, affecting 9.7% (16 of 165) of patients. Mild, moderate, or severe acute reactions occurred in 3.1% (15 of 479), 1.2% (six of 479), and 1.0% (five of 479) of infliximab infusions, respectively (74). Use of treatment protocols resulted in rapid resolution of all acute reactions to infliximab. All patients who experienced an initial mild or moderate acute reaction were able to receive additional infusions if the infusion was given over a longer time or together with anti-histamines or glucocor-ticoids. Four patients experienced a total of five severe acute reactions. Three patients were retreated: two patients had no further problems, whereas one patient had a second severe acute reaction that rapidly resolved with treatment. Delayed infusion reactions were rare, occurring in 0.6% (three of 479) of infusions. In our one year follow-up study of AS patients treated with infliximab two of the initial 70 patients had to discontinue treatment because of allergic reaction during infusion (37). In patients treated with etanercept, local injection side reactions occur frequently in about 30% of patients but do generally not cause severe or lasting problems (49).

New Occurrence of Psoriatic Skin Lesions

Despite a reported very good clinical efficacy of infliximab and etanercept for the treatment of synovitis, acne, pustalosis, hyperostosis and osteitis (SAPHO) syn-drome and PsA (65,75–78), three patients with AS developed palmoplantar pustulo-sis on infliximab therapy. We also observed recently the new occurrence of psoriatic skin lesions in four AS patients treated either with infliximab or etanercept (unpublished observations). At the moment there is no good explanation for this rather paradox finding. Whether there is a different pathogenetic mechanism for the psoriatic skin lesion which occurs during TNF-blocker treatment (as compared to normal psoriasis) has to be determined. All patients recovered from skin manifestations after TNF-blocker treatment was stopped.

New Occurrence or Exacerbation of IBD

Infliximab has been proven to be highly effective for induction and maintenance therapy of CD (19,20). This is of relevance because AS and the whole group of the SpA are associated with IBD, as such patients may develop AS and many patients with primary AS show histological gut lesions similar to CD (21). In contrast, etanercept, the 75 kDa TNF receptor fusion protein, seems not to work in CD (25,26). Interestingly, a new occurrence or exacerbation of IBD was reported in two and one respectively AS patients successfully treated with etanercept, and in one of the placebo-controlled AS studies with etanercept two patients treated with etanercept had to be withdrawn from the studies because of CD or ulcerative colitis (26,49,73). Thus, while infliximab is effective for gut manifestations occurring in association with AS, etanercept might even induce or worsen IBD. However, more data are necessary to exclude that such an association does not occur by chance.

Other Side Effects

Liver enzyme elevations and leucopenia and anemia occur but lead only rarely to discontinuation of TNF-blocker treatment.

ALTERATION OF CYTOKINE RESPONSE DURING TREATMENT WITH TNF-BLOCKERS

For the examination of cytokines in the serum different technologies have been used. While serum levels are usually measured by enzyme-linked immunosorbent assay techniques, there is also the possibility to analyze the capacity of peripheral blood or synovial fluid mononuclear cells (MNCs) for the secretion of cytokines. The advantage of the flow cytometry technique is the possibility to determine the potential of specific cells for the secretion of cytokines.

The effect of infliximab therapy on the T-cell cytokine profile was analyzed in two studies by using flow cytometry technology. The study in the Gent cohort documented that treatment with three infusions of infliximab in SpA patients resulted in an increase of the Th1 cytokines interferon-γ and interleukin (IL)-2, as measured by intracellular cytokine staining and quantified by flow cytometry (79). A reduction of IL-10-positive T cells was observed in those patients with high baseline values. However, this effect was mainly observed in the first four weeks.

In contrast, we obtained different data when the potential of the CD4+ and CD8+ T cells to produce cytokines during treatment with infliximab was analyzed at weeks 0, 6, and 12. The capacity of the T cells to produce IFN-γ and TNFα after in vitro stimulation went clearly down in the infliximab-treated group, but not in the placebo-treated group (80). The potential of monocytes derived from the peripheral blood to produce TNFα upon in vitro stimulation with LPS was not reduced after three months of infliximab treatment.

In a similar study peripheral blood MNCs from 10 patients with AS treated with etanercept and 10 patients with AS treated with placebo were investigated by flow cytometry (81). Twelve weeks of etanercept treatment induced a significant increase in the number of IFN-γ-positive and TNFα-positive CD4+ T cells and IFN-γ-positive and TNFα-positive CD8+ T cells after in vitro stimulation, but not in the placebo group. Thus, just neutralization of peripheral TNFα without affecting membrane bound TNFα, which happens probably during etanercept treatment, does not induce a downregulation of the ability of T cells to produce TNFα but rather an upregulation, possibly due to a counterregulatory mechanism. In contrasts, infliximab probably both neutralizes soluble TNFα and binds to cell-bound TNFα, with the possible consequence of deletion of TNFα-positive cells. These different effects of infliximab and etanercept on T cells might also explain the different side effects: TB occurring more often during infliximab therapy and IBD occurring more often during treatment with etanercept.

Do Anti-infliximab Antibodies Reduce Efficacy and Increase Allergic Reaction?

Anti-chimeric antibodies against infliximab seem to occur mainly if infliximab is given in a low dosage (82). In an early study this occurred predominantly in about 50% in the group receiving 1 mg/kg of infliximab alone (10). MTX or other immunosuppressive drugs have not yet been given additionally in AS studies because, as discussed above, its efficacy in AS is doubtful. Thus, at the moment there are no data whether such concomitant treatment can increase efficacy and/or decrease allergic reactions.

In a recent study in CD patients, parts of whom were treated with azathioprine in addition to infliximab, it was reported that not only fewer infusion reactions occurred but also the overall duration of the efficacy of infliximab doubled, if the immunosuppressive drug, mostly azathioprine, was coadministered (83). However, in contrast to treatment in AS many patients received only one infusion of infliximab which is more likely to induce antibodies (10). Nonetheless, this study provides arguments for a small but significant role for anti-infliximab antibodies and suggests that concomitant immunosuppressive therapy helps to prevent loss of efficacy and infusion reactions. No clinical effect of antibodies against etanercept has so far been reported.

The value of measuring infliximab serum levels and determining anti-infliximab antibodies is becoming clearer. MTX may reduce the clearance of infliximab from serum (84). In a recent analysis of data from the Anti-TNF Trial in Rheumatoid Arthritis with Concomitant Therapy (ATTRACT) trial, 26% of the subjects receiving 3 mg/kg infliximab every eight weeks had undetectable trough serum levels of infliximab at week 54 (85). A better response and a greater reduction of CRP levels were both associated with higher serum concentrations of infliximab, which supports the idea about a dose–response relationship. As predicted by pharmacokinetic models, decreasing the dosing interval from eight to six weeks would yield higher trough serum levels of infliximab than increasing the dose by 100 mg.

IDENTIFICATION OF PARAMETERS WHICH PREDICT RESPONSE TO ANTI-TNF THERAPY IN AS PATIENTS

Based on the data from our two placebo-controlled trials with infliximab and with etanercept we addressed the question whether a 50% improvement in the BASDAI can be predicted when parameters at study entry are analyzed (30,48). A univariate analysis revealed shorter disease duration, lower BASFI (meaning better function), younger age, and elevated erthryocyte sedimentation rate (ESR) or CRP as predictors for such a treatment response. Adjustment for disease duration revealed BASFI, ESR, and CRP, but not age to remain significantly associated (86). The best multivariate model built by stepwise regression contained the covariables: disease duration, BASFI, BASDAI, and CRP. Thus, indicators of shorter disease duration (disease duration, age, better function) and of higher disease activity (CRP and BASDAI) seem to predict a response best: 73% of patients with a disease duration of <10 years responded by 50% improvement while this level of response was only achieved by 31% of patients with a disease duration >20 years. Thus, these data indicate that a surprisingly high response rate can be expected if patients are carefully selected but, on the other hand, patients with advanced disease can also respond, but at a lower level. Preliminary data from Berlin suggest that in the case of CRP being negative MRI-positivity might also turn out to be a predictor of response (87).

WHICH AS PATIENT SHOULD BE TREATED WITH A TNF-BLOCKER?

The question of which AS patients to treat and which improvement criteria to use for follow-up has been recently addressed by an international consensus conference organized by the ASAS study group in January 2003 in Berlin (88). Recommendations were developed on the basis of this meeting which was prepared by a review of published reports in combination with a Delphi exercise. The final consensus comprises the following requirements for the initiation of anti-TNFα therapy: (*i*) a diagnosis of definitive AS, normally defined by the modified New York criteria; (*ii*) presence of refractory disease defined by failure of at least two NSAIDs during a three month period, in case of predominantly axial manifestations, unless contraindicated or not tolerated by the patient; in case of predominantly peripheral joint involvement a failure of sulfasalazine treatment in a dose up to 3 g/day over four months plus failure of intra-articular steroid injections should be demonstrated, unless contraindicated or not tolerated by the patient; in case of predominantly enthesitis, failure of local steroid injection should be present, unless this procedure is contraindicated or not tolerated; (*iii*) presence of active disease for at least four weeks as defined by both a sustained BASDAI of at least four and an expert opinion based on clinical features, acute phase reactants, and imaging modalities; and (*iv*) application and implementation of the usual precautions and contraindications for biological therapy.

For the monitoring of anti-TNFα therapy both the BASDAI and the ASAS core set for clinical practice should be followed regularly (89). A decision on further treatment with the TNF-blocker should be made after 6 to 12 weeks of treatment. Response was defined as improvement of at least 50% or two units (on a 0–10 scale) of the BASDAI, plus an expert opinion (normally a rheumatologist with experience with the disease and with TNF-blocker treatment) that treatment should be continued. It can be expected that more data will be available in the near future to become more precise about some of these points.

SOCIOECONOMICAL ASPECTS

Mainly because of the high costs for treatment with TNF-blockers the analysis of socioeconomical data for each disease separately is very important for the near future. Such investigations are currently underway calculating the decrease in direct and indirect costs and also the gain in quality of life in AS patients treated with TNF-blockers. We recently analyzed some of these effects in patients from our initially randomized placebo-controlled infliximab trial who were subsequently treated in an open fashion with infliximab 5 mg/kg body weight given every six weeks for two years (30). During the last 12 months before the screening visit, 41% of the completers had been hospitalized in contrast to only 10% after one or two years of treatment. This corresponded to a significant decrease in the mean number of inpatient days from 11.1 days per year before treatment to 0.6 day after one year and 2.9 days after two years. Similarly, the percentage of patients on sick leave and the number of work days missed by patients improved, also significantly, during infliximab therapy (90). More data on this subject will become available soon from the major placebo-controlled trials (41,49).

OTHER BIOLOGICS FOR THE TREATMENT OF AS

Two open studies have been published on the efficacy of the IL-1-receptor antagonist in AS (91,92). Compared to the striking efficacy seen with the TNF-blockers only a rather small improvement was observed. It will be interesting to see whether the rather great numbers of biologics which are now tested in other chronic inflammatory diseases such as RA will also be of use in AS.

REFERENCES

1. Braun J, Bollow M, Remlinger G, et al. Prevalence of spondylarthropathies in HLA B27-positive and negative blood donors. Arthritis Rheum 1998; 41:58–67.
2. Brandt J, Bollow M, Haberle J, et al. Studying patients with inflammatory back pain and arthritis of the lower limbs clinically and by magnetic resonance imaging: many, but not all patients with sacroiliitis have spondyloarthropathy. Rheumatology (Oxford) 1999; 38:831–836.
3. Gran JT, Husby G, Hordvik M. Prevalence of ankylosing spondylitis in males and females in a young middle-aged population of Tromso, Northern Norway. Ann Rheum Dis 1985; 44:359–367.
4. Saraux A, Guedes C, Allain J, et al. Prevalence of rheumatoid arthritis and spondyloarthropathy in Brittany, France. Societe de Rhumatologie de l'Ouest J Rheumatol 1999; 26:2622–2627.
5. Leirisalo-Repo M. Prognosis, course of disease, and treatment of the spondyloarthropathies. Rheum Dis Clin North Am 1998; 24(4):737–751.
6. Amor B, Dougados M, Khan MA. Management of refractory ankylosing spondylitis and related spondyloarthropathies. Rheum Dis Clin North Am 1995; 21(1):117–118.
7. van Tubergen A, Landewe R, van der Heijde D, Hidding A, Wolter N, Asscher M, Falkenbach A, Genth E, The HG, van der Linden S. Combined Spa-exercise therapy is effective in patients with ankylosing spondylitis: a randomized controlled trial. Arthritis Rheum 2001; 45(5):430–438.
8. Haibel H, Rudwaleit M, Lisitng J, Braun J, Sieper J. Six months open label trial of leflunomide in active ankylosing spondylitis. Ann Rheum Dis 2005; 64(1):124–126.
9. Braun J, Sieper J. Therapy of ankylosing spondylitis and other spondyloarthritides: established medical treatment, anti-TNF-alpha therapy and other novel approaches. Arthritis Res 2002; 4(5):307–321.

10. Maini RN, Breedveld FC, Kalden JR, Smolen JS, Davis D, Macfarlane JD, Antoni C, Leeb B, Elliott MJ, Woody JN, Schaible TF, Feldmann M. Therapeutic efficacy of multiple intravenous infusions of anti-tumor necrosis factor alpha monoclonal antibody combined with low-dose weekly methotrexate in rheumatoid arthritis. Arthritis Rheum 1998; 41(9):1552–1563.

11. Braun J, Sieper J. The sacroiliac joint in the spondyloarthropathies. Curr Opin Rheumatol 1996; 8(4):275–287.

12. McGonagle D, Gibbon W, O'Connor P, Green M, Pease C, Emery P. Characteristic magnetic resonance imaging entheseal changes of knee synovitis in spondylarthropathy. Arthritis Rheum 1998; 41:694–700.

13. Braun J, Bollow M, Eggens U, Konig H, Distler A, Sieper J. Use of dynamic magnetic resonance imaging with fast imaging in the detection of early and advanced sacroiliitis in spondylarthropathy patients. Arthritis Rheum 1994; 37:1039–1045.

14. Muche B, Bollow M, François RJ, Sieper J, Hamm B, Braun J. Which anatomical structures are involved in early and late sacroiliitis in spondyloarthritis—a detailed analysis by contrast enhanced magnetic resonance imaging. Arthritis Rheum 2003; 48(5):1374–1384.

15. Braun J, Bollow M, Neure L, et al. Use of immunohistologic and in situ hybridization techniques in the examination of sacroiliac joint biopsy specimens from patients with ankylosing spondylitis. Arthritis Rheum 1995; 38:499–505.

16. Laloux L, Voisin MC, Allain J, Martin N, Kerboull L, Chevalier X, Claudepierre P. Immunohistological study of entheses in spondyloarthropathies: comparison in rheumatoid arthritis and osteoarthritis. Ann Rheum Dis 2001; 60:316–321.

17. Bollow M, Fischer T, Reißhauer H, Sieper J, Hamm B, Braun J. T cells and macrophages predominate in early and active sacroiliitis as detected by magnetic resonance imaging in spondyloarthropathies. Ann Rheum Dis 2000; 59(2):135–140.

18. McCormack G, Moriarty D, O'Donoghue DP, McCormick PA, Sheahan K, Baird AW. Tissue cytokine and chemokine expression in inflammatory bowel disease. Inflamm Res 2001; 50(10):491–495.

19. Sandborn WJ. Anti-tumor necrosis factor therapy for inflammatory bowel disease: a review of agents, pharmacology, clinical results and safety. Inflamm Bowel Dis 1999; 5:119–133.

20. Hanauer SB, Feagan BG, Lichtenstein GR, et al. Maintenance infliximab for Crohn's disease: the ACCENT I randomised trial. Lancet 2002; 359:1541–1548.

21. Mielants H, Veys EM. HLA B27-related arthritis and bowel inflammation: sulfasalazine in HLA B27-related arthritis. J Rheumatol 1985; 12:287–293.

22. Van den Bosch F, Kruithof E, De Vos M, De Keyser F, Mielants H. Crohn's disease associated with spondyloarthropathy: effect of TNF-alpha blockade with infliximab on articular symptoms. Lancet 2000; 356(9244):1821–1822.

23. Sands BE, Tremaine WJ, Sandborn WJ, Rutgeerts PJ, Hanauer SB, Mayer L, Targan SR, Podolsky DK. Infliximab in the treatment of severe, steroid-refractory ulcerative colitis: a pilot study. Inflamm Bowel Dis 2001; 7(2):83–88.

24. Su C, Salzberg BA, Lewis JD, Deren JJ, Kornbluth A, Katzka DA, Stein RB, Adler DR, Lichtenstein GR. Efficacy of anti-tumor necrosis factor therapy in patients with ulcerative colitis. Am J Gastroenterol 2002; 97(10):2577–2584.

25. Sandborn WJ, Hanauer SB, Katz S, Safdi M, Wolf DG, Baerg RD, Tremaine WJ, Johnson T, Diehl NN, Zinsmeister AR. Etanercept for active Crohn's disease: a randomized, double-blind, placebo-controlled trial. Gastroenterology 2001; 121(5):1088–1094.

26. Marzo-Ortega H, McGonagle D, O'Connor P, Emery P. Efficacy of etanercept for treatment of Crohn's related spondyloarthritis but not colitis. Ann Rheum Dis 2003; 62(1):74–76.

27. Brandt J, Haibel H, Cornely D, Golder W, Gonzalez J, Sieper J, Braun J. Successful treatment of active ankylosing spondylitis with the anti-tumor necrosis factor alpha monoclonal antibody infliximab. Arthritis Rheum 2000; 43:1346–1352.

28. Garrett S, Jenkinson TR, Kennedy LG, Whitelock HC, Gaisford P, Calin A. A new approach to defining disease status in ankylosing spondylitis. The Bath AS disease activity index. J Rheumatol 1994; 21:2286–2291.

29. Brandt J, Haibel H, Reddig J, Sieper J, Braun J. Treatment of patients with severe ankylosing spondylitis with infliximab—a one year follow up. Arthritis Rheum 2001; 44(12):2936–2937.

30. Braun J, Brandt J, Listing J, Zink A, Alten R, Golder W, Gromnica-Ihle E, Kellner H, Krause A, Schneider M, Sörensen H, Zeidler H, Thriene W, Sieper J. Treatment of active ankylosing spondylitis with infliximab—a double-blind placebo controlled multicenter trial. Lancet 2002; 359:1187–1193.

31. Van den Bosch F, Kruithof E, Baeten D, De Keyser F, Mielants H, Veys EM. Effects of a loading dose regimen of three infusions of chimeric monoclonal antibody to tumour necrosis factor alpha (infliximab) in spondyloarthropathy: an open pilot study. Ann Rheum Dis 2000; 59:428–433.

32. Kruithof E, Van den Bosch F, Baeten D, Herssens A, De Keyser F, Mielants H, Veys EM. Repeated infusions of infliximab, a chimeric anti-TNFalpha monoclonal antibody, in patients with active spondyloarthropathy: one year follow up. Ann Rheum Dis 2002; 61:207–212.

33. Stone M, Salonen D, Lax M, Payne U, Lapp V, Inman R. Clinical and imaging correlates of response to treatment with infliximab in patients with ankylosing spondylitis. J Rheumatol 2001; 28(7):1605–1614.

34. Maksymowych WP, Jhangri GS, Lambert RG, Mallon C, Buenviaje H, Pedrycz E, Luongo R, Russell AS. Infliximab in ankylosing spondylitis: a prospective observational inception cohort analysis of efficacy and safety. J Rheumatol 2002; 29:959–965.

35. Breban M, Vignon E, Claudepierre P, Devauchelle V, Wendling D, Lespessailles E, Euller-Ziegler L, Sibilia J, Perdriger A, Mezieres M, Alexandre C, Dougados M. Efficacy of infliximab in refractory ankylosing spondylitis: results of a six-month open-label study. Rheumatology (Oxford) 2002; 41(11):1280–1285.

36. Collantes-Estevez E, Munoz-Villanueva MC, Canete-Crespillo JD, Sanmarti-Sala R, Gratacos-Masmitja J, Zarco-Montejo P, Torre-Alonso JC, Gonzalez-Fernandez C. Infliximab in refractory spondyloarthropathies: a multicentre 38 week open study. Ann Rheum Dis 2003; 62(12):1239–1240.

37. Braun J, Brandt J, Listing J, Zink A, Alten R, Burmester G, Golder W, Gromnica-Ihle E, Kellner H, Schneider M, Sorensen H, Zeidler H, Reddig J, Sieper J. Long-term efficacy and safety of infliximab in the treatment of ankylosing spondylitis: an open, observational, extension study of a three-month, randomized, placebo-controlled trial. Arthritis Rheum 2003; 48(8):2224–2233.

38. Temekonidis TI, Alamanos Y, Nikas SN, Bougias DV, Georgiadis AN, Voulgari PV, Drosos AA. Infliximab therapy in patients with ankylosing spondylitis: an open label 12 month study. Ann Rheum Dis 2003; 62(12):1218–1220.

39. Allali F, Roux C, Kolta S, Claudepierre P, Lespessailles E, Dougados M, Breban M. Infliximab in the treatment of spondylarthropathy, bone mineral density effect. Arthritis Rheum 2001; 44(9):S89.

40. Van den Bosch F, Kruithof E, Baeten D, Herseens A, De Keyser F, Mielants H, Veys EM. Randomized double-blind comparison of chimeric monoclonal antibody to tumour necrosis factor alpha (infliximab) versus placebo in active spondyloarthropathy. Arthritis Rheum 2002; 46:755–765.

41. van der Heijde D, Dijkmans B, Geusens P, Sieper J, De Woody K, Williamson P, Braun J. Efficacy and safety of infliximab in patients with ankylosing spondylitis: results of a randomized placebo-controlled trial (ASSERT). Arthritis Rheum 2005; 52(2):582–591.

42. D'Agostino MA, Breban M, Said-Nahal R, Dougados M. Refractory inflammatory heel pain in spondyloarthropathy: a significant response to infliximab documented by ultrasound. Arthritis Rheum 2002; 46:840–841.

43. Braun J, Baraliakos X, Golder W, Brandt J, Rudwaleit M, Listing J, Bollow M, Sieper J, Van Der Heijde D. Magnetic resonance imaging examinations of the spine in patients with ankylosing spondylitis, before and after successful therapy with infliximab: evaluation of a new scoring system. Arthritis Rheum 2003; 48(4):1126–1136.
44. Brandt J, Listing J, Alten R, Burmester G, Gromnica-Ihle E, Kellner H, Schneider M, Soerensen H, Zeidler H, Rudwaleit M, Sieper J, Braun J. Two-year follow-up results of a controlled trial of the anti-TNF alpha antibody infliximab in active ankylosing spondylitis. Arthritis Rheum 2003; 48:S172.
45. Brandt J, Haibel H, Reddig J, Sieper J, Braun J. Successful treatment of severe undifferentiated spondyloarthropathy with the anti-tumor necrosis factor α monoclonal antibody infliximab. J Rheumatol 2002; 29:118–122.
46. Marzo-Ortega H, McGonagle D, O'Connor P, Emery P. Efficacy of etanercept in the treatment of the entheseal pathology in resistant spondylarthropathy: a clinical and magnetic resonance imaging study. Arthritis Rheum 2001; 44(9):2112–2117.
47. Gorman JD, Sack KE, Davis JC. Treatment of ankylosing spondylitis by inhibition of tumor necrosis factor alpha. N Engl J Med 2002; 346(18):1349–1356.
48. Brandt J, Khariouzov A, Listing J, Haibel H, Sorensen H, Grassnickel L, Rudwaleit M, Sieper J. Six-month results of a double-blind, placebo-controlled trial of etanercept treatment in patients with active ankylosing spondylitis. Arthritis Rheum 2003; 48(6):1667–1675.
49. Davis JC Jr, Van Der Heijde D, Braun J, Dougados M, Cush J, Clegg DO, Kivitz A, Fleischmann R, Inman R, Tsuji W. Enbrel ankylosing spondylitis study group. Recombinant human tumor necrosis factor receptor (etanercept) for treating ankylosing spondylitis: a randomized, controlled trial. Arthritis Rheum 2003; 48(11):3230–3236.
50. Anderson JJ, Baron G, van der Heijde D, Felson DT, Dougados M. Ankylosing spondylitis assessment group criteria preliminary definition of short-term improvement in ankylosing spondylitis. Arthritis Rheum 2001; 44:1876–1886.
51. Marzo-Ortega H, McGonagle D, Haugeberg G, Green MJ, Stewart SP, Emery P. Bone mineral density improvement in spondyloarthropathy after treatment with etanercept. Ann Rheum Dis 2003; 62(10):1020–1021.
52. Dougados M, van der Linden S, Juhlin R, et al. The European spondylarthropathy study group preliminary criteria for the classification of spondylarthropathy. Arthritis Rheum 1991; 34(10):1218–1227.
53. Rudwaleit M, van der Heijde D, Khan MA, Braun J, Sieper J. How to diagnose axial spondyloarthritis early? Ann Rheum Dis 2004; 63:535–543.
54. Brandt J, Kariouzov A, Listing J, Haibel H, Soerensen H, Grassnickel L, Rudwaleit M, Sieper J, Braun J. Successful treatment of patients with severe undifferentiated spondyloarthritis with the anti-tumor necrosis factor α receptor fusion protein etanercept. J Rheumatol 2004; 31:531–538.
55. Dougados M, vam der Linden S, Leirisalo-Repo M, et al. Sulfasalazine in the treatment of spondylarthropathy. A randomized, multicenter, double-blind, placebo-controlled study. Arthritis Rheum 1995; 38(5):618–627.
56. Benitez-Del-Castillo JM, Garcia-Sanchez J, Iradier T, Banares A. Sulfasalazine in the prevention of anterior uveitis associated with ankylosing spondylitis. Eye 2000; 14: 340–343.
57. Smith JR, Levinson RD, Holland GN, Jabs DA, Robinson MR, Whitcup SM, Rosenbaum JT. Differential efficacy of tumor necrosis factor inhibition in the management of inflammatory eye disease and associated rheumatic disease. Arthritis Rheum 2001; 45(3):252–257.
58. Reiff A, Takei S, Sadeghi S, Stout A, Shaham B, Bernstein B, Gallagher K, Stout T. Etanercept therapy in children with treatment-resistant uveitis. Arthritis Rheum 2001; 44(6):1411–1415.
59. El-Shabrawi Y, Hermann J. Anti-tumor necrosis factor-alpha therapy with infliximab as an alternative to corticosteroids in the treatment of human leukocyte antigen B27-associated acute anterior uveitis. Ophthalmology 2002; 109(12):2342–2346.

60. Kruithof E, Kestelyn P, Elewaut C, Elewaut D, Van Den Bosch F, Mielants H, Veys EM, De Keyser F. Successful use of infliximab in a patient with treatment resistant spondyloarthropathy related uveitis. Ann Rheum Dis 2002; 61(5):470.

61. Fries W, Giofre MR, Catanoso M, Lo GR. Treatment of acute uveitis associated with Crohn's disease and sacroileitis with infliximab. Am J Gastroenterol 2002; 97(2):499–500.

62. Munoz-Fernandez S, Hidalgo V, Fernandez-Melon J, Schlincker A, Martin-Mola E. Effect of infliximab on threatening panuveitis in Behcet's disease. Lancet 2001; 358:1644.

63. Gomez-Reino JJ, Carmona L, Valverde VR, Mola EM, Montero MD. BIOBADASER Group. Treatment of rheumatoid arthritis with tumor necrosis factor inhibitors may predispose to significant increase in tuberculosis risk: a multicenter active-surveillance report. Arthritis Rheum 2003; 48(8):2122–2127.

64. Keane J, Gershon S, Wise RP, Mirabile-Levens E, Kasznica J, Schwieterman WD, Siegel JN, Braun MM. Tuberculosis associated with infliximab, a tumor necrosis factor alpha-neutralizing agent. N Engl J Med 2001; 345(15):1098–1104.

65. Baeten D, Kruithof E, Van den Bosch F, Van den Bossche N, Herssens A, Mielants H, De Keyser F, Veys EM. Systematic safety follow up in a cohort of 107 patients with spondyloarthropathy treated with infliximab: a new perspective on the role of host defence in the pathogenesis of the disease? Ann Rheum Dis 2003; 62(9):829–834.

66. Brown SL, Greene MH, Gershon SK, Edwards ET, Braun MM. Tumor necrosis factor antagonist therapy and lymphoma development: twenty-six cases reported to the food and drug administration. Arthritis Rheum 2002; 46(12):3151–3158.

67. Mohan N, Edwards ET, Cupps TR, Oliverio PJ, Sandberg G, Crayton H, Richert JR, Siegel JN. Demyelination occurring during anti-tumor necrosis factor alpha therapy for inflammatory arthritides. Arthritis Rheum 2001; 44(12):2862–2869.

68. Anker SD, Coats AJ. How to recover from renaissance? The significance of the results of recover, renaissance, renewal and attach. Int J Cardiol 2002; 86(2–3):123–130.

69. Chung ES, Packer M, Lo KH, Fasanmade AA, Willerson JT. Anti-TNF therapy against congestive heart failure investigators. Randomized, double-blind, placebo-controlled, pilot trial of infliximab, a chimeric monoclonal antibody to tumor necrosis factor-alpha, in patients with moderate-to-severe heart failure: results of the anti-TNF therapy against congestive heart failure (ATTACH) trial. Circulation 2003; 107(25):3133–3140.

70. Wolfe F, Michaud K. Congestive heart failure in rheumatoid arthritis: rates, predictors and the effect of anti-TNF therapy. Arthritis Rheum 2003; 48:S699.

71. Charles PJ, Smeenk RJ, De Jong J, Feldmann M, Maini RN. Assessment of antibodies to double-stranded DNA induced in rheumatoid arthritis patients following treatment with infliximab, a monoclonal antibody to tumor necrosis factor alpha: findings in open-label and randomized placebo-controlled trials. Arthritis Rheum 2000; 43(11):2383–2390.

72. De Rycke L, Kruithof E, Van Damme N, Hoffman IE, Van den Bossche N, Van den Bosch F, Veys EM, De Keyser F. Antinuclear antibodies following infliximab treatment in patients with rheumatoid arthritis or spondylarthropathy. Arthritis Rheum 2003; 48(4): 1015–1023.

73. Brandt J, Khariouzov A, Listing J, Haibel H, Soerensen H, Rudwaleit M, Schwebig A, Sieper J, Braun J. One year follow-up results of a controlled trial of a German double-blind placebo-controlled trial of etanercept in active ankylosing spondylitis. Arthritis Rheum 2003; 48:S173.

74. Cheifetz A, Smedley M, Martin S, Reiter M, Leone G, Mayer L, Plevy S. The incidence and management of infusion reactions to infliximab: a large center experience. Am J Gastroenterol 2003; 98(6):1315–1324.

75. Olivieri I, Padula A, Ciancio G, Salvarani C, Niccoli L, Cantini F. Successful treatment of SAPHO syndrome with infliximab: report of two cases. Ann Rheum Dis 2002; 61(4): 375–376.

76. Wagner AD, Andresen J, Jendro MC, Hulsemann JL, Zeidler H. Sustained response to tumor necrosis factor alpha-blocking agents in two patients with SAPHO syndrome. Arthritis Rheum 2002; 46(7):1965–1968.

77. Mease PJ, Goffe BS, Metz J, VanderStoep A, Finck B, Burge DJ. Etanercept in the treatment of psoriatic arthritis and psoriasis: a randomised trial. Lancet 2000; 356:385–390.
78. Antoni C, Dechant C, Hanns-Martin Lorenz PD, Wendler J, Ogilvie A, Lueftl M, Kalden-Nemeth D, Kalden JR, Manger B. Open-label study of infliximab treatment for psoriatic arthritis: clinical and magnetic resonance imaging measurements of reduction of inflammation. Arthritis Rheum 2002; 47(5):506–512.
79. Baeten D, Van Damme N, Van den Bosch F, Kruithof E, De Vos M, Mielants H, Veys EM, De Keyser F. Impaired Th1 cytokine production in spondyloarthropathy is restored by anti-TNFalpha. Ann Rheum Dis 2001; 60(8):750–755.
80. Zou J, Rudwaleit M, Brandt J, Thiel A, Braun J, Sieper J. Down-regulation of the non-specific and antigen-specific T cell cytokine response in ankylosing spondylitis during treatment with infliximab. Arthritis Rheum 2003; 48(3):780–790.
81. Zou J, Rudwaleit M, Brandt J, Thiel A, Braun J, Sieper J. Upregulation of the production of tumour necrosis factor alpha and interferon gamma by T cells in ankylosing spondylitis during treatment with etanercept. Ann Rheum Dis 2003; 62(6):561–564.
82. Wagner CL, Schantz A, Barnathan E, Olson A, Mascelli MA, Ford J, Damaraju L, Schaible T, Maini RN, Tcheng JE. Consequences of immunogenicity to the therapeutic monoclonal antibodies ReoPro and Remicade. Dev Biol (Basel) 2003; 112:37–53.
83. Baert F, Noman M, Vermeire S, van Assche G, D' Haens G, Carbonez A, Rutgeerts P. Influence of immunogenicity on the long-term efficacy of infliximab in Crohn's disease. N Engl J Med 2003; 348:601–608.
84. Schwab M, Klotz U. Pharmacokinetic considerations in the treatment of inflammatory bowel disease. Clin Pharmacokinet 2001; 40(10):723–751.
85. St Clair EW, Wagner CL, Fasanmade AA, Wang B, Schaible T, Kavanaugh A, Keystone EC. The relationship of serum infliximab concentrations to clinical improvement in rheumatoid arthritis: results from ATTRACT, a multicenter, randomized, double-blind, placebo-controlled trial. Arthritis Rheum 2002; 46(6):1451–1459.
86. Rudwaleit M, Listing J, Brandt J, Braun J, Sieper J. Prediction of a major clinical response (BASDAI 50) to TNF-α blockers in ankylosing spondylitis. Ann Rheum Dis 2004; 63:665–670.
87. Rudwaleit M, Brandt J, Braun J, Sieper J. Is there a role for MRI in predicting the clinical response to TNF alpha blockers in ankylosing spondylitis? Ann Rheum Dis 2003; 62(suppl 1):97.
88. Braun J, Pham T, Sieper J, Davis J, van der Linden S, Dougados M, van der Heijde D on behalf of the ASAS Working Group. International ASAS consensus statement for the use of anti-tumour necrosis factor agents in patients with ankylosing spondylitis. Ann Rheum Dis 2003; 62(9):817–824.
89. van der Heijde D, Bellamy N, Calin A, Dougados M, Khan MA, van der Linden S. Preliminary core sets for endpoints in ankylosing spondylitis. Assessments in ankylosing spondylitis working group. J Rheumatol 1997; 24:2225–2229.
90. Listing J, Brandt J, Rudwaleit M, Zink A, Sieper J, Braun J. Impact of anti-TNFα therapy on hospitalization and days on sick leave in patients with ankylosing spondylitis. Ann Rheum Dis 2004; 63:1670–1672.
91. Tan AL, Marzo-Ortega H, O' Connor, Fraser A, Emery P, McGonagle DG. Efficacy of anakinra in active ankylosing spondylitis: a clinical and magnetic resonance imaging study. Ann Rheum Dis 2004; 63(9):1041–1045.
92. Haibel H, Rudwaleit M, Braun J, Listing J, Sieper. Results of an open label study with Anakinra in active ankylosing spondylitis [abstr]. Ann Rheum Dis 2005; 64(2):296–298.

13

Physiotherapy Interventions for Ankylosing Spondylitis

Astrid van Tubergen
Division of Rheumatology, Department of Medicine, University Maastricht, Maastricht, The Netherlands

INTRODUCTION

Ankylosing spondylitis (AS) is associated with significant disability and increased socioeconomic costs (1). Until recently, available conventional therapies for AS were palliative at best, and often failed to control symptoms at the long run. With the introduction of the so-called "biologicals" that specifically inhibit mediators of inflammation, more promising effects in the long term may be expected. Physiotherapeutic interventions have always been considered as a necessary adjunct to drug therapy. But what is exactly meant by the word physiotherapy and how is it applied in AS? Traditionally, the mainstays of physiotherapy in the management of musculoskeletal conditions have been massage, manual therapy (manipulation and joint mobilization), electrotherapy (ultrasound, short-wave diathermy, or low-energy laser), and therapeutic exercises. In AS, various forms of physical therapy can be distinguished: supervised individualized physical therapy, unsupervised self-administered individualized physical therapy or exercises at home, and supervised group physical therapy. For each of these forms, physiotherapeutic interventions as described above may be applied, but also hydrotherapy (pool sessions) and patient education and information may be offered (Table 1). Special forms of physical therapy for AS are inpatient physiotherapy for two to four weeks at a specialized clinic consisting of daily physical exercises and pool sessions, but also education, and spa therapy consisting of a two to four week course of balneotherapy (bathing in mineral water), hydrotherapy [immersion of (parts of) the body in water], massages, physical exercises, mud applications, and education.

Patients recently diagnosed with AS may first receive a course of supervised individualized therapy. Afterwards, the patients are expected to exercise daily without supervision. They are often advised to join weekly group physical therapy sessions in order to enhance the effects of individual exercises. In addition, many patients attend annual courses of inpatient physiotherapy or spa therapy in combination with exercises.

Table 1 Spectrum of Physiotherapeutic Interventions for AS

Supervised exercises
  Individualized
  Group physical therapy
Unsupervised individualized exercises
  AS-specific exercises
  Recreational exercises
Manual therapy
Massage
Hydrotherapy
Electrotherapy
Warm and cold applications
Patient information and education
Inpatient physiotherapy
Spa therapy

Abbreviation: AS, ankylosing spondylitis.

AIMS OF PHYSICAL THERAPY IN AS

Pain and inflammation of muscles, joints, and connective tissue may lead to loss of muscle strength, range of motion, bone density, and endurance. The aims of physical therapy in AS in general are to: (i) maintain and improve mobility of the spine and peripheral joints, (ii) strengthen the muscles of the trunk, the legs, the back, and the abdomen, (iii) stretch the back, (iv) improve endurance, and (v) relax the body. These aims can be achieved by exercises, sporting activities, and hydrotherapy (2,3). Exercises may increase strength, mobility, and coordination, and thus improve joint stability. In hydrotherapy, the buoyancy of the water (law of Archimedes) reduces the relative weight of the body, and thus gravity on painful rheumatic joints (4,5). Warm water also provides muscle relaxation. The patient will experience a reduction in pain, which facilitates manipulating, mobilizing, and strengthening of affected joints and muscles, but also positively influences the patient's compliance (5,6).

   Although the aims of physiotherapeutic interventions may differ for individual persons, some general advices may be given. Exercises to improve mobility, strength, and endurance should always be at the basis of every exercise scheme. It is recommended to gradually increase the intensity and frequency of the exercises. Repeating the exercises, preferably up to the maximum level, is a requisite. If joint swelling or pain occurs, the intensity or frequency should be reduced. It is possible to perform exercises in several positions, such as standing erect, kneeling, sitting, and lying on the side, on the back, or prone. Variations in posture and type of exercises are important to maintain compliance. With the use of several materials the effects may also be enhanced. Detailed information on various forms of these physical exercises has been described in the literature, although no uniform protocol is yet available (3,6–10).

   Before starting an exercise program, it is important to realise that patient education plays a central role in successful management of AS. As soon as the diagnosis of AS is made, patients must be given clear explanations about the possible progression of their symptoms and other potential clinical features, as well as information about prognosis and treatment. Informing the patient about the possible occurrence of spinal ankylosis will enhance compliance with proposed treatments, especially physiotherapy. Besides, it is of great importance that the inflammation is reasonably controlled, for instance with NSAIDs, to maximize the effects of the treatment.

EXERCISE REGIMENS

Several exercise regimens for AS can be distinguished. In supervised individualized exercises, performed at a physiotherapy center or—to a lesser extent—at home, education plays a central role. The therapist teaches the patient how to move, how to rest in a particular position, and which sports are appropriate (badminton, volleyball, swimming, cross-country skiing) and which are not (horse riding, cycling, football). The aim of these exercises is to teach the patient an individual exercise program which he/she can subsequently continue daily unsupervised at home.

The unsupervised self-administered individualized exercises may consist of exercises learned in the supervised program, but may also include recreational exercises. These exercises should become a part of the patient's daily routine.

In practice, many patients find it difficult to perform daily exercises individually. Supervised group physical therapy is offered mainly to stimulate and motivate the patients to continue exercising, and to provide social contacts with fellow sufferers. Also, the supervising physiotherapist closely monitors the intensity of the exercises in order to achieve improvement. Group physical therapy usually consists of one hour of physical exercises, one hour of sports, and one hour of hydrotherapy.

Inpatient physiotherapy, consisting of two to four weeks daily exercising at a specialized clinic, is often offered to recently diagnosed patients or to patients experiencing a flare of their disease. Treatment usually consists of exercises and pool sessions, but also other treatment modalities (e.g., ice or heat applications, massages) may be applied. Also, education about the disease and the role of patient societies is provided.

A treatment at a spa center can be followed annually for two to four weeks. Beside balneotherapy, exercises (physical exercises and/or hydrotherapy) and relaxation, also massages, mud packs, and education may be offered. Patients may follow a course of spa treatment in a group or on an individual basis. Spa therapy is mostly supervised and takes place (at least partly) in-house.

ASSESSMENT OF EFFECTIVENESS OF PHYSIOTHERAPEUTIC INTERVENTION IN AS

As described, physical therapy for AS comprises a whole spectrum of therapeutic interventions. These interventions are usually not standardized and applied by nonstandardized physiotherapists to different patients whose disease (AS) might differ in important aspects such as activity, severity or stage of the condition to be treated. Patients may have varying degrees of involvement of the axial skeleton ranging from radiographic changes limited to the sacroiliac joints to complete fusion of the spine. Also, features such as peripheral arthritis, enthesitis, anterior uveitis, or organ involvement may or may not be present. All these stages may be associated with different degrees of functional limitations or disability and may require different physiotherapeutic approaches. Thereby, one should have realistic expectations if one prescribes physiotherapy to patients with AS, not only with respect to the sorts of effects of the different interventions, but also to the horizon of these effects. In fact, we are dealing with a whole array of possible interventions (Table 1) and many possible outcomes (or prevention of certain outcomes) over considerable periods of time. In order to promote standardization in this field and allow comparison among studies, the international Ankylosing Spondylitis Assessment working group (ASAS) has selected "core sets" of outcome measures to be used in different kinds of trials in AS. The core set for the assessment of effectiveness of physical therapy consists of: physical function, pain, stiffness, patient global assessment, and spinal mobility (Schober test, occiput-to-wall distance, and chest expansion) (11). Studies assessing the effectiveness of several forms of physical therapy in AS are now being judged on these outcome measures.

EVIDENCE FOR BENEFITS OF PHYSICAL THERAPY

A Cochrane review on physiotherapeutic interventions for AS summarized the available scientific evidence on effectiveness of physiotherapy interventions in AS (12). Randomized and quasi-randomized studies were included if at least one of the comparison groups received some kind of physiotherapy. Altogether 43 studies were considered for inclusion in this review. Thirty-seven studies were excluded due to inappropriate study design, being a follow-up study or absence of full reports. Six randomized controlled trials (RCTs) met the inclusion criteria (2,6,13–16). The reviewers concluded that a home exercise program is better than no program, supervised group physical therapy is better than home exercises, and that combined in-patient spa-exercise therapy followed by supervised weekly group physical therapy is better than group physical therapy alone. The results of the best evidence studies will be discussed in more detail below and are shown in Table 2.

Supervised Individualized Exercises

One RCT, with an additional follow-up period, assessed the effects of supervised individualized physical exercises (13,17). Patients were randomly allocated to either physiotherapy and disease education at home ($n = 26$) or to no treatment ($n = 27$). After four months, the patients from the control group were also offered physiotherapy sessions at home. In comparison with the control group, the intervention group

Table 2 Effects of Several Forms of Physical Therapy in AS Judged According to the ASAS Core Set of Outcome Measures

Treatment modality (reference number)	Patient global	Function	Pain	Stiffness	Spinal mobility
Supervised individual exercises (13,17)	n.a.	+	0	0	0
Unsupervised individual exercises (15)	0	0	0	n.a.	n.a.
Group physical therapy (2,16,18)	+	+	0	0	+
Inpatient physiotherapy (6)	n.a.	n.a.	+	+	0
Spa therapy (14)	+	+	+	0	n.a.

Note: +, Improvement; 0, no change in intervention group compared with a control group; n.a., not assessed.
Abbreviations: AS, ankylosing spondylitis; ASAS, ankylosing spondylitis assesment working group.

showed at four months (end of trial period) statistically significantly more improvement in finger-to-floor distance (mean between-group improvement $= 42\%$) and function (23%). At eight months (end of open follow-up period), only function had significantly changed in both study groups compared with results at four months. Interestingly, the intervention group showed significantly more improvement at four months in comparison with the control group at eight months. This reduced treatment effect might be explained by the fact that the intervention group had received more therapy sessions in the first four months compared with the controls in the second period of four months, implying that more therapy given on a regular basis will be more effective.

Unsupervised Self-Administered Individualized Exercises

The effects of unsupervised self-administered individualized exercises at home was assessed in one RCT (15). Patients were randomly selected from a database and randomized to either individual exercises and disease education at home ($n = 100$) or to no treatment ($n = 100$). After an intervention of six months, a completer analysis was performed. The home-based exercise intervention package significantly improved self-efficacy for exercise and self-reported levels of exercise, but no significant differences between the two groups were found with respect to function, disease activity, and global well-being.

Supervised Group Physical Therapy

The efficacy of weekly supervised group physical therapy has been investigated in an RCT (2), and extended by a second RCT examining the effects of continuation of this therapy (18). In the first study, patients were randomly allocated to a group that followed weekly group physical therapy in addition to daily unsupervised exercises at home ($n = 68$) or to a group that only exercised daily at home ($n = 76$) (2). After nine months, statistically significantly more improvement in favor of the intervention group was found for thoracolumbar flexion and extension (mean between-group improvement $= 7\%$), physical fitness (5%), and global health (28%). In a second, consecutive study, the intervention group was randomized again into a group continuing weekly group physical therapy for another nine months ($n = 30$), and a group discontinuing this ($n = 34$) (18). Both groups were advised to continue exercising at home. After nine months, statistically significantly more improvement was found in the continuation group compared with the discontinuation group in global health (28%). Function did not improve much in the continuation group (4%), but deteriorated significantly in the discontinuation group (-28%). During the study period, the time spent on exercises at home appeared to be significantly higher in the continuation group than in the discontinuation group. An explanation for this could be peer pressure and encouragement by the supervisor of the continuation group stimulating home exercising (18). This may consequently also have had effects on the outcomes of the study.

More recently, another RCT reported the effects of supervised group physical therapy in AS (16). Patients were randomly allocated to a group that followed an intensive group exercise program three days a week for six weeks ($n = 27$) or to a group that performed exercises individually at home ($n = 24$). After six weeks and three months, only change in spinal flexion was significantly greater in the intervention group than the control group. No significant differences in pain, stiffness, and function between the two groups were found, although the intervention group had shown significant improvements in within-group comparisons.

Inpatient Physiotherapy

One RCT reported the effects of inpatient physiotherapy (6). Three groups of patients were studied: group A ($n = 15$) followed three weeks of intensive inpatient physiotherapy, group B ($n = 15$) followed during a six-week period twice weekly hydrotherapy sessions and performed individual exercises twice daily at home, group C ($n = 14$) only performed individual exercises at home. All groups were advised to continue exercising at home after the treatment period. Significant differences among the three groups were found immediately after treatment (i.e., at six weeks) in pain, stiffness, and cervical rotation, with most improvement found in the two intervention groups. However, at six months no significant differences were found between the groups in any of the outcome measures.

Spa Therapy

One RCT evaluated the effects of three weeks of spa therapy in combination with exercises as an adjunct to standard treatment with drugs and weekly group physical therapy in patients with AS (14). Two groups of 40 patients each received treatment at two different spas (in Austria and The Netherlands, respectively) for three weeks, and subsequently followed weekly group physical therapy for 37 weeks. A control group ($n = 40$) stayed at home and received weekly group physical therapy for 40 weeks. An aggregate score of questionnaires on function, patient global well-being, pain, and duration of morning stiffness was used to evaluate effects. Immediately after the spa treatment, both intervention groups showed significant improvements in this score compared with the control group. Benefit was maintained over the 40-week study period in patients receiving spa-exercise therapy, although at 40 weeks, the improvement in the aggregate score had lost statistical significance, as compared with controls. The maximum between-group improvements were 24% for functioning, 30% for pain, and 33% for global well-being.

OPTIMUM THERAPEUTIC REGIMEN FOR INDIVIDUAL PATIENTS

Who will benefit most from exercise therapy and how much would be the optimum? To assess whether patients with particular characteristics would benefit more from physical therapy than others, several studies performed additional subgroup analyses. Most studies reported no influence on treatment effect by the duration of the disease (19), disease severity (6), a reduction in range of motion (6), the degree of chest expansion or restrictive lung disease (20,21). Also, improvements were equally found in men and women in one study (22), whilst others found a trend for women to improve more than men, and moreover, patients who had attended fewer courses of inpatient physiotherapy tend to achieve more improvement, and younger patients appeared to do better than older patients (23).

One study reported that in patients with <15 years of AS, performing recreational exercises—but not back exercises—was associated with improvement in pain and stiffness, but not function (24). Among patients with more than 15 years of AS, performing back exercises—but not recreational exercises—was associated with improvement in pain and function. It is recommended to exercise at least 30 minutes a day, at least five days a week, and to perform back exercises rather than recreational exercises, because these were associated with better functional outcome in the long term (24).

Another study assessed the effects of the intensity and frequency of exercises (including sports, AS-specific exercises, and hydrotherapy) on disease activity and function (25). Exercising at a moderate level was associated with improved function and lower disease activity, and exercising at an intensive level was associated with improved function, but not disease activity. It may be concluded that consistency rather that quantity is of most importance (25).

ADVANTAGES AND DISADVANTAGES OF EXERCISE THERAPIES

Each treatment modality has its advantages and disadvantages. The advantages of supervised individualized exercises are personal contact with a therapist and possibility to adapt an exercise program to individual needs. However, a disadvantage may be decreased motivation because of long-lasting and monotonous treatment. Unsupervised individual exercises can be performed at any time of the day and may consist of AS-specific exercises or sporting activities. Also with individual exercises, it may be difficult to maintain discipline, and patients may get bored of the same, repeating exercises. Team sporting activities are often not suitable for a patient with AS, because of the competitive elements that may cause injuries to an individual with AS.

Advantages of group physical therapy over unsupervised exercises alone are mutual encouragement, increased motivation to carry out home exercises, exchange of experience, contact with fellow sufferers, and personal feedback (2). Patients attending group physical exercises tend to spend more time on individual exercises compared with those who do not participate in group programs (18). However, there are also several disadvantages: motivation and energy may not be optimal after working hours, and for practical, logistic reasons (group therapy is usually provided only once or twice a week) patients may decide not to participate (2).

Advantages of two to four weeks of inpatient physiotherapy or spa therapy are intensive supervision, together with education, and encouragement of the patients, and the possibility to achieve improvements in a short term (6). The main disadvantages are high costs and difficulties patients who are employed may encounter in being absent from work.

IMPLICATIONS FOR PRACTICE

Physical therapy plays a central role in the overall management of patients with AS. Although the evidence for efficacy of physical therapy in AS is scanty, in general, it seems that physical therapy might be effective and would be beneficial to all kinds of patients. Patients should consider exercising as part of their daily routine. Depending on their personal needs and preferences, disease activity and severity, patients may opt for unsupervised (recreational or AS-specific) exercises alone or may also attend group physical therapy sessions. If necessary, they may follow an inpatient course of physiotherapy or engage in spa therapy. The paucity of data makes it difficult to identify the best administration mode of these interventions based upon scientific evidence today.

Self-management of the patient is a prerequisite to success, with the basis lying initially at the treating physician convinced of the need of exercising and referring the patient to a physiotherapist. Inspired and motivated by the physiotherapist to follow a time-consuming exercise program, the patient may eventually benefit from a better disease outcome (26).

REFERENCES

1. Boonen A. Socioeconomic consequences of ankylosing spondylitis. Clin Exp Rheumatol 2002; 20(suppl 28):S23–S26.
2. Hidding A, van der Linden S, Boers M, et al. Is group physical therapy superior to individualized therapy in ankylosing spondylitis? A randomized controlled trial. Arthritis Care Res 1993; 6:117–125.
3. Viitanen JV, Suni J. Management principles of physiotherapy in ankylosing spondylitis—which treatments are effective? Physiotherapy 1995; 81:322–329.
4. McNeal RL. Aquatic therapy for patients with rheumatic disease. Rheum Dis Clin North Am 1990; 16:915–929.
5. Machtey I. Hydrotherapy and balneotherapy: state of the art. In: Balint G, Gömör B, Hodinka L, eds. Rheumatology, State of the Art. Amsterdam: Excerpta Medica, 1992: 390–392.
6. Helliwell PS, Abbott CA, Chamberlain MA. A randomised trial of three different physiotherapy regimens in ankylosing spondylitis. Physiotherapy 1996; 82:85–90.
7. Simon L, Blotman F. Exercise therapy and hydrotherapy in the treatment of rheumatic diseases. Clin Rheum Dis 1981; 7:337–347.
8. Rasmussen JO, Hansen TM. Physical training for patients with ankylosing spondylitis. Arthritis Care Res 1989; 2:25–27.
9. Gall V. Exercise in the spondyloarthropathies. Arthritis Care Res 1994; 7:215–220.
10. Stucki G, Kroeling P. Physical therapy and rehabilitation in the management of rheumatic disorders. Baillieres Best Pract Res Clin Rheumatol 2000; 14:751–771.
11. van der Heijde D, Calin A, Dougados M, Khan MA, van der Linden S, Bellamy N. Selection of instruments in the core set for DC-ART, SMARD, physical therapy, and clinical record keeping in ankylosing spondylitis. Progress report of the ASAS Working Group. J Rheumatol 1999; 26:951–954.
12. Dagfinrud H, Hagen K. Physiotherapy interventions for ankylosing spondylitis. Cochrane Database Syst Rev 2004; 4:Cd002822. pub 2.
13. Kraag G, Stokes B, Groh J, Helewa A, Goldsmith C. The effects of comprehensive home physiotherapy and supervision on patients with ankylosing spondylitis—a randomized controlled trial. J Rheumatol 1990; 17:228–233.
14. van Tubergen A, Landewe R, van der Heijde D, et al. Combined spa-exercise therapy is effective in patients with ankylosing spondylitis: a randomized controlled trial. Arthritis Rheum 2001; 45:430–438.
15. Sweeney S, Taylor G, Calin A. The effect of a home based exercise intervention package on outcome in ankylosing spondylitis: a randomized controlled trial. J Rheumatol 2002; 29:763–766.
16. Analy Y, E. O, Karan A, Diracoglu D, Aydin R. The effectiveness of intensive group exercise on patients with ankylosing spondylitis. Clin Rehabil 2003; 17:631–636.
17. Kraag G, Stokes B, Groh J, Helewa A, Goldsmith CH. The effects of comprehensive home physiotherapy and supervision on patients with ankylosing spondylitis—an 8-month follow-up. J Rheumatol 1994; 21:261–263.
18. Hidding A, van der Linden S, Gielen X, de Witte L, Dijkmans B, Moolenburgh D. Continuation of group physical therapy is necessary in ankylosing spondylitis: results of a randomized controlled trial. Arthritis Care Res 1994; 7:90–96.

19. Hidding A, van der Linden S, de Witte L. Therapeutic effects of individual physical therapy in ankylosing spondylitis related to duration of disease. Clin Rheumatol 1993; 12:334–340.
20. Fisher LR, Cawley MI, Holgate ST. Relation between chest expansion, pulmonary function, and exercise tolerance in patients with ankylosing spondylitis. Ann Rheum Dis 1990; 49:921–925.
21. Seckin U, Bolukbasi N, Gursel G, Eroz S, Sepici V, Ekim N. Relationship between pulmonary function and exercise tolerance in patients with ankylosing spondylitis. Clin Exp Rheumatol 2000; 18:503–506.
22. Tomlinson MJ, Barefoot J, Dixon ASJ. Intensive in-patient physiotherapy courses improve movement and posture in ankylosing spondylitis. Physiotherapy 1986; 72: 238–240.
23. Band DA, Jones SD, Kennedy LG, et al. Which patients with ankylosing spondylitis derive most benefit from an inpatient management program? J Rheumatol 1997; 24:2381–2384.
24. Uhrin Z, Kuzis S, Ward MM. Exercise and changes in health status in patients with ankylosing spondylitis. Arch Intern Med 2000; 160:2969–2975.
25. Santos H, Brophy S, Calin A. Exercise in ankylosing spondylitis: how much is optimum? J Rheumatol 1998; 25:2156–2160.
26. Calin A. Can we define the outcome of ankylosing spondylitis and the effect of physiotherapy management? J Rheumatol 1994; 21:184–185.

14

Anesthesiological Considerations for the Ankylosing Spondylitis Patient

Jaap J. de Lange and Wouter W. A. Zuurmond
*Department of Anesthesiology, VU University Medical Center,
Amsterdam, The Netherlands*

Ankylosing spondylitis (AS) is an inflammatory systemic disease affecting the sacroiliac joints and spine leading to ankylosis and "bamboo spine," and adjacent soft tissues. Systemic involvement may result in weight loss, fatigue, low-grade fever, conjunctivitis, uveitis, pulmonary fibrosis in the upper lobes, aortic regurgitation due to thickening of the valve cusps, dilatation of the valve annulus, and cardiac conduction abnormalities.

Human leucocyte antigen (HLA)-B27 may be positive in more than 90% of the patients, which may explain the high familial incidence. The inflammatory disease may affect 1.6% of the population, four times as many males as females. The severity of AS varies from mild stiffness and pain in the sacroiliac joints to severe systemic abnormalities and deformities especially of the cervical and thoracic spinal joints (1–3). Anesthesia in patients with AS poses a number of specific problems.

PREOPERATIVE CONSIDERATIONS

Predictability and Handling of Musculoskeletal Involvement

Upper Airway

What are the possible risk factors and available tests for diagnosing airway difficulty (4,5)?

Ankylosing of the Cervical Spine. Cervical spine stiffness interferes with the flexion and extension of the neck.

During the preoperative visit of the patient suffering from AS, evaluation of the upper airway has to be performed meticulously. Diagnosing an obvious difficulty for intubation is mostly easy and this makes the anesthesiologist aware of the problems which may arise during intubation.

Relative Tongue/Pharyngeal Size, the Mallampati Test (6). The size of the tongue in relation to the size of the oral cavity can be simply and visually graded by how much of the pharynx is obscured by the tongue.

The purpose of the test is:

- classifying the view of pharyngeal structures,
- defining the size of the tongue in relation to the size of the oral cavity, and
- visually grading how much the pharynx is obscured by the tongue.

The test is performed by asking the patient to maximally protrude the tongue from a fully open mouth while sitting upright. The pharyngeal structures are inspected and classified into four grades:

Class I: faucial pillars, soft palatine and uvula are visible,
Class II: faucial pillars and soft palatine can be visualized, but the uvula is—partially—masked by the base of the tongue,
Class III: only the soft palatine and the base of the uvula can be visualized, or
Class IV: soft palatine is not visible.

Class III and Class IV are associated with increasing difficulty to intubate.

Atlanto-occipital Joint Extension and Flexion. When the neck is slightly to moderately flexed on the chest and the atlanto-occipital joint is well extended, resulting in an extended head on the neck, the oral, pharyngeal, and laryngeal axes are brought more nearly into a straight line, the well-known "sniffing-the-morning-air-position." In this position less of the tongue will obscure the view of the larynx and, consequently, there will be much less need for strenuous effort to bring the tongue forward. In healthy people, a mean extension of 25–35 grades occurs at level C1–C2. However, to consider movement between C0–C1 and C1–C2 as separate would be inappropriate. The extension takes place at C0–C2 and amounts to 35°.

The patient has to be evaluated by sitting straight with head held erect and facing directly to the front. In this position the occluded surface of the upper teeth is horizontal and parallel to the ground. The patient then extends the atlanto-occipital joint as much as possible and the examiner measures the angle traversed by the occluded surface of the upper teeth. Any reduction in extension can be as a fraction of the normal.

When the atlanto-occipital gap cannot be extended, the laryngoscopist will cause an increase in the convexity of the cervical spine, which will bring the larynx further forward. Patients who suffer with rheumatoid disease of the neck or degenerative spinal diseases often have reduced neck mobility making intubation harder.

The Space Anterior to the Larynx, the So-called "Mandibular Space." The mandibular space can be measured by a ruler or by a number of finger breadths. The thyromental distance, the distance between the inside of the mandible to the hyoid bone has to be >6 cm or two fingers or more. The horizontal length of the mandible has to be >9 cm. These measurements are tightly associated with a low tongue/pharyngeal size classification and strongly suggest that direct laryngoscopy will be easy. When there is a large mandibular space, the tongue is easily compressed into a large compartment and does not have to be pulled maximally forward in order to reveal the larynx.

Jaw Movement. Two aspects of jaw movement are significant when assessing difficult intubation:

- The interdental gap—mouth opening permits adequate insertion of the laryngoscope and tube. Limited movement of the mandible is a recognized cause of difficult intubation. This may be related to temporomandibular dysfunction or trismus. In AS patients the incidence of temporomandibular joint involvement varies between 10% and 40%. Cricoarythenoid involvement may be expected if dyspnea or hoarseness occurs (1).

- Subluxation of the jaw—the maximal forward protrusion of the lower incisors beyond the upper incisors. Good forward protrusion of the mandible provides additional space for forward displacement of the tongue.

View Obstruction. *Dentition*: unusually long upper incisors, the so-called buck teeth, may adversely affect the position of the upper end of the line of sight. In addition, a receding mandible may indicate that the tongue is positioned more at the back than usually, blocking the view. Finally, a body weight more than 110 kg or a Quetelet index >30 may interfere with intubation.

The above mentioned tests and limitations cannot be seen alone and a combination of the above tests is better than using only one to predict difficulties in intubation.

Anesthesia in patients with AS with a difficult airway may lead to the following complications:

- Direct trauma

    the airway and surrounding tissues
    upper airway resulting in hemorrhage, lacerations and subsequent tissue emphysema and risk of infection
    chipped or broken teeth
    fracture of the facial bones
    fracture-subluxation of the cervical spine

- Directly mediated reflexes

    laryngovagal (airway spasm, apnea, bradycardia, arrhythmia, or hypotension)
    laryngosympathetic (tachycardia, tachyarrhythmia, or hypertension)
    laryngospinal (coughing, vomiting, or bucking)

- Interruption of the gas exchange

    hypoxia and hypercapnia which may cause brain injury, myocardial infarction and death

Both direct trauma and morbidity from airway obstruction may range from minor to major and life threatening. Criteria during difficult intubation are classified according to Cormack and Lehane (7). These criteria are defined for the patient in position supine with the head in the sniffing position. Grades 1 and 2 are considered to be adequate exposure and grades 3 and 4 inadequate exposure.

Grade 1: Glottis including anterior and posterior commissures could be fully exposed
Grade 2: Glottis could be partly exposed and anterior commissure could not be visualized
Grade 3: Glottis could not be exposed, corniculate cartilages only could be visualized
Grade 4: Glottis including corniculate cartilages could not be exposed.

Difficult Intubation Strategies

In the United States, guidelines for difficult airway management were developed by a nine-person task force appointed by the American Society of Anesthesiologists

(ASA) Ad Hoc Committee on Practice Parameters (8). A difficult intubation drill was introduced. Three basic problems may occur alone or in combination: difficult intubation, difficult ventilation, and/or difficulty with patient cooperation or consent.

Difficult intubation may or may not be accompanied with difficulty in mask ventilation. In these cases, we have to consider the relative merits and feasibility of basic management choices:

- use of nonsurgical techniques versus surgical technique,
- preservation of spontaneous ventilation during intubation versus ablation of spontaneous ventilation during intubation attempts, and
- awake intubation versus intubation attempts after induction of anesthesia. Concerning awake intubation preoperative preparation and information of the patient combined with local anesthetic techniques may facilitate this procedure.

Awake Intubation. During awake intubation, intravenous sedation may be administered. However, respiratory depression or losing verbal contact with the patient has to be prevented.

There are two important nerve blocks for decreasing discomfort of the patient during awake intubation: the bilateral blockage of the lingual branch of the IX nerve and the superior laryngeal block. First, the bilateral blockage of the lingual branch of the IX nerve eliminates the gag reflex. The tongue of the patient is gently retracted laterally, exposing the palatoglossal arch. The palatoglossal arch is pierced approximately 0.5 cm from the lateral margin of the root of the tongue at the point at which it joins the floor of the mouth. The needle is inserted 0.5 cm and 2 mL of 2% lidocaine is inserted after a negative aspiration test.

Secondly, the internal branch of the superior laryngeal nerve can be blocked. The superior laryngeal block consists of application of local anesthetic superficial and deep to the inferior lateral cornu of the hyoid bone. The nerve pierces the membrane at this point and can be blocked at either sides of the membrane. Furthermore topical spray (lidocaine 10%) may be applied.

Intubation Techniques

- Orally with direct laryngoscopy, the conventional technique. In many countries modifications on the normal laryngoscope have been commercially available, for example, the Bullard (9). New types of laryngoscopes and new techniques should not be practiced for the first time during a difficult intubation. All new inventions have to be evaluated thoroughly.
- Orally over a guiding stylet. A modification on the guiding stylet is the illuminating stylet.
- Nasal intubation with laryngoscope.
- Nasal intubation after first oral attempt.
- Blind nasal intubation.
- Laryngeal mask (10,11).
- Intubation with flexible bronchoscope. A flexible laryngoscope is the most useful aid to awake intubation in the patient with the difficult airway. Fiber-optic-aided intubation can be performed using the oral or nasal route. After successful passage through the vocal cords, a tube can be inserted over the fiberscope (12).

- It is recommendable to use a mask with a hole to permit passage of the fiberscope.
- Retrograde translaryngeal-guided intubation.

Retrograde intubation techniques have been in use for several decades. Retrograde intubation seems to be an underused elective or emergency intubation technique in the management of the difficult airway.

After properly positioning the patient, the skin and underlying tissue have to be infiltrated with local anesthetics and punctured, two segments lower than the cricothyroid membrane at an angle of 30°. The puncture pressure may be high and care must be taken to prevent piercing the opposite side of the trachea. A simple way to detect the airway can be utilized to connect the needle with the capnograph.

An epidural set may be used. After insertion of the epidural needle, a catheter has to be inserted and guided to the mouth. If nasal intubation is demanded, a nasal airway may guide the epidural catheter to the entrance of the nose (13).

Learning this technique could be a problem: for ethical reasons, it is not usual to perform these techniques in normal patients:

- coniotomy and high frequency ventilation, or
- tracheotomy.

Conclusion. The prediction of difficult intubation preoperatively may save lives in the future. An emergency drill has to be available. Techniques for difficult intubation have to be learned. The choice of the intubation technique depends mainly on the experience of the anesthesiologist.

Spinal Involvement

The entire ankylosed spine in these patients needs special attention. It is mandatory to prevent excessive manipulation of the cervical spine, especially during intubation and positioning of the patient, to prevent fracture of the spine and subsequent spinal cord injury. A difficult position for the AS patient is the prone position. Meticulous attention should be paid to maintain the patient's own posture. It is extremely important not to offend patients' "own anatomy." Positioning of the patient should be a close collaboration between anesthesiologist and surgeon.

A consequence of thoracic spinal involvement may be a "stiff thorax" with decreased rib cage movement resulting in impaired lung function. Preoperative evaluation of lung function is essential. The abnormalities in the spine may sometimes shut the door on performing regional anesthesia (epidural and/or spinal) due to limited joint mobility and closed interspinous spaces (14). An increased risk of epidural hematoma in patients with AS may be present especially in multiple attempts either to puncture or to place the catheter (15). External cardiac massage may be hindered by the "stiff thorax."

Predictability and Handling of Respiratory System Involvement

The upper lobe pulmonary fibrosis may be diagnosed by chest X-ray. The X-ray findings may not be mistaken for tuberculosis (2). Postoperatively special attention should be paid to the respiratory parameters in case of impairment of the lung function.

Predictability and Handling of the Cardiovascular System Involvement

Preoperative evaluation of the cardiovascular system has to be done to exclude extension of the disease to the connective tissue of the aorta and aortic valve cusp resulting in aortic valve insufficiency and heart rhythm disturbances. Stoke Adams attacks may occur due to conduction defects (1–3): preoperative examination involves EKG to detect left ventricular hypertrophy and conduction defects and echocardiography to detect aortic valvular disease.

Predictability and Handling of the Neurological System Involvement

Neurological deficits are common in patients suffering from AS. Meticulous preoperative neurological evaluation is mandatory not only for achieving adapted proper positioning during anesthesia and operation, but also for forensic reasons, especially when regional techniques are performed.

Predictability and Handling of Concomittant Problems

Patients suffering from AS may have impaired renal function due to amyloidosis and/or due to chronic use of nonsteroidal anti-inflammatory drugs (NSAIDs). Preoperative full blood count, urea and electrolytes, and clotting time have to be investigated term NSAID's prescriptions.

INTRAOPERATIVE CONSIDERATIONS

Anesthetic Technique

The anesthetic technique for the AS patient is not different from other patients and should be tailor-made to the patient's condition, and the extent of the operation. However, as mentioned before special attention should be paid to proper positioning of the patient, intubation possibilities and conditions, and postoperative respiratory problems and pain relief.

Blood Loss

Intraoperatively, the anesthesiologist has to deal with blood loss during spinal surgery. To prevent and/or treat excessive blood loss the following special measures could be performed:

1. Prevention and immediate treatment of clotting disorders.
2. Applying cell saver techniques.
3. Sampling and storing of autologous blood in the preoperative period.
4. Pretreatment of the patient by means of erythropoietine (16). This should be planned three to four weeks before the surgical procedure.
5. Controlled hypotension during moments of the excessive blood loss. This technique is controversial, because it depends on the patient's condition: disturbed neuroautoregulation of the central nervous system and hypotension is not a preferable combination and may lead to neurological deficits. For this reason the decision to apply controlled hypotension should be made carefully.

Spinal Cord Monitoring

The development of spinal cord monitoring techniques has replaced the old fashioned "wake up test" during spinal surgery. To detect spinal threatening due to surgery two techniques are available:

1. Monitoring somatosensory evoked potentials (SSEP), or
2. Transcranial electro-motor evoked potentials.

Most experience has been achieved with SSEP. By electrical stimulation of a peripheral nerve (e.g., the post-tibial nerve) the response in the cerebral cortex is monitored. Interruption of the signal indicates threatening of spinal damage and immediate restoration of spinal cord function may be still possible. With this technique one monitors the integrity of the somatic sensory system, thus the dorsal part of the medulla. Applying the second technique the integrity of the motor system of the medulla (the ventral part) is monitored. This technique is especially suitable for monitoring the function of the spinal cord during aortic surgery.

Both techniques demand a standardized anesthetic technique. All inhaled anesthetic agents cause a marked dose-related depression of the signal; nitrous oxide does not influence latency time, but depresses the amplitude of the signal by 50%. Continuous infusion of an opioid combined with propofol has proven to be the preferable anesthetic technique, because propofol shows more stability of the signal (17,18).

Monitoring of SSEP has to be started in the awake patient to obtain reference values. During the crucial moments of surgery the anesthesia has to be performed smoothly by continuous infusion without top up doses.

POSTOPERATIVE CONSIDERATIONS

Respiratory Aspects

Postoperative artificial ventilation is needed if the respiratory function is marginal and a smooth recovery is demanded. In AS patients, extubation should be performed if the patient has fully recovered from anesthesia, because the necessity to re-intubate could be disastrous.

Pain Relief

Special attention should be paid to proper postoperative pain relief: insufficient pain relief may result in hypoventilation and too high doses of opioids may result in oversedation, respiratory depression, and insufficient coughing. Tailor-made analgesia may be achieved by personal attention and patient controlled analgesia with opioids.

Administering NSAIDs is only indicated in patients without renal impairment or excessive blood loss. Epidural analgesia is preferable, but often not technically feasible. Sometimes it is possible to place an epidural catheter during the operation by the surgeon.

REFERENCES

1. Campbell A, Hamilton-Davies C. Ankylosing spondylitis. In: Pollard BJ, ed. Handbook of clinical anaesthesia. 2nd. London: Churchill Livingstone, 2004:232–234.

2. Stoelting RK, Dierdorf SF. Anaesthesia and co-existing disease. Chapter 26. Skin and musculoskeletal diseases. 4th ed. London: Churchill Livingstone, 2002:532.

3. Allman KG, Wilson IH. Ankylosing spondylitis. Oxford Handbook of Anaesthesia. Oxford: Oxford University Press, 2001:163.

4. Benumof JL. Management of the difficult airway. With special emphasis on awake tracheal intubation. Anesthesiology 1991; 75:1087–1110.

5. Benumof JL. Airway management. Principles and practice. St Louis: Mosby-Year Book 1996.

6. Mallampati SR, Gatt SP, Gugino LD, et al. A clinical sign to predict difficult tracheal intubation. A prospective study. Can J Anaesth 1985; 32:429–434.

7. Cormack RS, Lehane J. Difficult tracheal intubation in obstetrics. Anaesthesia 1984; 39:1105–1111.

8. Practice guidelines for management of the difficult airway: a report by the American society of anesthesiologists task force on management of the difficult airway: Anesthesiology 1993; 78:597–602.

9. King TA, Adams AP. Failed tracheal intubation. Br J Anaesth 1990; 65:400–414.

10. Lu PP, Brimacombe J, Ho AC, Shyr MH, Liu HP. The intubating laryngeal mask airway in severe ankylosing spondylitis. Can J Anaesth 2001; 48(10):1015–1019.

11. Ferson DZ, Rosenblatt WH, Johansen MJ, Osborn I, Ovassapian A. Use of the intubating LMA-Fastrach in 254 patients with difficult-to-manage airways. Anesthesiology 2001; 95(5):1175–1181.

12. Ovassapian A. Fiberoptic endoscopy and the difficult airway. Philadelphia: Lippincott-Raven, 1996.

13. Bourke D, Levesque PR. Modification of retrograde guide for endotracheal intubation. Anesth Analg 1974; 53:1013–1014.

14. Schelew BL, Vaghadia H. Ankylosing spondylitis and neuraxial anaesthesia—a 10 year review. Can J Anaesth 1996; 43(1):65–68.

15. Gustafsson H, Rutberg H, Bengtsson M. Spinal haematoma following epidural analgesia. Report of a patient with ankylosing spondylitis and a bleeding diathese. Anaesthesia 1988; 43:220–222.

16. Faris PM, Ritter MA, Abels RI. The effects of recombinant human erythropoietin on perioperative transfusion requirements in patients having a major orthopaedic operation. J Bone Joint Surg Am 1996; 78:62–72.

17. Kalkman CJ, Traast H, Zuurmond WWA, Bovill JG. Differential effects of propofol and nitrous oxide on posterior tibial nerve somatosensory cortical evoked potentials during alfentanil anaesthesia. Br J Anaesth 1991; 66:483–489.

18. Scheepstra GL, De Lange JJ, Booij LHDJ, Ros HH. Median nerve evoked potentials during propofol anaesthesia. Br J Anaesth 1989; 62:92–94.

15

Lumbar Osteotomy in Ankylosing Spondylitis: A Structured Review of Three Methods of Treatment

Arthur de Gast
Department of Orthopaedic Surgery, VU University Medical Center,
Amsterdam, The Netherlands

INTRODUCTION

Ankylosing spondylitis (AS) mainly affects the synovial joints and soft tissue structures of the axial skeleton. Inflammatory processes in the intervertebral joints eventually lead to ankylosits, which together with ossification of the anterior and posterior longitudinal ligaments render the spine into a rigid beam. Despite maximum conservative treatment, stiffening of the spine in an advert position can occur. In AS, this mostly is a combination of a thoracic hyperkyphosis and flattening of the lumbar lordosis: a thoracolumbar kyphotic deformity (TLKD) (1–5).

A severe TLKD can prevent the patient from sitting, standing, or lying comfortably, especially if the TLKD is accompanied by a flexion contracture of the hip joints that adds up to the total flexion deformity of the patient's body. Also, patients with a TLKD lose the ability to see straight forward to the horizon. Obviously, the physical posture and impairments caused by a TLKD also have strong psychological and social implications (Fig. 1) (67,68).

A corrective spinal osteotomy may be considered in selected cases. The main goal of a corrective spinal osteotomy is to restore the patient's spinal balance and the restoration of a horizontal view angle (Fig. 2). Positive side effects of a corrective spinal osteotomy are to relieve compression of the abdominal viscera by the margin of the inferior rib cage, and improvement of diaphragmatic respiration.

The TLKD is best corrected by a lordosating osteotomy of the lumbar spine, as thoracic correction is strongly limited by ankylosis of the costovertebral joints (3,4,6–11). Furthermore, the overall correction is greatest when the intervention is performed at the lowest possible level of the lumbar spine (7,9,12,13). In addition, the relative narrow thoracic spinal canal renders the mid-thoracic spinal cord more vulnerable to perioperative injury than the cauda equina in its spacious spinal canal.

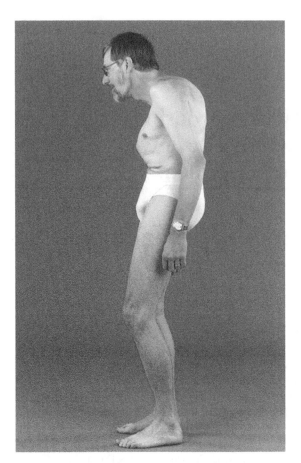

Figure 1   Clinical photograph of a patient with a severe TLKD due to AS. Note the extension of the hip joints, the kyphotic deformity of the spine, and the inability to look straight forward. *Abbreviations*: TLKD, thoracolumbar kyphotic deformity; AS, ankylosing spondylitis.

Reports on lumbar osteotomies for correction of TLKD attributable to AS are limited. Most authors reported results of only few patients (7,14–25). Few authors, however, have experience with more than 50 patients (9,12,26–28,66).

HISTORY AND CURRENT OPTIONS FOR SURGICAL TREATMENT

There are a number of descriptions of operative techniques for the correction of TLKD. Still, these descriptions can be reduced to three basic operative techniques to correct TLKD resulting from AS at the level of the lumbar spine: opening wedge osteotomy, polysegmental wedge osteotomies, and closing wedge osteotomy (Figs. 3–5).

Opening Wedge Osteotomy

The original technique is commonly credited to Smith-Petersen et al. (10), who reported an anterior opening wedge osteotomy in six patients in 1945. This technique involves two- and three-level osteotomies removing the articular processes of L1,

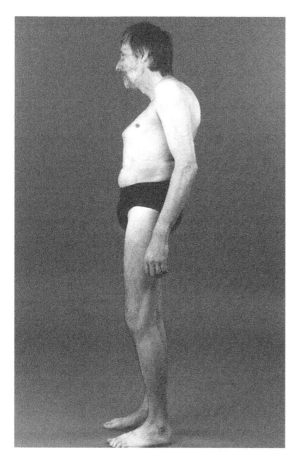

Figure 2 Clinical photograph of the same patient after surgical correction of the patient's posture by means of an extending lumbar osteotomy (in this case a single-level closing wedge osteotomy). Note among others, the restoration of the patient's view angle as compared with Figure 1.

L2, and L3 (10). Correction of the kyphotic deformity was then achieved by forceful manual extension of the lumbar spine in an attempt to close the posterior wedge osteotomies. Obviously, this forceful manipulation must cause a disruption of the anterior longitudinal ligament and vertebral structures to create an anterior mono-segmental intervertebral opening wedge with elongation of the anterior column (Fig. 6).

In the same period, the Dutch orthopedic surgeon La Chapelle (20) described a two-stage anterior opening wedge osteotomy for correction of TLKD in one patient. First of all he removed the lamina of L2 under local anesthesia, followed two weeks later by an anterior release and resection of the intervertebral disc between L2 and L3. The anterior osteotomy was then wedged open and grafted with a bone block. Since then, many modifications of this anterior opening wedge osteotomy have been described (1,3–6,11,12,15,26,27,29–39,67). The sharp lordotic angle and elongation of the anterior column resulting from this procedure were believed to be associated with serious vascular and neurological complications (6,12,19,24,26,33,36,38). To avoid such complications, polysegmental posterior wedge osteotomies and closing wedge posterior osteotomies of the lumbar spine were introduced.

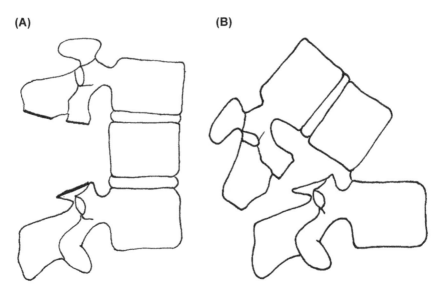

Figure 3 Diagrams of the OWO. (**A**) Lateral view outlining the bone block to be resected. (**B**) Postoperative lateral view showing how correction is achieved by closure of the posterior elements, and creating an open wedge of the anterior column. *Abbreviation*: OWO, opening wedge osteotomy.

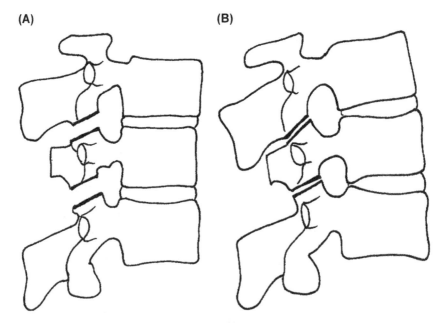

Figure 4 Diagrams of the PWO. (**A**) Lateral view outlining the bone blocs to be resected through the original facet joints in the direction of the interspinal foramen. (**B**) Postoperative lateral view showing how correction is achieved by closure of the posterior osteotomies. *Abbreviation*: PWO, polysegmental wedge osteotomies.

(A) (B)

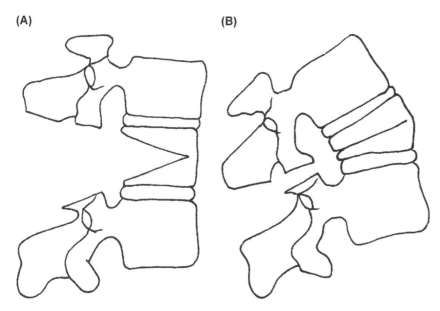

Figure 5 Diagrams of the CWO. (**A**) Lateral view outlining the bone block to be resected. (**B**) Postoperative lateral view showing how correction is achieved by closure of the intravertebral osteotomy. *Abbreviation*: CWO, closing wedge osteotomy.

Polysegmental Wedge Osteotomy

In 1949, Wilson and Turkell (25) were the first to report a patient with TLKD attributable to AS treated by polysegmental lumbar posterior wedge osteotomies. Correction was achieved by extending the lumbar spine after multiple lumbar posterior closing wedge osteotomies, including removal of tissues in the interlaminar space and the inferior and superior articular processes. This method provides a more gradual correction without rupturing of the anterior longitudinal ligament (Fig. 4). In the 1980s, Zielke (40–44) also advocated polysegmental lumbar posterior wedge osteotomies, but, in contrast to his predecessors, with the use of internal fixation. He and his colleagues first used Harrington rods and laminar hooks, and later, transpedicular screws (9).

Closing Wedge Osteotomy

Correction of TLKD due to AS by a monosegmental intravertebral closing wedge osteotomy of the lumbar spine was first described by Scudese in 1963 (22) and later by Ziwjan in 1982 (28) and by Thomasen in 1985 (45). This technique encompasses the resection of the posterior elements of one vertebra, including the lamina, articular processes, and pedicles, in combination with the posterior wedge of the vertebral body. Correction is then achieved by passive extension of the lumbar spine, thus closing the posterior osteotomy with an anterior hinge (Fig. 5). A variety of methods of internal fixation such as wiring, metal plates, or transpedicular fixation have been used to ensure immediate stability and rapid consolidation of the osteotomy site (13,17,45,46).

The above mentioned three basic surgical techniques are in use to treat TLKD caused by AS (13,27,35,41,47). Currently, authors prefer polysegmental lumbar

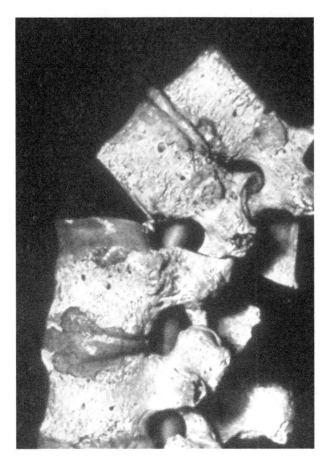

Figure 6 Model representation of OWO in a spine. Note the resection of the adjacent articular processes of the vertebra. Considerable elongation of the anterior column occurs after opening the osteotomy. Note that this model does not show a bamboo spine as is the case in ankylosing spondylitis. *Abbreviation*: OWO, opening wedge osteotomy.

posterior wedge osteotomies or a monosegmental or closing wedge posterior osteotomy above anterior opening wedge osteotomy because of the high complication and mortality rate associated with the latter (2,9,13,16,17,22,35). Nevertheless, the association of open wedge osteotomy (OWO) with a high vascular and neurological complication rate is challenged by several others (6,11,27,29,47).

In an attempt to offer the readers of this book a rationale for decision making on the surgical technique that yields the best technical results for the correction of TLKD associated with AS, a structured review of the literature will be presented in this chapter.

For the purpose of clarity and uniformity in this chapter, the operative technique of an anterior opening wedge osteotomy according to Smith-Petersen is referred to as OWO (Fig. 3). The technique of polysegmental lumbar posterior wedge osteotomies is referred to as polysegmental wedge osteotomies (PWO) (Fig. 4), and the monosegmental posterior closing wedge osteotomy is referred to as closing-wedge osteotomy (CWO) (Fig. 5).

LITERATURE REVIEW

A comprehensive search of all journal articles (referred to as reports) was performed. All reports written in English, French, and German, published between 1966 and 2003 and referenced on Medline, concerning lumbar osteotomies for the correction of TLKD because of AS, were included in this systematic review. The reference lists of all reports were also scanned in order to find other reports. From different reports with an overlap in the patient groups (that is, same patients described in both reports) only the report with the most detailed data was used. From each report, only the data of patients with TLKD attributable to AS treated by a surgical correction of the lumbar spine were analyzed. Reports with at least 10 patients and sufficient clinical information were analyzed for demographic data. After a preliminary review of all reports, a list of six data categories was developed, considered by the author as the minimum requirements for meaningful data interpretation. These categories are: (i) at least four patients treated by the same method, (ii) age and sex of patients, (iii) a comprehensible description of the surgical procedure, (iv) radiographic assessment of the correction in degrees, (v) complications, and (vi) subjective (patient-reported) outcomes. Only reports analyzable on all six data categories were included for further analysis. The reports were further divided in three groups according to the surgical techniques used (i.e., OWO, PWO, and CWO). From the reports, the degree of postoperative correction, degree of correction at follow-up, loss of correction, superficial infection, deep infection, re-operation, pseudarthrosis, neuropraxia, retrograde ejaculation, paralysis, and implant failure were recorded and referred to as the technical outcome data. In order to be able to make a comparison of the technical outcome data of the three surgical techniques, the results were graded good, fair, and poor according to Table 3.

RESULTS

Search of the Literature

An extensive search of the literature revealed 61 citations. Of these, 43 reports could be included for further analysis (Table 1). The reasons for exclusion of 18 reports were overlap of patient groups (41–44,48–52) and absence of clinical results (6,8,53–59). Halm et al. (40,41) reported functional outcome analysis using a subjective score. The technical outcome data of these patients are described in more detail in a referred textbook (60). Another author reports on a prospective study with emphasis on clinical outcome data (66). In another report, the results of two surgical methods were presented (35). Because of insufficient clinical data in most of the reports, statistical meta-analysis of the technical outcomes of the three surgical techniques was not feasible, let alone of the clinical outcome data.

Patient Series and Treatment Groups

The 43 reports describe 979 patients treated by lumbar osteotomy for TLKD resulting from AS; the data are presented in Table 1. In 451 patients (46%; 29 studies) an OWO was performed. A PWO, reported in five studies, was performed in 249 patients (25%). In ten studies, 297 patients (30%) were treated by CWO. Sixteen reports, including 712 (73%) patients, met the criteria for demographic analysis.

Table 1 Data in Series of 979 Patients Treated by Lumbar Wedge Osteotomies for TLKD Because of AS

References	Patients (n)	Open wedge osteotomies	Polysegmental wedge osteotomies	Closing wedge osteotomies	Mortality
Bossers (1)	4	4			
Bradford et al. (29)	8	8			
Briggs et al. (30)	5	5			
Camargo et al. (12)	66	66			1
Chapchal (14)	2	2			1
Chen (2)	16		16		
Chen et al. (66)	78			78	
Dawson (7)	2	2			1
Donaldson (31)	6	6			1
Emnéus (15)	3	3			
Goel (3)	11	11			
Halm et al. (40)	34		34		2
Hähnel (16)	2			2	
Hehne et al. (9)	177		177		4
Herbert (32)	4	4			4
Herbert (33)	30	30			4
Jaffray et al. (17)	3			3	
Junghanns (34)	12	12			
Kallio (18)	1	1			
Kim et al. (67)	45			45	
Klems (19)	1	1			1
La Chapelle (20)	1	1			
Law (26)	120	120			10
Lazennec et al. (35)	31	19		12	
Lichtblau and Wilson (36)	5	5			1
McMaster and Coventry (4)	17	17			2
McMaster (11)	14	14			
McMaster (37)	15	15			1
Schubert and Polak (21)	2	2			
Scudese and Calabro (22)	1			1	
Simmons (5)	19	19			
Smith-Petersen et al. (10)	6	6			
Stuart and Rose (23)	1	1			
Styblo et al. (38)	20	20			
Thiranont and Netrawichien (46)	6			6	
Thomasen (45)	11			11	
Thompson and Ingersoll (39)	5	5			
Van Royen and Slot (13)	22			22	
Van Royen et al. (62)	21		21		
Weale et al. (27)	50	50			2
Weatherley et al. (24)	2	2			2
Wilson and Turkell (25)	1		1		
Ziwjan (28)	99			99	2
Total	979	451	249	297	34

Table 2 Demographic Data of Series with More Than 10 Patients

References	Patients (*n*)	Mean age (range)	Male	Female
Camargo et al. (12)	66	34 (19–55)	59	7
Chen (2)	16	40 (24–63)	14	2
Chen (78)	78	37 (19–63)	74	4
Goel (3)	11	33 (23–46)	10	1
Halm et al. (40)	34	41 (24–57)	31	3
Hehne et al. (9)	177	41 (24–65)	15621	
Kim et al. (67)	45	35 (17–55)	43	2
Lazennec et al. (35)	31	44 (32–61)	26	5
McMaster and Coventry (4)	17	42 (31–49)	11	6
McMaster (11)	14	42 (31–66)	11	3
Styblo et al. (38)	20	41 (19–57)	19	1
Thomasen (45)	11	38 (28–56)	8	3
Van Royen and Slot (13)	22	48 (27–70)	18	4
Van Royen et al. (62)	21	42 (19–61)	16	5
Weale et al. (27)	50	43 (26–57)	44	6
Ziwjan (28)	99	41 (21–56)	97	2
Combined data	589	40 (17–70)	637	75

The mean age at the time of operation was 41 years (range 19–73). The male–female ratio was 7.5:1 (Table 2). Eighteen reports, including 646 patients (66%), were analyzed for technical outcome data. Of these, nine reports [including 224 patients (34%)] deal with OWO (3–5,11,12,27,29,35,38), four reports [including 248 patients (38%)] with PWO (2,9,40,62), and six [including 174 patients (26%)] with CWO (13,35,45,46,66,67).

Preoperative, Operative, and Postoperative Approaches

Few authors describe their preoperative assessment, i.e., measurement of the severity of the TLKD and the degree of correction needed to obtain an appropriate sagittal balance of the spinal column (29,48,61,62,67). Böhm (48) designed a pair of glasses to measure the view angle in relation to the plumb line. Other authors advise to assess the deformity preoperatively by the chin–brow to vertical angle (61,62,67), or by the C7 plumb line on a standing sagittal radiograph of the whole spine (29,67).

General anesthesia and fiber optic intubations are the most commonly used techniques during the operative procedure; however, some authors (5,14,15,20) advocated local anesthesia. Whereas a prone position of the patient is generally advocated, Adams (6) and Simmons (5) described a surgical technique with the patient in a lateral decubitus position. Some authors advised an anterior release prior to or after the osteotomy but before correction in cases of osteoporotic bone, considerable disk calcification, and ossification of the anterior longitudinal ligament (5,20,32,33,35,38,62). To prevent neurological complications, gradual plaster correction have been advocated in OWO (4,12,15) and CWO (Fig. 7) (16). Neural monitoring (35) and the use of a wake-up test (2,11,29) have been reported sparsely in the earlier reports, but these modalities are used more routinely in present-day procedures (66,67).

In early reports no internal fixation was used (1,3,6,10,38,39). Briggs et al. (30) were the first to use a spinal implant, the Wilson spinous process plate. Subsequently, internal wire loop (5,7,22,27,31,34,45,46,49,53), Luque rectangle (5,46), Harrington

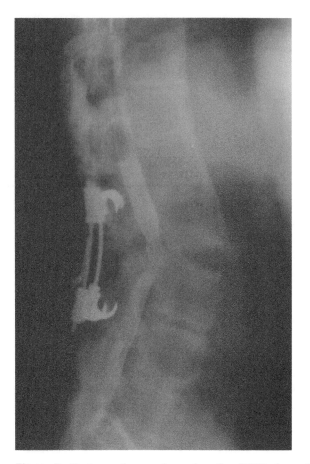

Figure 7 Postoperative myelography after OWO shows the course of the dural sac in the spinal canal. Besides a static angular deformation no significant narrowing occurs. *Abbreviation*: OWO, opening wedge osteotomy.

(11,29,38,40,43), and Wisconsin (27,38) posterior compression instrumentation have been used. Recently, pedicle screw fixation has been used to ensure immediate stability (66,67). Some authors performed lumbar osteotomies both with and without instrumentation (26,27,35,38,45,61).

For postoperative treatment, all authors advocated a plaster thoracolumbar sacral orthosis (TLSO) immobilization with one leg included. To prevent a contracture of the immobilized hip joint in patients with inflammatory involvement of the hip joints, changing the side of immobilization of the leg after two months has been advised (13). The total duration of immobilization depended on the surgical technique, the use of internal fixation, the postoperative stability, and the quality of bone. It ranges from two to four months in CWO and 6 weeks to 15 months in OWO and PWO.

Mortality

Perioperative mortality was reported in 3.5% (34 of 979 patients), mostly (76%; 26 of 34 patients) caused by postoperative pulmonary and intestinal problems, cardiac failure, and septicemia. There were 26 fatal perioperative complications in OWO, six in PWO, and two in CWO. Thus the incidence of perioperative mortality in OWO was 2.7%, in PWO 0.6%, and in CWO 0.2% (Table 1). The remaining 8 deaths out of 979 reported patients (0.8%) could be attributed to vascular complications. One patient died after a high aortic rupture because of adhesions between the aortic arch and the trachea at the level of a tracheotomy, another one died after erosion of a lumbar artery related to chronic osteomyelitis, and one died of uncontrollable bleeding from small vessels (4,12,27). In one patient, a retroperitoneal hematoma caused compression of the vena cava inferior, which led to a fatal Budd–Chiari syndrome (40). Fatal aortic rupture has been reported in four patients, all associated with anterior lengthening of the lumbar spine (19,36,24). Of these, three patients were treated by OWO (19,24). In the fourth patient, a fatal rupture of the aorta occurred after manipulation and nonsurgical correction of a severe kyphotic deformity in a patient who had been treated previously with radiation therapy for AS (36).

Technical Outcome Data Analysis

The technical outcome data of 646 patients presented in 18 reports were analyzed. For the overall technical outcome data, see Tables 3–6. For a comparison of the technical outcomes of OWO, PWO, and CWO, see Table 7. In 453 patients, the degree of surgical correction was reported. The average postoperative correction achieved in the lumbar spine ranged from 37° to 40° for the three surgical techniques (Fig. 8).

The desired angular correction of the lumbar spine with the use of PWO was not always achieved resulting in a decreased correction (Fig. 9). Unintentionally, the correction appeared to be monosegmental in several cases (2,9,40,62). Halm (40) reported a monosegmental or bisegmental correction in 19 of the 34 patients (56%), and Hehne and Zielke (9) reported a monosegmental correction in 27% of their patients. Insufficient correction or no correction at all has been reported in PWO, especially in patients with osteoporotic bone and calcification of the anterior longitudinal ligament (62). Loss of correction has been reported especially in OWO and PWO, whereas minimal loss of correction occurred in CWO (Tables 4–6). In reports with loss of correction occurring in only one or two patients, this was averaged over all reported patients (4,29). Five authors discussed lumbar osteotomy both with and without internal fixation (26,27,35,38,45). They all observed loss of correction related to patients treated without instrumentation.

Many complications have been reported. Duramater lacerations, most likely because of adhesion to the ossified ligamentum flavum in AS, were frequently reported in all surgical techniques (2,11–13,15,38,46). Transient nerve root dysfunction was

Table 3 Technical Outcome Grading Criteria

Good	Fusion and consolidation
	Loss of correction up to 10°
	No implant failure
Fair	Pseudarthrosis or loss of correction >10°
	Neuropraxia, deep infection, or re-operation
	Implant failure
Poor	No correction achieved, recurrent deformation
	Paralysis, vascular complications or fatal complications

Table 4 Comparison of Good vs. Fair and Poor Postoperative Technical Outcomes for the Open Wedge Osteotomy for Reports Fulfilling the Inclusion Criteria. The Mean Postoperative Correction, Correction at Follow-Up, and the Loss of Correction in Degrees. Range and Median in Parentheses

References	Patients (n)	Results			Correction		
		Good	Fair	Poor	Postoperative	Follow-up	Loss
Bradford et al. (29)	8	2	5	1	31 (21–41/29.5)	28 (2–41/29.5)	3.1 (0–25/0)
Camargo et al. (12)	66	62	2	2	? (22–55/?)	?	?
Goel (3)	11	9	2	0	39 (25–60/35)	?	?
Lazennec et al. (35)	19	6	12	1	41 (?/?)	?	?
McMaster (11)	14	13	1	0	37.6 (26–48/37.5)	32.9 (20–45/32.5)	4.7 (0–12/4.5)
McMaster and Coventry (4)	17	12	2	3	39[a] (20–50/36.5)	?	?
Simmons (5)	19	19	0	0	47 (30–60/?)	?	?
Styblo et al. (38)	20	13	7	0	44.4[b] (30–60/42)	39.9[b] (19–55/40)	4.5[b] (−5–40/0)
Weale et al. (27)	50	28	19	3	38.7 (15–64/?)	?	4.8 (0–20/?)
Total Mean	224	164	50	10	40.3	35.3	3.9

[a]Data reported in 16 patients.
[b]Unpublished data, personal communication.

Table 5 Comparison of Good vs. Fair and Poor Postoperative Outcomes for the Polysegmental Osteotomies for Reports Fulfilling the Inclusion Criteria. The Mean Postoperative Correction, Correction at Follow-Up, and the Loss of Correction in Degrees. Range and Median in Parentheses

		Results			Correction		
References	Patients (n)	Good	Fair	Poor	Postoperative	Follow-up	Loss
Chen (2)	16	0	6	0	26.7 (10–50/25.6)	25.8 (10–50/24)[a]	0.9
Hehne et al. (9)	177	140	29	8	46[b] (?/?)	39[b]	7[b]
Halm et al. (40)	34[c]	16	13	4	40.4 (23–67/?)	36.4	4
Van Royen et al. (62)	21	4	14	3	35.9 (0–68/36)	25.3	10.7
Total	248	170	62	15			
Mean					40.3	34.2	6.0

[a]Range between brackets.
[b]Data reported in 53 patients.
[c]No data of one patient died after two years.

Table 6 Comparison of Good vs. Fair and Poor Postoperative Outcomes for the Closing Wedge Osteotomy for Reports Fulfilling the Inclusion Criteria. The Mean Postoperative Correction, Correction at Follow-Up, and the Loss of Correction in Degrees. Range and Median in Parentheses

		Results			Correction		
References	Patients (n)	Good	Fair	Poor	Postoperative	Follow-up	Loss
Cheng et al. (66)	78	76	2	0	34.5[a] (15–60)	?	?
Kim et al. (67)	45	40	5	0	34.0	?	?
Lazennec et al. (35)	12	6	6	0	47.4 (?/?)	?	?
Thiranont and Netrawichien (46)	6	6	0	0	33.2 (20–45/33.5)	?	?
Thomasen (45)	11	10	1	0	28.3[b] (12–50/20)	?	?
Van Royen (13)	22	18	4	0	35.1[c] (25–54/34.5)	32.4	2.7
Total	174	156	18	0			
Mean					35.4	?	?

[a]Amount of correction in one-level-osteotomies, the author reported a mean correction of 62.2 (39–100) in two-level-osteotomies.
[b]Data reported in nine patients.
[c]Unpublished data.

Table 7 Surgical Technique: Comparison of the Neurological Complications and Comparison of Good vs. Fair and Poor Postoperative Outcomes for the Different Surgical Techniques of the Reports Fulfilling the Inclusion Criteria

Surgical technique	Reports (*n*)	Patients (*n*)	% Neuro-Praxia	Paralysis	Results Good	Results Fair + poor
Opening wedge osteotomy	9	224	8.5	3.1	73	27
Polysegmental osteotomies	4	247	11.3	2.0	69	31
Closing wedge osteotomy	6	174	3.6	0.6	194	18

reported equally in all surgical techniques; however, permanent neurological complications have been reported only in OWO (3.1%; 7 of 224) and PWO (2.0%; 5 of 247) (Fig. 10) (Table 7). Transient and permanent retrograde ejaculation has been reported in seven patients in OWO (27,38). Implant breakage and loosening of the rod–screw

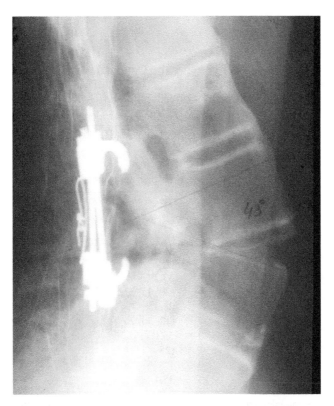

Figure 8 Postoperative lateral radiograph of the spine after OWO shows a correction of the TLKD by 43°. *Abbreviations*: OWO, opening wedge osteotomy; TLKD, throcolumbar kyphotic deformity.

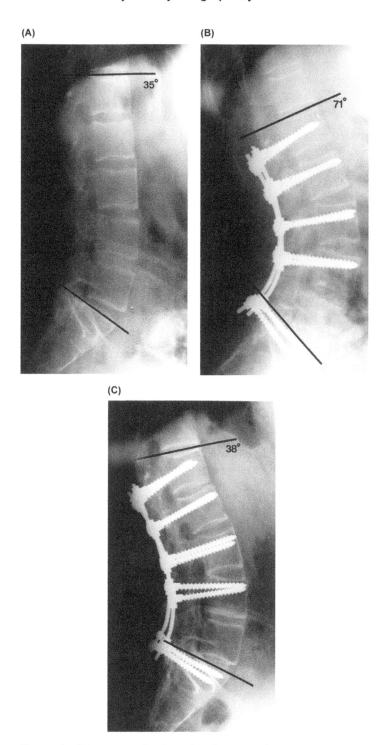

Figure 9 (**A**) Preoperative lateral radiograph of the lumbar spine from a patient with AS. (**B**) Postoperative lateral radiograph after PWO with USIS-instrumentation shows a correction of 36°. (**C**) After 82 months there is a loss of correction of 33°. Note the rod breakage at the highest two levels and failure at the junction of pedicle screw and the rod in the lowest level. *Abbreviation*: PWO, polysegmental wedge osteotomies.

(A)   (B)

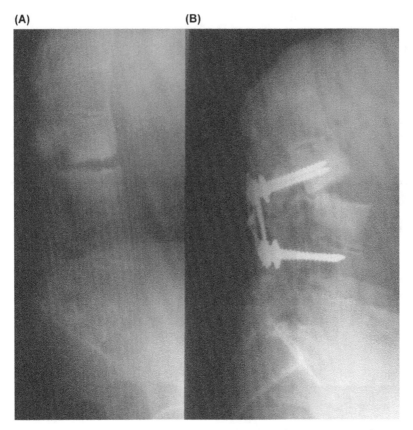

Figure 10 (**A**) Preoperative lateral radiograph of the lumbar spine from a patient with a typical Andersson lesion in AS. (**B**) Postoperative situation after OWO with unintentional retro-
listhesis at the level L2–L3. In such circumstances significant narrowing of the spinal canal and
the intervertebral foramina may occur. It is to be noted, however, that since the spine is a rigid
beam in AS, the neurological consequences of such a narrowing usually prove better than
expected. *Abbreviations*: AS, ankylosing spondylitis; OWO, opening wedge osteotomy.

connection has been reported in OWO (3.6%; 8 of 224 patients), PWO (6.5%; 16 of 248
patients) and CWO (1.7%; 3 of 174 patients). Screw breakout of the pedicle during
correction in PWO has been reported in patients with osteoporotic bone (62). Re-
operations have been reported in seven patients (3.1%) in OWO, 24 patients (9.7%)
in PWO, and four patients (2.3%) in CWO. The indication for re-operation was
neurological injury, implant failure, nonunion, deep infection, and progressive loss
of correction. Deep and superficial infections reported in some reports were as high
as 43% (3,4,13,27,35,62).

DISCUSSION

Three operative techniques have been described to correct TLKD because of AS at
the level of the lumbar spine. Which technique can be recommended? Evidence
based medicine requires the choice of a surgical technique that provides the best risk
to benefit ratio. Therefore, a reliable comparison of outcomes of the three techniques
is necessary. However, such a comparison has not yet been reported.

The most important result to emerge from the above review is that it cannot be concluded that one surgical technique is preferable over the other. This conclusion is based on the fact that there were no appreciable differences in mean postoperative correction and complication rates among the three surgical techniques. The present analysis showed that the average postoperative correction achieved in CWO was 3.8° less than in OWO or PWO; however, meaningful interpretation of this difference is not feasible because of the great range of the amount of correction presented. Another reason was insufficiently reported correction at final follow-up in 9 out of the 18 analyzed reports.

It should be noted also that in the last decade there are no more reports on OWO, and surgeons focused their attention on CWO.

Complications

Three types of complications were associated with lumbar osteotomy for the correction of TLKD in AS: (i) loss of correction, (ii) vascular complications, and (iii) neurological complications. Firstly, AS related osteoporosis increases the chance of loss of correction or insufficient correction by implant loosening, implant failure, and pull-out of the laminar hooks and screw breakout of the pedicle (27,29,38,62). These complications have been reported in OWO and PWO especially (Fig. 9) (3,29,33,34,50,62). Theoretically, this may be explained by a technique related lack of primary anterior stability. In case of insufficient correction, the center of gravity of the thorax will remain too far anterior of the spine. As a result, the posterior fusion zone and implants are placed under considerable tension. This increases the risk of implant failure, delayed union or nonunion, and inevitable loss of spinal correction. Secondly, the risk of rupture of the aorta or its branches associated with the anterior lengthening of the lumbar spine in OWO is mentioned in many reports (1,6,9,13,17). Although this risk showed to be small (0.9%; 4 of 450 patients), it cannot be ignored (19,24,36). Vascular injury has been reported if the opening wedge was performed at the level L1–L2 and L2–L3. However, no vascular injury has been reported in association with procedures below level L3. Thirdly, lumbar osteotomy inevitably carries the risk of neurological complications. Displacement of a vertebral body causing a neurological deficit has been referred as a potential risk in lumbar osteotomy (6,26,30,45,49). This has been reported in six patients treated by OWO (2.7%) and in one patient (0.6%) treated by CWO (35,45,53). In these patients, no or insufficient internal fixation was mentioned as the cause of vertebral displacement.

Do the results of this study imply that there is no preference at all for one of the surgical techniques? In my opinion the answer to this question is no. Although this review showed no differences between the corrections achieved by the three surgical techniques, the technical outcome data showed that with the use of CWO there is a tendency toward less serious complications. Permanent neurological complications were not reported in CWO. In addition, it should be noted that in the past years several authors have reported on CWO, not only for AS but also for angular kyphotic deformities (69,70). Such is the case after trauma, congenital deformity, infection, or spinal tumors. The technique described in these reports is a method transpedicular to CWO that has been technically refined and it avoids the use of sudden forces in correcting the spine. It is rather a closing osteoclasis than an opening wedge. Furthermore, loss of correction in CWO was minimal, most probably because of the two cancellous surfaces of the vertebral osteotomy ensuring a rapid consolidation after closure. However, the maximum correction achieved with this technique is restricted by the anatomical limitations of one vertebral body. This showed to be about 35° (15–54°) (Fig. 8). Interestingly, some authors report a correction as high as 75° in CWO (35). The only way to explain such a correction by CWO is by fracturing of the anterior hinge of the osteotomy, thus transforming it into OWO. In these instances, additional benefit may be obtained from pedicle screw fixation, since this will lock the corrected position like a tension band (17).

Another important result of this study is that the indications for operative treatment were generally poorly defined. Preoperative clinical or radiographic assessment of the kyphotic deformity was mentioned in few (5 of 41) reports, and one referred textbook (13,29,38,48,61,62). This is not surprising, as there are no standardized parameters for the preoperative and postoperative evaluation of the severity of TLKD due to AS. Different authors suggest different parameters. Assessment of the chin–brow to vertical angle is easy to use; however, its reproducibility and reliability are not known (61,62). Another method is the assessment of TLKD on a standing lateral radiograph of the whole spine (29). On these radiographs, measurements of the horizontal distance from S1 to the sagittal vertical axis or the C7 plumb line are suggested. These measurements, however, are found to differ depending on small changes of the angles of the hip, knee, and ankle joints and therefore are not accurate (63). Furthermore, the exact position of landmarks C7 and S1, and the position of the long cassette film to the horizon are also not known.

One recent report presented patients treated by OWO and CWO (35). However, the authors did not compare the results of these two techniques. It can be questioned why there are no studies available comparing different techniques of lumbar osteotomy in AS. The explanation is twofold. Firstly, the number of patients treated by lumbar osteotomy for TLKD due to AS is low and decreasing, most probably because of successful conservative treatment. Our study showed that reports on lumbar osteotomy are sparse indeed, and that only few authors have experience with a larger number of patients. Secondly, there are no standardized methods for assessing the sagittal deformity of the spine, and accurate preoperative planning including the degree of correction required and the level to operate on (for further details on deformity planning in AS see chap. 10). As a result, investigators simply lack adequate data to perform a reliable comparative study.

Functional outcome analysis and measuring quality of life is important in surgery for TLKD because of AS. Only two authors reported functional and clinical outcome data in spinal osteotomy (41,67). Halm (40,41) used a questionnaire to study retrospectively patients treated in the 1970s and 1980s. Kim (67) prospectively studied 45 patients treated with a CWO, offering the most detailed clinical outcome study so far. All other reports focus on operative technique, degree of correction, and complication rate. Ideally, a study should evaluate the outcome of the operative procedure on the effect it produces on the patient's quality of life. However, workable methods to assess quality of life in patients with AS have only been developed recently (64,65,67). In line with the technical developments in spinal surgery and the present-day relative constancy of the spinal correction achieved, it is to be expected that future studies will put more emphasis on clinical outcome than on technical outcome (67).

CONCLUSIONS

The structured review of the literature concerning three methods of lumbar osteotomy for correction of TLKD attributable to AS showed that the number of reliable reports is limited and that they provide scant information on clinical data. Statistical analysis of the technical outcome data from these surgical methods was therefore not possible. Although the available data from the current literature suggest that CWO causes less serious complications and has better results, these data are not suitable yet for decision-making with regard to which surgical treatment is preferable. Furthermore, there is a need for a generally accepted clinical score that encompasses accurate measurements needed for preoperative and postoperative assessment of the spinal deformity in these patients. Such scores are under development at the present time.

REFERENCES

1. Bossers GT. Columnotomy in severe Bechterew kyphosis. Acta Orthop Belg 1972; 38: 47–54.
2. Chen PQ. Correction of kyphotic deformity in ankylosing spondylitis using multiple spinal osteotomy and Zielke's VDS instruments. J Formos Med Assoc 1988; 87:692–698.
3. Goel MK. Vertebral osteotomy for correction of fixed flexion deformity of the spine. J Bone Joint Surg 1968; 50-A:287–294.
4. McMaster MJ, Coventry MB. Spinal osteotomy in ankylosing spondylitis: technique, complications, and long-term results. Mayo Clin Proc 1973; 48:476–487.
5. Simmons EH. Kyphotic deformity of the spine in ankylosing spondylitis. Clin Orthop 1977; 128:65–77.
6. Adams JC. Technique, dangers and safeguards in osteotomy of the spine. J Bone Joint Surg 1952; 34-B:226–232.
7. Dawson CW. Posterior elementectomy in ankylosing arthritis of the spine. Clin Orthop 1957; 10:274–281.
8. Gerscovich EO, Greenspan A, Montesano PX. Treatment of kyphotic deformity in ankylosing spondylitis. Orthopedics 1994; 17:335–342.
9. Hehne HJ, Zielke K, Böhm H. Polysegmental lumbar osteotomies and transpedicular fixation for correction of long-curved kyphotic deformities in ankylosing spondylitis. Report on 177 cases. Clin Orthop 1990; 258:49–55.
10. Smith-Petersen MN, Larson CB, Aufranc OE. Osteotomy of the spine for correction of flexion deformity in rheumatoid arthritis. J Bone Joint Surg 1945; 27:1–11.
11. McMaster MJ. A technique for lumbar spinal osteotomy in ankylosing spondylitis. J Bone Joint Surg 1985; 67-B:204–210.
12. Camargo FP, Cordeiro EN, Napoli MM. Corrective osteotomy of the spine in ankylosing spondylitis. Experience with 66 cases. Clin Orthop 1986; 208:157–167.
13. Van Royen BJ, Slot GH. Closing-wedge posterior osteotomy for ankylosing spondylitis. Partial corporectomy and transpedicular fixation in 22 cases. J Bone Joint Surg 1995; 77-B: 117–121.
14. Chapchal G. Operative treatment of severe kyphosis as the result of Bechterew's disease. Arch Chir Neerl 1949; 1:57–63.
15. Emnéus H. Wedge osteotomy of spine in ankylosing spondylitis. Acta Orthop Scand 1968; 39:321–326.
16. Hähnel H. Erste Erfahrungen mit operativen Kyphosekorrekturen bei M. Bechterew und M. Scheuermann. Beitr Orthop Traumatol 1988; 35:153–160.
17. Jaffray D, Becker V, Eisenstein S. Closing wedge osteotomy with transpedicular fixation in ankylosing spondylitis. Clin Orthop 1992; 279:122–126.
18. Kallio KE. Osteotomy of the spine in ankylosing spondylitis. Ann Chir Gynaec Fenn 1963; 52:615–619.
19. Klems VH, Friedebold G. Ruptur der Aorta abdominalis nach Aufrichtungs-operation bei Spondylitis Ankylopoetica. Z Orthop 1971; 108:554–563.

20. La Chapelle EH. Osteotomy of the lumbar spine for correction of kyphosis in a case of ankylosing spondylarthritis. J Bone Joint Surg 1946; 28:851–858.

21. Schubert T, Polak K. Ergebnisse der operativen Behandlung von Patienten mit Spondylarthritis ankylopoetica. Beitr Orthop Traumatol 1988; 5:290–295.

22. Scudese VA, Calabro JJ. Vertebral wedge osteotomy. Correction of rheumatoid (ankylosing) spondylitis. J Am Med Assoc 1963; 186:627–631.

23. Stuart FW, Rose GK. Ankylosing spondylitis treated by osteotomy of the spine. Br Med J 1950; 1:165–166.

24. Weatherley C, Jaffray D, Terry A. Vascular complications associated with osteotomy in ankylosing spondylitis: a report of two cases. Spine 1988; 13:43–46.

25. Wilson MJ, Turkell JH. Multiple spinal wedge osteotomy. Its use in a case of Marie Strümpell spondylitis. Am J Surg 1949; 77:777–782.

26. Law WA. Osteotomy of the spine. Clin Orthop 1969; 66:70–76.

27. Weale AE, Marsh CH, Yeoman PM. Secure fixation of lumbar osteotomy. Surgical experience with 50 patients. Clin Orthop 1995; 321:216–222.

28. Ziwjan JL. Die behandlung der Flexionsdeformitäten der Wirbelsäule bei der Bechterewschen Erkrankung. Beitr Orthop Traumatol 1982; 29:195–199.

29. Bradford DS, Schumacher WL, Lonstein JE, Winter RB. Ankylosing spondylitis: experience in surgical management of 21 patients. Spine 1987; 12:238–243; Erratum: 590–592.

30. Briggs H, Keats S, Schlesinger PT. Wedge osteotomy of the spine with bilateral, intervertebral foraminotomy: correction of flexion deformity in five cases of ankylosing arthritis of the spine. J Bone Joint Surg 1947; 29:1075–1082.

31. Donaldson JR. Osteotomy of the spine for kyphus due to Marie-Strümpell's arthritis. Indian J Surg 1959; 21:400–402.

32. Herbert JJ. Vertebral osteotomy, technique, indications and results. J Bone Joint Surg 1948; 30-A:680–689.

33. Herbert JJ. Vertebral osteotomy for kyphosis, especially in Marie-Strümpell Arthritis. J Bone Joint Surg 1959; 41-A:291–302.

34. Junghanns H. Operative rehabilitation bei spondylitis ankylopoetica. Therapiewoche 1971; 24:1835–1838.

35. Lazennec JY, Saillant G, Saidi K, et al. Surgery of deformities in ankylosing spondylitis: our experience of lumbar osteotomies in 31 patients. Eur Spine J 1997; 6:222–232.

36. Lichtblau PO, Wilson PD. Possible mechanism of aorta rupture in orthopaedic correction of rheumatoid spondylitis. J Bone Joint Surg 1956; 38-A:123–127.

37. McMaster PE. Osteotomy of the spine for fixed flexion deformity. J Bone Joint Surg 1962; 44A:1207–1216.

38. Styblo K, Bossers GT, Slot GH. Osteotomy for kyphosis in ankylosing spondylitis. Acta Orthop Scand 1985; 56:294–297.

39. Thompson WAL, Ingersoll RE. Osteotomy for correction of deformity in Marie-Strümpell arthritis. Surg Gynecol Obstet 1950; 90:552–556.

40. Halm H, Metz-Stevenhagen P, Schmidtt A, Zielke K. Operatieve Behandlung kyphotischer Wirbelsäulendeformitäten bei der Spondylitis ankylosans mit dem Harrington-Kompressions system: Langzeitergebnisse auf der Basis der MOPO-Skalen im Rahmen einer retrospektiven Fragenbogenerhebung. Z Orthop 1995; 133:141–147.

41. Halm H, Metz-Stevenhagen P, Zielke K. Results of surgical correction of kyphotic deformities of the spine in ankylosing spondylitis on the basis of the modified arthritis impact measurement scales. Spine 1995; 20:1612–1619.

42. Hehne HJ, Becker HJ, Zielke K. Die Spondylodiszitis bei kyphotischer Deformität der Spondylitis ankylosans und ihre Ausheilung durch dorsale Korrekturosteotomien. Bericht über 33 Patienten. Z Orthop 1990; 128:494–502.

43. Püschel J, Zielke K. Korrekturoperation bei Bechterew-Kyphose. Indikation, Technik, Ergebnisse. Z Orthop 1982; 120:338–342.

44. Zielke K, Rodegerds U. Operative Behandlung der fixierten Kyphose bei "Spondylitis ankylosans". Indikation, Komplikationen und Ergebnisse. Vorläufiger Bericht über 78 Fälle. Z Orthop 1985; 123:679–682.
45. Thomasen E. Vertebral osteotomy for correction of kyphosis in ankylosing spondylitis. Clin Orthop 1985; 194:142–152.
46. Thiranont N, Netrawichien P. Transpedicular decancellation closed wedge vertebral osteotomy for treatment of fixed flexion deformity of spine in ankylosing spondylitis. Spine 1993; 18:2517–2522.
47. Simmons EH. Relation of vascular complication to the level of lumbar extension osteotomy in ankylosing spondylitis. Presented at the 61st Annual Meeting of the American Academy of Orthopaedic Surgeons, New Orleans, USA, Feb 25, 1994.
48. Böhm H, Hehne HJ, Zielke K. Die Korrektur der Bechterew Kyphose. Orthopäde 1989; 18:142–154.
49. Law WA. Lumbar spine osteotomy. J Bone Joint Surg Br 1959; 41-B:270–278.
50. Law WA. Osteotomy of the spine. J Bone Joint Surg Am 1962; 44-A:1199–1206.
51. Püschel J. Korrekturosteotomien beim M. Bechterew-Kyphose. Technik, Ergebnisse. Z Orthop 1981; 119:823–824.
52. Roy-Camille R, Henry P, Saillant G, Doursounian L. Chirurgie des grandes cyphoses vertebrales de la spondylarthrite ankylosante. Rev Rhum Mal Osteoartic 1987; 54:261–267.
53. Chapchal G. Columnotomy in severe Bechterew kyphosis. Acta Orthop Belg 1972; 38:55–58.
54. Dahmen G. Operative Behandlung der Bechterewschen Erkrankung. Med Monatsschr 1972; 26:194–201.
55. Junghanns H. Aufrichtungsoperation bei spondylitis ankylopoetica (Bechterew). Dtsch Med Wochenschr 1968; 93:1592–1594.
56. Junghanns H. Operative Behandlung schwerer Kyphosen und Hüftarthrosen bei ankylosierender Spondylitis. Verh Dtsch Ges Rheumatol 1969; 1:171–178.
57. Law WA. Surgical treatment of the rheumatic diseases. J Bone Joint Surg Br 1952; 34-B:215–225.
58. Law WA. President's address. Ankylosing spondylitis and spinal osteotomy. Proceedings of the Royal Society of Medicine 1976; 69:715–720.
59. Morscher E, Müller W. Operative Korrektur fixierter Kyphosen. Orthopäde 1973; 2:193–200.
60. Hehne HJ, Zielke K. Die Kyphotische Deformität bei Spondylitis ankylosans. Klinik, Radiologie und Therapie. In: Schulitz KP, ed. Die Wirbelsäule in Forschung und Praxis Vol. 112. Stuttgart: Hippocrates Verlag, 1990:32–69.
61. Simmons EH. Ankylosing spondylitis: surgical considerations. In: Rothman RH, Simeone FA, eds. The Spine, Vol. 2. 3rd ed. Philadelphia: WB Saunders, 1992:1447–1511.
62. Van Royen BJ, De Kleuver M, Slot GH. Polysegmental lumbar posterior wedge osteotomies for correction of kyphosis in ankylosing spondylitis. Eur Spine J 1998; 7:104–110.
63. Van Royen BJ, Toussaint HM, Kingma I, et al. Accuracy of the sagittal vertical axis in a standing lateral radiograph as a measurement of balance in spinal deformities. Eur Spine J 1998; 7:408–412.
64. Abbott CA, Helliwell PS, Chamberlain MA. Functional assessment in ankylosing spondylitis: evaluation of a new self-administered questionnaire and correlation with antropometric variables. Br J Rheumatol 1994; 33:1060–1066.
65. Kennedy LG, Jenkinson TR, Mallorie PA, Whitelock HC, Garrett SL, Calin A. Ankylosing spondylitis: the correlation between a new metrology score and radiology. Br J Rheumatol 1995; 34:767–770.
66. Cheng I-H, Chien J-T, Yu T-C. Transpedicular wedge osteotomy for correction of thoracolumbar kyphosis in ankylosing spondylitis. Spine 2001; 26:354–360.

67. Kim K-T, Suk K-S, Cho Y-J, Hong G-P, Park B-J. Clinical outcome results of pedicle subtraction osteotomy in ankylosing spondylitis with kyphotic deformity. Spine 2002; 27:612–618.
68. Suk K-S, Kim K-T, Lee S-H, Kim J-M. Significance of chin–brow vertical angle in correction of kyphotic deformity of ankylosing spondylitis patients. Spine 2003; 28: 2001–2005.
69. Kawahara N, Tomita K, Baba H, Kobayashi T, Fujita T, Murakami H. Closing–opening wedge osteotomy to correct angular kyphotic deformity by a single posterior approach. Spine 2001; 4:391–402.
70. Bridwell KH, Lewis SJ, Edwards C, et al. Complications and outcomes of pedicle subtraction osteotomies for fixed sagittal imbalance. Spine 2003; 18:2093–2101.

16

Image-Based Planning and Computer Assisted Surgery in Ankylosing Spondylitis

Michael Ruf, Viktor Moser, and Jürgen Harms
Department of Spinal Surgery, Klinikum Karlsbad-Langensteinbach, Karlsbad, Germany

INTRODUCTION

Ankylosing spondylitis is a chronic inflammatory disease leading to increasing stiffness and kyphotic deformity of the spine. Conservative treatment, especially intensive physiotherapy, is necessary to keep patients mobile and to prevent deformity as long as possible. Despite these efforts, in many patients ankylosis progresses from the lumbar and thoracic spine to the cervical spine. These patients end up in a fixed kyphosis of the thoracolumbar spine without the possibility to compensate in the cervical region.

The horizontal gaze becomes increasingly difficult for the patient. To obtain an upright position, the patient tilts his pelvis back with retroversion of the sacrum. This compensatory rotation of the pelvis leads to a continuous hyperextension of the hip joints, which may cause additional pain. Besides, this hyperextension is often limited by an accompanying coxarthritis in the ankylosing spondylitis patient. The patient then has to bend his knees in an attempt to assume the upright position.

Surgical therapy has to facilitate the patient's life with his stiff spine. The aims of surgical therapy, therefore, are:

- To restore the sagittal profile,
- To normalize the gravity line,
- To normalize the position of the sacrum and pelvis, and
- To normalize the position of the head.

Normalization of the pelvic tilt reduces the stress in the hip joints due to hyperextension. The normalization of the gravity line reduces the muscle strain that is necessary to balance the trunk in an upright standing position. Normalization of the head position allows for a horizontal gaze without painful hyperextension of the possibly still flexible cervical spine.

To meet these requirements and to achieve predictable surgical results with optimal correction of the malformation, precise preoperative planning and exact surgical realization is required.

Since the spine in an advanced ankylosing spondylitis is a rigid piece of bone, the effect of a defined correction osteotomy on the overall sagittal profile is predictable by simple mathematical calculations. The angle and the level of this calculated correction osteotomy is then realized during surgery. The ideal device to transfer the preoperative planning to surgery is an appropriate navigation system. The data of the calculated osteotomy are entered into the navigation system, and the system allows precise corrective procedures along premarked lines with image guided tools.

A technique of preoperative planning and surgical realization, and results thereof in patients afflicted by ankylosing spondylitis has been described below (1).

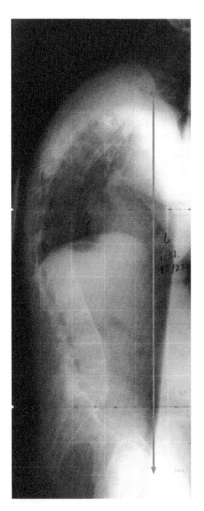

Figure 1   Lateral radiograph of a 40-year-old patient with ankylosing spondylitis in standing position.

PREOPERATIVE PLANNING

Preliminary Remarks

Planning of the correction should consider the following aspects:

- Effect on the position of the head (line of vision),
- Effect on the gravity line,
- Effect on the position of the sacrum and the pelvis, and
- Technical requirements.

Two variables have to be determined:

1. The level of the osteotomy and
2. The angle of correction.

When we select the level of the osteotomy we have to consider its influence on the overall sagittal profile as well as its technical requirements. Correction with a predetermined angle via a fulcrum close to the sacrum has more impact on the gravity line than correction with the same angle via a more cranial pivot. The impact on the inclination of the head, which depends only on the angle of correction, is affected similarly. To achieve a maximum effect on the gravity line, the osteotomy should be performed as caudally as possible. Furthermore, an osteotomy in the lumbar spine is technically less demanding and associated with minor neurological risk

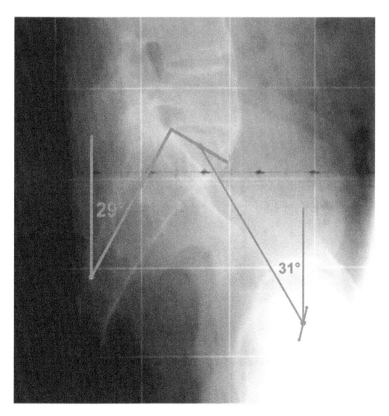

Figure 2   The pelvis is rotated backwards to allow an upright standing position: sacral slope 29°, sacrofemoral tilt 31°.

in comparison with osteotomy in the thoracic spine. On the other hand, a certain distance of the osteotomy from the sacrum is required for sufficient distal fixation in the usually osteoporotic bone. Accordingly, L3 is usually the favored osteotomy site. This level has sufficient effect on the gravity line and concurs ideally with the technical requirements. There are, however, a few cases that require an osteotomy in the thoracic or cervical spine, mostly in posttraumatic cases or patients with Anderson lesions.

The selection of the correction angle has to consider its influence on the overall sagittal profile, especially gravity line, head inclination, and tilt of the pelvis. We have to normalize the gravity line to enable the patient to stand upright comfortably in a position where muscle activity is minimized. The optimal gravity line in ankylosing spondylitis patients is not yet well defined. In our opinion the plumb line from the center of the vertebral body of C7 should fall behind the center of the femoral heads through the endplate of S1 close to the anterior edge of S1. Equally important is normalization of sacral inclination to avoid continuous hyperextension of the hip

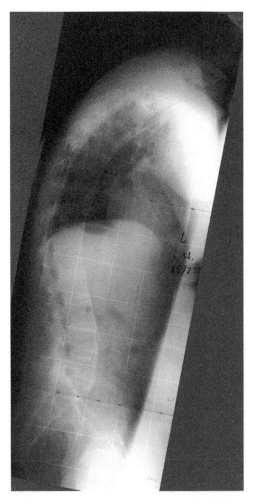

Figure 3 The radiograph is rotated (11° clockwise) to achieve a normal sacral slope of 40°. The pivot is defined at the level of L3.

joints or, what is worse, the bending of knees while standing. The head should obtain a neutral or slightly anteflexed position to allow the patient to observe his feet.

Preoperative Planning

Anteropostero and lateral radiographs of the entire spine including sacrum and hip joints were obtained in a standing position (Figs. 1 and 2).

The first step of the planning procedure is virtual correction of the retroversion of the sacrum, thereby achieving correction of the pelvic tilt. The lateral radiograph of the whole spine is digitized and entered into a computer drawing program. The radiograph is then rotated to a normal sacral slope of 40–45°. The level of osteotomy is defined, in most cases at the level L3 (Fig. 3).

In a second step, the upper part of the radiograph (above the osteotomy level) is rotated backwards. The fulcrum of this rotation is situated near the superior–anterior cortex of the predetermined vertebra at the osteotomy level. This fulcrum

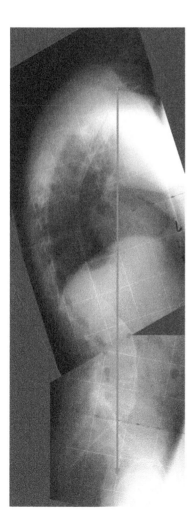

Figure 4   The upper part of the spine (above L3) is rotated backwards, until the gravity line is normalized: 28° anticlockwise. This represents the planned correction angle.

corresponds to the tip of the wedge in a closing wedge resection. The virtual reclination is continued until the gravity line is normalized, i.e., until the plumb line from the center of C7 passes behind the centers of the hip joints near the anterior edge of the sacral endplate (Fig. 4). The angle of rotation of the upper part of the radiograph which is necessary to achieve normalization of the gravity line is the planned angle for surgical correction (correction angle). Thus, the correction angle comprises anterior rotation of the pelvis and posterior rotation of the spine above the osteotomy. Indeed, animation allows for assessment of the expected postoperative overall sagittal profile and for the prediction of head inclination.

Correction angle should not exceed 35° per osteotomy level. Otherwise, the common foramen of the two nerve roots around the osteotomy will become too narrow. If more correction is necessary, a second osteotomy should be planned.

Transfer to the Navigation System

The correction angle is then transferred to the navigation system (Brainlab™). For this, computed tomography (CT) of the level of the osteotomy and the adjacent vertebrae is performed. The CT scans are entered into the computer of the

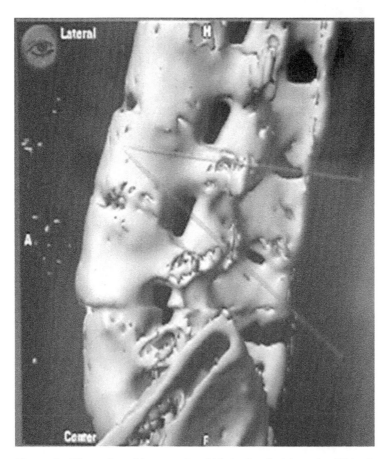

Figure 5   The wedge with an angle of 28° is sketched into the CT in the navigation system. *Abbrevation*: CT, computed tomography.

navigation system. The navigation system allows for three-dimensional preoperative planning. The dimensions of the wedge to be resected is sketched in the CT scans of the patient (Fig. 5). The tip of the wedge is situated approximately 5 mm behind the anterior cortex of the osteotomy vertebra. The upper osteotomy plane is parallel to the upper endplate a few millimeters below this endplate. The lower osteotomy plane descends from the tip with the calculated correction angle, thus creating a posterior based wedge. This wedge includes the pedicles of the osteotomy vertebra.

IMAGE-GUIDED SURGICAL PROCEDURE

During surgery, the patient is placed in a prone position supported at the pelvis and the upper rib cage. A posterior approach is performed, exposing the posterior aspect of the osteotomy vertebra including the transverse processes and the adjacent verte-brae. After fixing the reference array, registration of the patients' spine into the navi-gation system is performed. This may be more difficult due to the shape of the spine

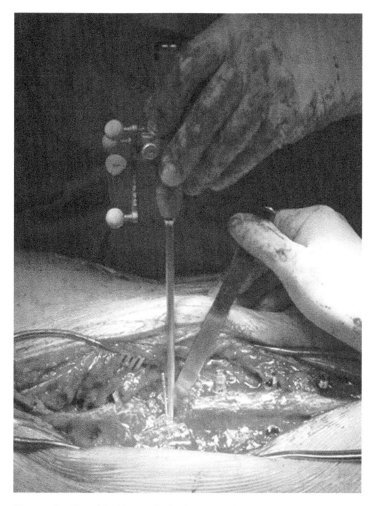

Figure 6   The chisel is marked with the reflector array of the navigation system.

and the synostosis of the vertebrae. CT-fluoro matching is usually impracticable, since anteropostero X-ray images of the kyphotic spine with the decreased inner width of the C-arm due to the registration kit is impossible. In our experience, best results are obtained by surface matching. Once registration is performed, the navigation system can be used with good precision along the entire ankylosed spine. Pedicle screws are inserted in the vertebrae adjacent to the osteotomy level, usually three vertebrae above and three vertebrae below.

Correction is achieved by a pedicle subtraction closing wedge osteotomy (2,3). After resection of the posterior elements of the vertebra, the dura and nerve roots are identified. The pedicles and the transverse processes are removed, and the lateral aspect of the vertebral body is exposed. The wedge osteotomy of the vertebral body is performed with assistance of the navigation system. An image-guided chisel is advanced along the preplanned osteotomy planes, and the calculated posterior based wedge of the vertebra is removed (Figs. 6 and 7). The guided cut on each side of the spinal cord creates identical wedges in the same plane. These even resection planes fit perfectly on each other when correction is performed. During resection at one side, a rod is fixed at the contralateral side for stabilization. After complete resection of the calculated wedge, the created gap is closed completely by compression via the rods, and the preplanned correction is achieved (Figs. 8–12).

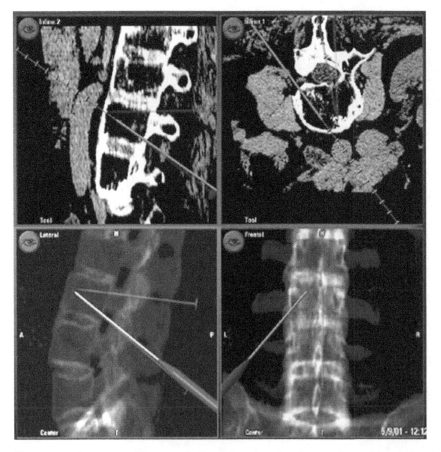

Figure 7 The osteotomies are performed under visual control on the screen along the marked lines, thus creating a wedge of exactly 28°.

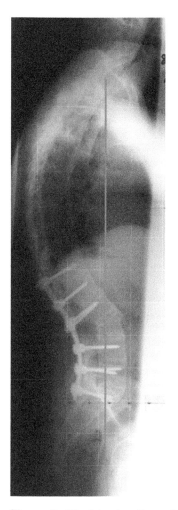

Figure 8 The lateral radiograph postoperatively with normalized gravity line.

RESULTS

Seven patients with ankylosing spondylitis underwent posterior lumbar pedicle subtraction osteotomies with the assistance of a navigation system between November 2000 and September 2003 at the Department for Orthopaedics, Center for Spinal Surgery, Klinikum Karlsbad-Langensteinbach. Six patients were male, one patient was female. Average age at time of surgery was 44 years (range, 40–56 years). Osteotomy was performed at L3 in all patients; in one case an additional osteotomy was performed at T12. Segmental transpedicular instrumentation was performed from T12 to S1 in three patients, from T10 to S1 in two patients. In one patient with additional osteotomy at T12, the instrumentation was extended from T8 to S1; in one patient with additional Anderson lesion at T11/12 the instrumentation was performed from T9 to S1. The average operation time was 306 minutes (range, 230–445 minutes), the average blood loss was 2740 mL (range, 1000–6000 mL). All patients were mobilized within the first postoperative week. A brace or cast was used for 12 weeks. A solid fusion without any loss of correction was achieved in

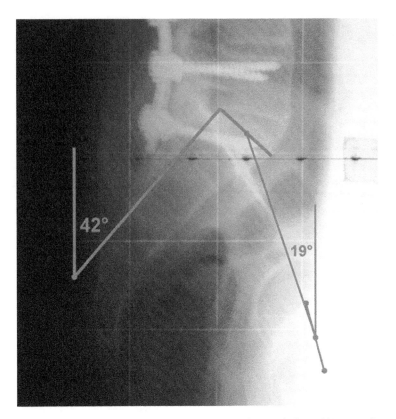

Figure 9 The pelvic parameters are corrected: sacral slope 42°, sacrofemoral tilt 19°.

all patients. There was no neurologic deficit. In two patients there were liquor effusions that required revision surgery with closure of the dural tear. Follow-up time
averaged 10 months (range, 2–25 months).

The preoperative calculation of the planned correction angle at the level of L3
varied between 24 and 35° (Table 1). In the patient with 35°, a second osteotomy was
planned at the level of T12 for complete correction of the gravity line. These angles
were marked in the sagittal CT reconstruction and entered into the navigation
system. Registration of the CT scans in the operating room was performed by surface matching in four patients, and by CT-fluoro matching in one patient. In two
early cases, navigation was performed in a lateral fluoro image.

Postoperatively, radiographs of the whole spine in a standing position were
taken. The real correction angle at the osteotomy level was evaluated and compared
to the preoperative planned angle. In all patients, the measured correction angle
corresponded to the planned angle within a range of few degrees. The difference
between real and planned angle had an average of 3° (range, 1–6°).

Corresponding to the realization of the scheduled wedge osteotomy, the overall
sagittal profile and the posture of the patients improved. The sacral slope and the
sagittal alignment (gravity line from the center of C7 in relation to the posterior
superior aspect of S1) were measured on whole spine radiographs in standing
position. Patients were asked to stand in their usual posture. Preoperatively, the
average sacral slope was 23° (range, −6° to 40°), improved to 40° postoperatively
(range, 27–49°), and was 41° at latest follow-up (range, 27–48°). The gravity line

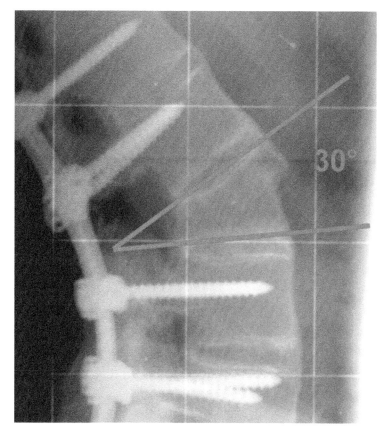

Figure 10 A wedge of 30° has been resected.

averaged 112 mm preoperatively (range, 47–196 mm), 31 mm postoperatively (range, −7 mm to 135 mm), and 35 mm at latest follow-up (range, −44 mm to 137 mm).

DISCUSSION

Surgical treatment of the fixed thoracolumbar kyphosis in ankylosing spondylitis is still a challenging problem. Various techniques have been described: opening wedge osteotomies (4–7), polysegmental osteotomies (8,9), and closing wedge osteotomies (2,3,10–12). An excellent lordosating effect with a minimum of neurologic risk is achieved by lumbar closing wedge osteotomies.

But up to now there is no generally accepted procedure for planning the level and angle of the correction osteotomy. It is necessary to predict the effect of the surgical procedure on the overall postoperative posture. A good clinical outcome requires normalization of the position of the pelvis, balance of the trunk over the hip joints, and horizontalization of the line of vision. A measurable parameter for the pelvic tilt is the sacral slope angle; a parameter for the balance is the gravity line. These parameters are taken from a lateral radiograph of the whole spine in standing position. It is more difficult to assess the head position, mainly, the line of vision.

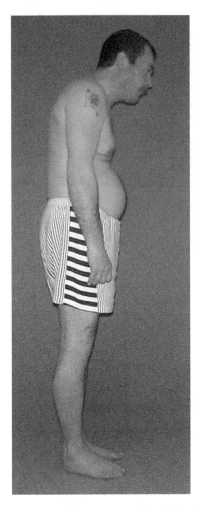

Figure 11   The preoperative clinical picture of the same patient as in the radiographs.

A measurable parameter is the chin–brow to vertical angle. This angle, however, is taken from a clinical picture, and not directly related to the radiographic findings (13).

The technique described above allows for an exact preoperative planning with predictable results regarding pelvic tilt and balance of the trunk. The exact surgical realization of the planned correction osteotomy is as important as the meticulous planning. The connecting link between planning and surgery is the navigation system. By means of image-guided tools, the surgeon is enabled to resect precisely the preoperatively planned wedge. Shape, angle, and localization of the wedge in relation to the spine are shown on the screen. The surgeon is able to control continuously, if the wedge he is going to excise corresponds to the sketched wedge on the screen. He further controls the assumed pivot at the tip of the wedge. In addition, the navigation facilitates the resection of identical wedges at both sides of the dura. By closing the created gap completely the precalculated correction angle is achieved.

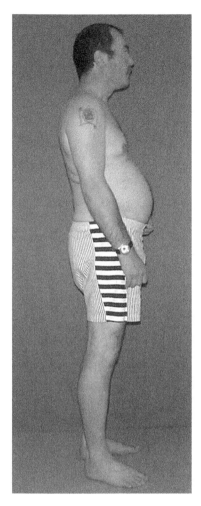

Figure 12 The postoperative standing position is much more relaxed, the gaze is horizontal.

In our patient group we achieved a good correction of the line of vision. But we are aware of the fact that the head position, for example, chin–brow angle, is not taken into consideration in the planning procedure described above. In cases with a fixed cervical spine, the following procedure would be applicable: An additional lateral radiograph (film with grid) of the spine is performed with the patient asked to keep his head in the upright position he likes to have postoperatively (similar to the technique described by Van Royen) (14). The trunk leans back in standing or sitting position to achieve this desired head position. The angle of the spine on this radiograph is compared to the angle of the upper part of the spine on the preoperative plan described above. If there is more reclination desired to restore the head position, a more cranial osteotomy level should be considered; a more cranial pivot requires a greater angle to restore the gravity line and therefore has more impact on the head position. If less reclination of the head is desired, a more caudal pivot is useful. In case these angles are difficult to reconcile, a second osteotomy at the cervical spine should be considered (15).

Table 1 Pre- and Postoperative Angle of the Osteotomy, Gravity Line and Sacral Slope

	Age/ sex	Osteotomy level	Instrumentation	Nav.-registration	Angle of wedge osteotomy				Gravity line (C7-post. edge S1)			Sacral slope		
					Planned	Postop.	Follow-up	Diff.	Preop.	Postop.	Follow-up	Preop.	Postop.	Follow-up
1	47/M	L3, D12	D8-S1	Lat. fluoro	35	41	41	6	196	135	137	−6	44	45
2	42/M	L3	D10-S1	Lat. fluoro	30	26	26	4	102	34	34	16	27	27
3	42/M	L3	D10-S1	Surface matching	29	27	27	2	47	−7	15	18	39	42
4	56/F	L3	D12-S1	CT-fluoro matching	24	22	21	2	85	7	18	40	49	48
5	41/M	L3	D12-S1	Surface matching	24	28	27	4	60	0	−44	23	38	34
6	40/M	L3	D12-S1	Surface matching	28	29	30	1	110	14	9	29	43	42
7	42/M	L3	D9-S1	Surface matching	30	31	32	1	184	37	78	40	42	46
Average					29	29	29	3	112	31	35	23	40	41

Abbreviation: CT, computed tomography.

CONCLUSION

The technique described is a reliable procedure to plan and realize a precise correction osteotomy in ankylosing spondylitis. A balanced spinal profile with restoration of the pelvic tilt and horizontalization of the line of vision is achieved. The use of a navigation system increases the precision and safety of the osteotomy.

REFERENCES

1. Ruf M, Moser V, Harms J. Posterior lumbar pedicle subtraction osteotomy—preoperative planning and image guided surgery. Poster Presented at the 8th International Meeting on Advanced Spine Techniques, Nassau, Bahamas, July 12–14, 2001.
2. Lehmer SM, Keppler L, Biscup RS, Enker P, Miller SD, Steffee AD. Posterior transvertebral osteotomy for adult thoracolumbar kyphosis. Spine 1994; 19(18):2060–2067.
3. Thomasen E. Vertebral osteotomy for correction of kyphosis in ankylosing spondylitis. Clin Orthop 1985; 194:142–151.
4. Smith-Peterson MN, Larson CB, Aufranc OE. Osteotomy of the spine for correction of flexion deformity in rheumatoid arthritis. J Bone Joint Surg 1945; 27:1–11.
5. Simmons EH. Kyphotic deformity of the spine in ankylosing spondylitis. Clin Orthop 1977; 128:65–77.
6. McMaster MJ. A technique for lumbar spinal osteotomy in ankylosing spondylitis. J Bone Joint Surg Br 1985; 67:204–210.
7. Camargo FP, Cordeiro EN, Napoli MM. Corrective osteotomy of the spine in ankylosing spondylitis: Experience with 66 cases. Clin Orthop 1986; 208:157–167.
8. Hehne HJ, Zielke K, Bohm H. Polysegmental lumbar osteotomies and transpedicled fixation for correction of long-curved kyphotic deformities in ankylosing spondylitis. Report on 177 cases. Clin Orthop 1990; 258:49–55.
9. Halm H, Metz-Stavenhagen P, Zielke K. Results of surgical correction of kyphotic deformities of the spine in ankylosing spondylitis on the basis of the modified arthritis impact measurement scales. Spine 1995; 20:1612–1619.
10. Jaffray D, Becker V, Eisenstein S. Closing wedge osteotomy with transpedicular fixation in ankylosing spondylitis. Clin Orthop 1992; 279:122–126.
11. Chen IH, Chien JT, Yu TC. Transpedicular wedge osteotomy for correction of thoracolumbar kyphosis in ankylosing spondylitis: experience with 78 patients. Spine 2001; 26: E354–E360.
12. Van Royen BJ, De Gast A. Lumbar osteotomy for correction of thoracolumbar kyphotic deformity in ankylosing spondylitis. A structured review of three methods of treatment. Ann Rheum Dis 1999; 58:399–406.
13. Suk KS, Kim KT, Lee SH, Kim JM. Significance of chin-brow vertical angle in correction of kyphotic deformity of ankylosing spondylitis patients. Spine 2003; 28(17): 2001–2005.
14. Van Royen BJ, De Gast A, Smit TH. Deformity planning for sagittal plane corrective osteotomies of the spine in ankylosing spondylitis. Eur Spine J 2000; 9(6):492–498.
15. Sengupta DK, Khazim R, Grevitt MP, et al. Flexion osteotomy of the cervical spine: A new technique for correction of iatrogenic extension deformity in ankylosing spondylitis. Spine 2001; 26:1068–1072.

17

Polysegmental Wedge Osteotomy for Thoracolumbar Kyphosis in Ankylosing Spondylitis

Heinrich Boehm and Hesham El Saghir
*Department of Orthopaedics, Spinal Surgery and Paraplegiology,
Zentralklinik Bad Berka, Bad Berka, Germany*

INTRODUCTION

In spite of the great advances in medicine, there is no effective conservative or operative method that can succeed in halting the ankylosing process in the spine of ankylosing spondylitis (AS) patients. Moreover, there is no known effective joint replacement in the field of the spine that can restore part of the lost spinal movements in those patients. The main role of surgery is in restoring a balanced spine by recreating an acceptable sagittal contour.

As early as 1945 a publication by Smith-Petersen et al. (1) published a method of posterior osteotomies: in the region of laminae and obliterated joints L2/3 or L1/2 osteotomies were performed, followed by an extension maneuver that yielded correction via lordotic angulation of the spine. Postoperatively the patients spent weeks in a plaster bed, followed by immobilization in a plaster cast for one year and a corset for another two years. Of the six cases reported—the follow-up ranged from 6 to 18 months—no information is given about complications or amount of correction. La Chapelle (2) in 1946 proposed a two stage procedure: in the first step, the lamina of L2 and the joints L2/3 were removed under local anesthesia. In the second step, from an anterior lumbotomy, the former disk was osteotomized. After manual correction of the spine, the interbody defect was bridged by graft from the tibia. No follow-up information of this case was given.

A third principle of correction, to our knowledge first performed by Zivian (3), consists of a posterior approach with laminectomy, pediculectomy, and—from the posterior—creating a wedge vertebra by decancellation of the posterior wall. "Egg shell procedure" or "pedicle subtraction osteotomy" are modern terms denoting this selective weakening of the posterior column that allows angular correction and preservation of some spinal stability by hinging in the anterior portion. All methods had one thing in common—they lacked internal stabilization.

Larger series of the Smith-Petersen method by Law (4) or the La Chapelle method by Herbert (5) revealed tremendous complications including paraplegia and death rates around 10%.

The advent of spinal implants improved the outcome markedly, in particular when transpedicular anchoring was made possible after development/application of rod–screw systems (Roy Camille Rodegerts, Zielke).

THE POLYSEGMENTAL TECHNIQUE OF CORRECTION (ZIELKE)

Zielke et al. analyzed the causes of failures and the high complication rate in large series of AS reported by other authors (1,4–7). They found a high mortality rate up to 10% in one series, persistence or even development of neurological deficits after correction of the deformity, loss of the achieved correction due to reliance completely on external immobilization, or the application of inadequate internal fixation like hooks. The principle in the other studies was to do overcorrection at one segment to compensate for a deformity involving multiple segments. The kyphosis in ankylosing spondylitis is, however, a global deformity. It begins mainly at the thoracolumbar junction with or without increase of the thoracic kyphosis and flattening of the lumbar lordosis.

Boehm et al. (8) tried to overcome all shortcomings of other procedures by introducing the so-called dorsal lordosing spondylodesis (DLS). The procedure entails polysegmental posterior osteotomies, segmental instrumentation using pedicle screw–rod system (Ulrich System at that time), and—if the osteotomies close as hoped by the surgeon—harmonious correction of the deformity over several segments.

Operative Technique

The operation is done in the prone position under hypotensive general anesthesia. A midline incision is done extending from D8 to S1. The spine is explored in the usual way adopted by Stagnara. Using special osteotomes, five to seven osteotomies are done (Fig. 1A). The osteotomy is V-shaped and includes removal of the commonly ossified ligamentum flavum, the fused facet joints, and part of the laminae. Care should be taken because the dura in AS is commonly very thin and adherent at the lamina. The size of the osteotomy should be fashioned to meet the requirements for slight overcorrection of the segmental kyphosis so that the overall correction through five to seven osteotomies can compensate for the increased thoracic kyphosis, possible cervicothoracic kyphosis and an expected partial loss of correction during the period of follow-up. The borders of the osteotomy should be trimmed in a way that protects the dura at the time of closing the osteotomy. Generally speaking, the osteotomy—when closed—should not result in foraminal or spinal canal stenosis. As a rule, all segments between D11–D12 and L3–L4 should be osteotomized. According to Zielke technique an anterior osteotomy is not needed. Polysegmental fixation is done using screw–rod system. In the original work of Zielke et al. top loading screws and threaded rod (USIS: Universal Spine Instrumentation System) were applied. The correction is achieved by gradual segmental compression until closure of the osteotomy (Fig. 1B, D). The operative table should be tilted cranially and caudally in a direction that suits the new and desired sagittal profile. This titratable segmental correction can be utilized to correct an associated scoliosis by adapted width of the osteotomy and applying

(A)

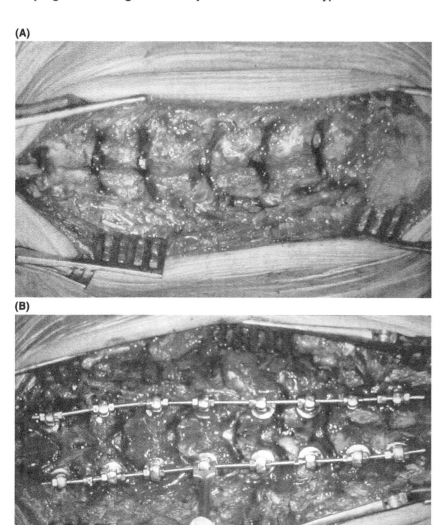

(B)

Figure 1   (A) Oligosegmental posterior osteotomies. In a V-shaped manner a gap of 6 mm is taken out of the posterior elements starting from the 11th thoracic vertebra extending to L4. (B) Threaded rods of 3.2 mm are inserted in the screwheads of transpedicular screws. By gradual zentripetal tightening of the nuts the osteotomies are closed and correction of kyphosis via shortening is achieved. (C) Lumbar lordosis is reached by the Zielke method of closing several posterior osteotomies. The implant, by which correction has been reached, remains for stabilization. Bone from the osteotomies is used to enhance posterior bridging and fusion. (D) Idealized schematic of oligosegmental correction of kyphosis in AS. *Abbreviation*: AS, ankylosing spondylitis.

more compressive forces on the convex side. An experienced anesthetist can guess the time needed for his patient to be ready for the wake up test at the moment of correction of the deformity. The posterior bony structures are then decorticated for the posterior fusion. Bone chips gained from the osteotomy and the spinal

(C)

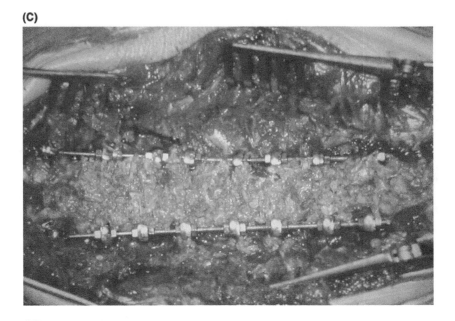

(D)

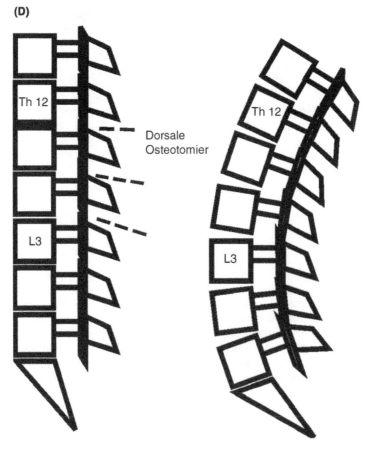

Th 12

L3

Dorsale
Osteotomier

Th 12

L3

Figure 1 *(Continued)*

processes are added to augment the fusion (Fig. 1C). As a prophylactic measure against decompensation at a higher level, exposure of the spine is extended to D3 and non-instrumented fusion in situ is done above the instrumented region. Closure of the wound is done in layers after inserting a suction tube.

Postoperative Treatment

External immobilization using a plaster jacket is applied and the patient is allowed to ambulate one week after the operation. According to Zielke, the duration of the plaster jacket should last for six months and be replaced after this period by a Stagnara orthosis for another six months (Fig. 2C). Plain X-rays (anterior/posterior, lateral, and oblique views) are done at the immediate postoperative period and at three months interval in the first year after the operation. Further follow-up is done on prolonged intervals (once yearly).

(A)

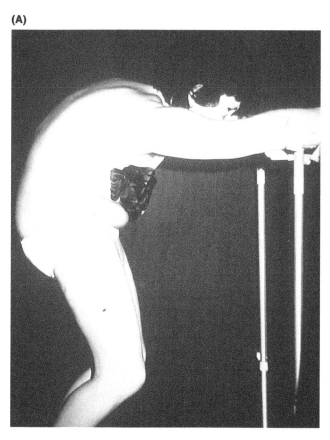

Figure 2 (A) Preoperative status of a 32-year-old female with a 13-year history of AS. (B) Standing X-rays pre- and postoperatively of a 32-year-old female, corrected by oligosegmental posterior osteotomies. In addition to the Zielke method the anterior opening defect of an Andersson-lesion at L4–L5 had been addressed by an additional anterior surgery. (C) One year after oligosegmental posterior osteotomies with subsequent six months immobilization in a cast. *Abbreviation*: AS, ankylosing spondylitis.

(B)

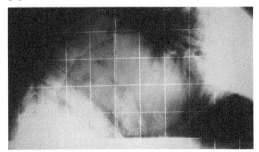
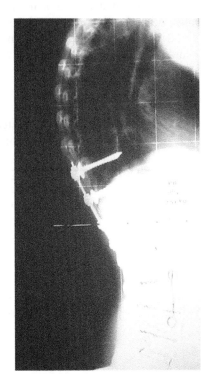

Figure 2   (*Continued*)

Results of the Original Polysegmental Procedure of Zielke

Evaluation of the results of the Zielke technique in 172 patients with mean age of
41 years showed better and move harmonious correction and a lower rate of complications in comparison to other series reported in the literature. An average correction
of 43.4° in the instrument at the immediate postoperative period with a mean loss of
8° three years after the operation yielded harmonic correction of the kyphosis in
70% of the cases and nonharmonic correction in the remaining 30%. The main
obstacle for failure to achieve harmonic lordosis was the presence of bamboo spine (8).
A low mortality rate of 2.3% was reported and was not directly related to the
operation. Reversible neurological deficits affecting one root were encountered in
18%, while irreversible neurological deficits were encountered in 2.3%; one of them
had paraplegia.

Limitations of the Zielke Procedure

- Failure to achieve harmonic lordosis in 30% of the cases or failure to achieve
  correction at all, particularly in those patients having a bamboo spine (9).
- The rods are used for two purposes: as a means to achieve correction and
  for stabilization. For the first action they need to be flexible. Since the same
  rods are remaining in place, they are underdimensioned for the function as
  permanent stabilizers. This leads to an unacceptable high rate of implant
  failures (10).

(C)

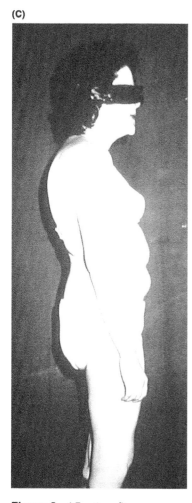

Figure 2   (*Continued*)

- Long period of postoperative external immobilization in spite of the internal fixation.
- Avoiding pedicular fixation above D10 with possibility of decompensation above this level due to absence of the hardware.

Overcoming the Limitations of the Zielke Technique: The Bad Berka Concept

The Smith-Peterson (1) osteotomy and the multiple osteotomies of Zielke et al. are based upon one concept, which is disruption of the anterior syndesmophytes through extension of the spine. Being associated with polysegmental transpedicular instrumentation with harmonious correction of the deformity in the sagittal plane, the Zielke technique offered substantial therapeutic progress. Two conditions have remained as an obstacle for the use of this technique as a standard one at the thoracolumbar spine: the bamboo spine and the presence of giant Andersson's lesion. Correction of the deformity in the bamboo spine necessitates an anterior osteotomy, while a large anterior defect as in Andersson's lesion left without reconstruction will transfer huge loads on the posterior instrumentation with eventual metal failure and loss of correction. For these reasons the need for anterior surgery is frequently mandatory. Although the anterior release or reconstruction can be done through a posterior approach, the risks of neurological deficits and the increased blood loss due to epidural bleeding make an anterior approach wiser to perform, particularly at the thoracolumbar spine. The inability to perform the anterior and posterior surgery with great safety in one position and the non-optimum reconstruction when the patient position is changed once during surgery made some surgeons prefer changing the position of the patient twice: to start posteriorly and end posteriorly (dorso-ventro-dorsal reconstruction) or start anteriorly and end anteriorly (ventro-dorso-ventral reconstruction). Owing to the increased blood loss, the prolonged operative time, and the protracted postoperative course, this modality has been often modified, where part of the procedure is abandoned to be done in a separate session. The Bad Berka concept simplifies the complexity of the dorso-ventro-dorsal correction in ankylosing spondylitis. The ability to perform the anterior and posterior procedures in the prone position along with reducing the trauma of the anterior approach due to the use of the endoscope has obvious advantages in shortening the operative time, reducing the blood loss, optimizing the correction and reconstruction, facilitating the postoperative course, and reducing the overall costs of treatment (11,12).

Minimal Invasive Technique of Corrective Osteotomy at the Thoracolumbar Spine

The procedure is performed in the prone position and done in steps.

Step 1: Posterior Multiple Osteotomies and Implantation of Transpedicular Fixation Screws

Posterior exposure of the spine is done in the normal way described by Stagnara. Transpedicular screws are inserted and fluoroscopy is then done to assure optimal placement and length of the screws. Multiple V-shaped osteotomies are done at the most commonly involved segments in the kyphosis; this is commonly the thoracolumbar junction. The part to be removed is dictated by the amount of correction needed. Care should be taken in fashioning the osteotomy so that it can be closed safely without compressing any neural structure.

Step 2: Anterior Endoscopically Assisted Osteotomy and Fusion

A keyhole incision (3 cm) is placed opposite the apex of the kyphosis at the level of the posterior axillary line. A second portal (1.5 cm) is used for insertion of the endoscope (Fig. 3A). A special set of instruments is used to retract lung and aorta and for keeping an adequate and safe access to the target. In the spondylarthritic ossification type, correction of the deformity is usually achieved through the posterior osteotomies and the role of the minimal invasive anterior procedure is just to decorticate the end plates and to restore the anterior spinal column for rapid bony consolidation. This is particularly needed in those cases with Anderson's lesions where the correction of the deformity accentuates the anterior gap. In the bamboo spine, anterior osteotomy is necessary to achieve correction of the spine. After meticulous division of all bony elements anterior to the spinal cord, the trunk is gradually extended to correct the deformity. The created gap(s) are then filled with bone graft or cage filled with cancellous bone. In cases of severe instability, additional fixation devices from

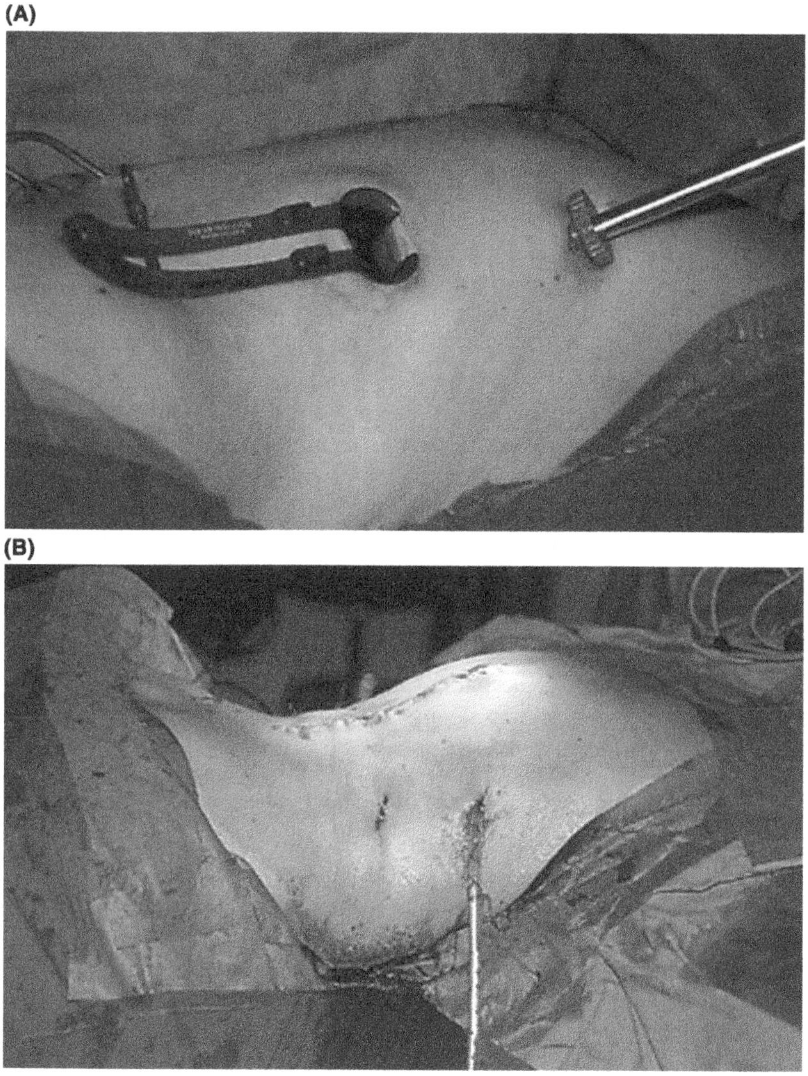

(A)

(B)

Figure 3 (**A**) Simultaneous front and back approach for global kyphosis in AS. Patient positioned prone on the operative table. After posterior release some correction already is achieved. Keyhole approach to anterior spine in prone position for anterior osteotomy and fusion under endoscopic control. (**B**) Normal S-shaped of the spine is reconstructed after posterior correction osteotomy combined with thoracolumbar endoscope-assisted anterior osteotomy and correction. *Abbreviation*: AS, ankylosing spondylitis.

the anterior might be needed. They can be applied in the same minimally invasive technique. For locations caudal to L2, the anterior spine is similarly treated via a retroperitoneal mini-approach.

Step 3: Completion of the Posterior Spondylodesis
The rods are inserted and tightened under compression at the heads of the screws. Posterior spondylodesis augmented with bone chips is then done and the wound is

closed in layers. Intraoperative somatosensory evoked potential (SEP) monitoring and wake up tests are routine measures to assure safety of the procedure (Fig. 3B).

RESULTS

In the period between 1996 and 2003, 112 patients (mean age: 50.5, male:female = 8:1) were treated by the aforementioned technique for kyphosis at the thoracolumbar spine. It was possible to do the anterior spinal procedure with the aid of the endoscope through a keyhole incision in all the patients. In no case was it necessary to abandon part of the procedure. Post-thoracotomy syndrome was not seen. The postoperative degree of correction of the thoracic kyphosis was 48.6° and reached 42.2° at the end of the follow-up period. A mean gain of 34.5° was achieved at the immediate postoperative period and showed a mean loss of 4.8° at the end of the follow-up period. Revision surgery was needed on two occasions because of graft resorption in one and the need to extend the fusion from L4 to S1 in the other. Irreversible neurological complications in the form of paraplegia were encountered in one patient.

The minimally invasive technique for the anterior surgery combined with the multiple posterior wedge osteotomies has the following advantages:

- It avoids repositioning of the patient and redraping for correction of the deformity. In this way it is time saving and more safe than a technique that needs intraoperative change of the patient's position.
- The anterior procedure is done in a minimally invasive way using keyhole incision. This decreases the incisional morbidity and at the same time avoids potential problems associated with conventional thoracotomies and thoraco-lumbotomies.
- The only way which ensures that circumferential release is adequate is a technique which offers the surgeon the possibility of having both anterior and posterior accesses to the target simultaneously. Actually, this is the main advantage in the strategy of correction of kyphosis.
- Contrary to Zielke's method, where closure of all osteotomies rarely could be reached, the additional anterior intervention facilitates it.
- Biomechanically speaking after anterior osteotomy the axis of rotation is shifted toward the posterior wall, allowing a higher angle of correction without stretching or compressing the spinal canal.
- The technique offers a reasonable solution for kyphosis of the bamboo spine where the multiple posterior osteotomy technique of Zielke frequently fails.
- Should—as often in longstanding Anderson's lesions—the cord need anterior decompression, this can be performed safely and effectively under endoscopic vision and control.

CONCLUSION

Most of the traditionally performed old procedures for osteotomies at the thoracolumbar spine are considered formidable. Introduction of minimally invasive techniques and availability of better implants have allowed a dramatic improvement in the results of surgical treatment.

REFERENCES

1. Smith-Peterson MN, Larson CB, Aufranc OE. Osteotomy of the spine for correction of flexion deformity in rheumatoid arthritis. J Bone Joint Surg 1945; 27:1.
2. La Chapelle EH. Osteotomy of the lumbar spine for correction of kyphosis in case of ankylosing spondyloarthritis. J Bone Joint Surg 1946; 28:851–858.
3. Zivian Ja L. Lumbar correcting vertebrotomy in ankylosing spondylarthritis (in Russian). Khirurgia (Mosk.) 1971; 47:47.
4. Law WA. Osteotomy of the spine. J Bone Joint Surg Br 1959; 41:270.
5. Herbert JJ. Vertebral osteotomy for kyphosis especially in Marie-Strümpell arthritis. J Bone Joint Surg Am 1959; 41:291–302.
6. Scudese V, Calabro JJ. Vertebral wedge osteotomy. J Am Med Assoc 1963; 186:627.
7. Thomasen E. Vertebral osteotomy for correction of kyphosis in ankylosing spondylitis. Clin Orthop 1985; 194:142.
8. Boehm H, Hehne HJ, Zielke K. Correction of Bechterew kyphosis. Orthopade 1989; 18(2):142–154.
9. Van Royen BJ, De Gast A. Lumbar osteotomy for correction of thoracolumbar kyphotic deformity in ankylosing spondylitis. A structured review of three methods of treatment. Ann Rheum Dis 1999; 58:399–406.
10. Van Royen BJ, de Kleuver M, Slot GH. Polysegmental lumbar posterior wedge osteotomies for correction of kyphosis in ankylosing spondylitis. Eur Spine J 1998; 7:104–110.
11. Boehm H. Zugangswege zur Wirbelsäule in Plastische und Wiederherstellungschirurgie In: Schmelzle R, Bschorer R, eds. Unimed Verlag, 1996:638–646.
12. Boehm H. Simultaneous front and back surgery: a new technique with a thoracoscopic or retroperitoneal approach in prone position. Fourth International Meeting on Advanced spine techniques, Bermuda, 1997.

18

The Closing Wedge Osteotomy for Thoracolumbar Deformity in Ankylosing Spondylitis

Sigurd H. Berven and David S. Bradford
Department of Orthopaedic Surgery, University of California, San Francisco, California, U.S.A.

INTRODUCTION

Ankylosing spondylitis (AS) is an important cause of fixed sagittal plane deformity of the spine. AS is a seronegative spondyloarthropathy with a high specificity for involvement of the spinal entheses, or attachments of joint capsules, ligaments, and tendons into bone. Characteristically, the axial skeleton including the sacroiliac joints and the spinal motion segments are affected by sterile inflammation, erosion, fibrosis, and ossification. Ankylosis of the spine results in significant and measurable disability and compromise of quality of life (1). There are three recognized phases of disease progression: inflammation, flexion deformity, and bony ankylosis (2). Medical management and postural exercises have not reliably changed the natural history of deformity progression, although new therapies including tumor necrosis factor-alpha inhibition have improved symptoms and pain (1). Spinal deformity in AS most commonly affects the thoracolumbar spine with flattening of lumbar lordosis and kyphosis across the mobile thoracolumbar junction. Cervical and upper thoracic deformity is present in 30% of cases, and involvement of these regions is more common in women (3). In the absence of a reliable medical intervention for the management of progressive spinal deformity in AS, surgical care remains an important consideration for the cohort of patients with AS and disabling spinal deformity. The purpose of this article is to review the surgical care of kyphotic deformity at the thoracolumbar spine using the closing wedge osteotomy.

INDICATIONS FOR SURGICAL CORRECTION OF KYPHOTIC DEFORMITY

The natural history of AS is variable, but appears to follow a predictable pattern after the first 10 years of involvement with patients having severe spinal restriction progressing to severe deformity and disability (4). The age of onset of AS has been

255

shown to have an inverse correlation with the severity of disease, with patients with a younger age at onset demonstrating more severe disability than those with onset at a later age (5). AS is a diagnosis that is often delayed due to the insidious onset of symptoms, and the nonspecific involvement of the axial skeleton (6). With the development of new medications and disease modifying agents that may positively affect the natural history of disease progression in AS, early detection may be an important goal.

Progressive deformity of the spine is characteristic of patients with an early onset of disease and with severe symptoms of inflammation and stiffness early in the course of disease. Sagittal imbalance and progressive kyphosis at the thoracolumbar spine is the most characteristic deformity of the patient with AS. Neutral sagittal alignment follows a vertical axis from C2, in front of T7, behind L3, and across S2 (7,8). There is significant normal variation of lumbar lordosis and thoracic kyphosis in maintaining overall sagittal balance (3). Sagittal balance is important for biomechanical optimization of forces at segmental interspaces. Sagittal plane malalignment is most often clinically significant when there is loss of normal lordosis of the lumbar and cervical spine. Excessive kyphosis across these mobile, unsupported segments increases intradiscal pressures and compromises the mechanical advantage of the erector spinae musculature (9). Clinically, the patient with fixed sagittal deformity presents with intractable pain, early fatigue, and a subjective sense of imbalance and leaning forward and difficulty with horizontal gaze. AS results in a global fixed kyphosis, with the occiput and cervical spine displaced anteriorly to the sacrum. Glassman et al. demonstrated that displacement of the spine more than 4 cm anterior to the anterior sacral prominence is the most significant radiographic determinant of health status in patients with spinal deformity, exceeding the influence of coronal plane imbalance, curve magnitude, and rotational deformity (10). Global sagittal imbalance is distinct from localized kyphosis. Focal kyphosis caused by disorders such as infection or fracture generally result in maintenance of global sagittal balance due to the capacity of the remaining mobile spine to compensate with hyperlordosis, or hypokyphosis. In AS, a fundamental aspect of the spinal pathology is the absence of mobile segments capable of compensating for deformity. The extra axial skeleton may be able to compensate for global spinal kyphosis, specifically through extension of the hips and flexion of the knees. This compensation occurs at the cost of fatigue and decreased standing and walking tolerance. The patient with AS is again compromised in his ability to compensate using the hips and knees due to the high prevalence of concurrent peripheral arthropathy, and hip flexion contracture.

The indications for surgical correction of fixed spinal deformity in AS are:

1. progression of sagittal plane deformity,
2. impairment of forward gaze and visual field (chin–brow angle),
3. inability to stand erect, or balance during gait,
4. compromise of thoracic and abdominal capacity due to kyphotic deformity, and
5. concern about physical appearance and deformity.

Progression of sagittal plane deformity is due to both the progression of disease intrinsic to the spine, and the loss of compensatory mechanisms in the hips and knees. Patients may become more symptomatic with aging despite relative stability of the spinal deformity. Impairment of forward gaze is a significant disability for patients with AS. The angle of the line between the chin and brow and the vertical is a quantifiable measure of fixed kyphotic deformity (Fig. 1). A chin–brow vertical angle that fixes the patient's gaze in a downward posture significantly impacts the

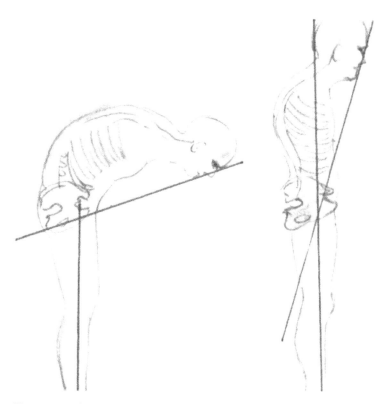

Figure 1 Chin–brow vertical angle.

patient's abilities in interpersonal communications, driving, personal hygiene, and walking. Correction of chin–brow vertical angle to neutral is an important determinant of clinical outcome and patient satisfaction after corrective osteotomy of the spine (11). Lumbar hypolordosis and kyphosis at the thoracolumbar spine may significantly compromise diaphragmatic excursion and respiratory capacity. In the patient with AS, costochondral and costovertebral ossification significantly limit chest expansion and forced vital capacity. The addition of compromise in diaphragmatic excursion may lead to measurable compromise in pulmonary function. Similarly, compromise of abdominal capacity by deformity is associated with poor appetite and compromised access to the abdomen for elective or emergent surgery to the upper abdominal region. Finally, patient appearance and perception of deformity is an important determinant of self-image and social function. The surgical correction of sagittal deformity may have an important impact on self-image and mental health in patients with AS.

AN OVERVIEW OF SURGICAL CORRECTIVE TECHNIQUES

The goals of surgical correction of fixed kyphotic decompensation of the spine in patients with AS are:

1. safety with protection of neural and vascular structures,
2. restoration of a normal angle for forward gaze (chin–brow angle), and
3. restoration of the sagittal alignment of C7 with the sacral prominence.

Surgical strategies for the correction of thoracolumbar kyphosis in anklyosing spondylitis have included posterior and combined anterior and posterior approaches. The surgical correction of fixed sagittal deformity in AS was first reported by Smith-Peterson et al. (12) in 1945. The Smith-Peterson osteotomy described pivots on the posterior longitudinal ligament, with consequent lengthening of the anterior column through the disk space (13). The technique is well suited for patients with flexible disks anteriorly and posterior pseudarthrosis at multiple levels. Anterior column distraction can compromise intra-abdominal and retroperitoneal structures. Complications include vascular insult, paraplegia, gastrointestinal obstruction, and death (1,14–20).

Combined anterior and posterior surgery offers the advantage of a controlled manipulation of the anterior column, and fusion with structural graft. La Chapelle described a combined anterior and posterior osteotomy for the management of AS that involved cutting the anterior column directly, followed by grafting in order to avoid risks of an anterior opening wedge (21). The combined anterior and posterior osteotomy for the correction of iatrogenic lumbar kyphosis has led to good restoration of lumbar lordosis, maintained at greater than two year follow-up (6,22). However, in fixed kyphotic deformity due to AS, the anterior approach is limited due to ankylosis of the anterior column, requiring a difficult access to the posterior vertebral body, and often involving significant anterior column bleeding.

There are several advantages of a posterior only approach to correction of sagittal deformity, including single stage surgery, reduced morbidity compared with combined surgery, addressing the deformity at the apex, creation of compressive forces at the osteotomy site, and maximal correction with a minimal number of osteotomies (23). Posterior surgical options can be categorized by the fulcrum across which correction is achieved. Posterior osteotomies that hinge on the posterior longitudinal ligament cause opening of the anterior column (i.e., Smith-Peterson). Opening the anterior column may compromise bone healing, distract neural, vascular and visceral structures, and is associated with limited corrective potential. Closing wedge osteotomies effectively shorten the spine and, therefore, protect the neural elements. Similarly, the anterior column of the spine including vascular and visceral structures are unaffected by a posterior closing wedge. Spinal shortening osteotomies gain sagittal plane correction without distraction of the anterior column. Heinig's eggshell decancellation procedure includes a controlled compression fracture of the anterior column with differentially more closure posteriorly. In contrast, the Thomasen osteotomy maintains the height of the anterior column and hinges on the anterior longitudinal ligament. The Thomasen osteotomy is a circumferential wedge excision rather than a decancellation and compression with vertebral body collapse. The transpedicular approach places the apex of correction anteriorly, serving to shorten the spine, and avoid anterior column lengthening. Advantages of this technique include the prevention of neural compression by creation of a large, shared neural foramen through removal of the pedicles, limited stretch on anterior structures, and cancellous bone healing (24–26). There are many reports of posterior procedures for the management of AS including opening and closing wedge procedures (11,12,14,16,18,21,27–34). The closing wedge osteotomies permit greater potential for sagittal plane correction with osteotomy at a single level than multiple opening wedges, and overall offer greater safety and less complications. A meta-analysis review of the literature on outcomes after posterior osteotomies for the treatment of AS demonstrated less loss of correction in osteotomies that hinge on the anterior longitudinal ligament, with little difference in overall correction and complications (34).

TECHNIQUE OF THE TRANSPEDICULAR WEDGE RESECTION (THOMASEN OSTEOTOMY)

The transpedicular wedge resection osteotomy was described by Thomasen for the correction of deformity secondary to AS (33). This technique is the most effective surgical approach to the management of fixed thoracolumbar kyphosis in AS.

Positioning

The patient with a fixed sagittal plane deformity presents a challenge for positioning in both the supine and the prone position. In the supine position for intubation, the patient will require head support and elevation because the shoulders will be elevated from the table. Fiber-optic nasotracheal intubation facilitates visualization of the true vocal cords and airway placement in the patient with significant deformity and rigidity in the cervicothoracic region.

In the prone position, the patient will not fit well on a standard four poster frame as this will lead to significant point contacts at the chest and iliac crest. We prefer to use a technique with two separate posts, one each for the chest and the pelvis. In separating the posts, we may flex the operating room table to accommodate the preoperative deformity and permit the chest and pelvis to be congruent with the contour of the post (Fig. 2). The hips are positioned in full extension, with care to keep pressure off the patella and other bony prominences including the elbows and periorbital region. After the osteotomy is complete, reversal of the flexion of the table permits and facilitates a controlled closure of the wedge resection.

Surgical Approach

The posterior approach to the spine is standard. The spine is exposed at least from a level four segments above the planned osteotomy to the mid-sacrum below because stable internal fixation requires instrumentation to these levels at a minimum. A sub-periosteal dissection is completed to the level of the transverse process tips of the segments to be fused. Decompression of the spinal canal begins at the lamina of the

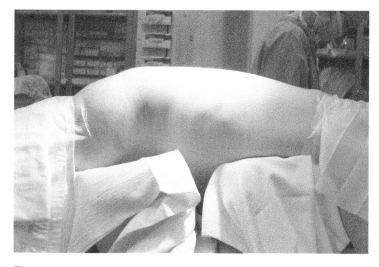

Figure 2

vertebra to be osteotomized. It is important to extend the decompression to at least one level above and one level below the pedicle subtraction, meaning a complete laminectomy of L3 and L5 if the L4 pedicle is to be resected. If a wide decompression is not accomplished, the posterior elements will impinge upon the spinal canal with the wedge closure, so an adequate decompression is important to protect the neural elements. The undersurface of L2 may be further undercut in order to prevent infolding of ligamentum flavum and bone onto the neural elements. Transient neurologic deficits have been reported in up to 20% of transpedicular wedge resection osteotomies, and an adequate decompression is important in reducing the incidence of this complication.

After a wide midline decompression, remaining posterior elements (the superior facet, the inferior facet, and the pars) of the vertebra to be osteotomized are removed. During the removal of the superior facet, the medial half of the transverse process is removed to permit access to the lateral wall of the vertebral body. Extension of the facetectomy to include a portion of the inferior facet of the level above and a portion of the superior facet of the level of the pedicle below effectively creates a single foramen shared by the nerve root above the osteotomy and the nerve root at the level of the osteotomy. After removal of the posterior elements, the remaining pedicle is visible as are the nerve roots above and below (Fig. 3). Fat and perineurium should be left around the nerve roots during this exposure. Hemostasis is maintained by bipolar electrocautery. We have found the Floseal Matrix Hemostatic Sealant (Baxter International, Jersey City, New Jersey, U.S.) and bovine collagen matrices to be useful in the maintenance of hemostasis during the bony resection portion of the procedure.

After completion of the decompression, pedicle screws are placed at the levels above and below the osteotomy, encompassing at least three segments above and below (Fig. 4). In order to include three segments below the osteotomy, the instrumentation may extend to include the ilium using an iliac screw (Galveston technique).

Pedicle Subtraction Technique

Removal of the pedicle and decancellation of the vertebral body is a portion of the procedure in which the neural elements are at risk of injury and bleeding may be

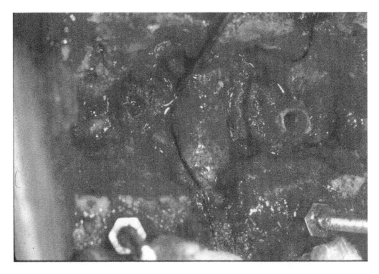

Figure 3

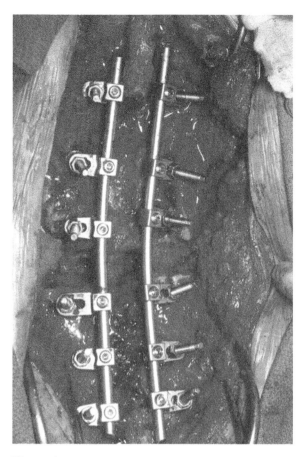

Figure 4

quite brisk. In order to protect the neural elements, we use two hand held brain
retractors positioned for each pedicle. A sharp periosteal elevator is used to dissect
the soft tissue laterally to the base of the pedicle and anteriorly approximately 2 cm
along the outer wall of the vertebral body, taking great care to avoid injury to the
nerve roots. The medial wall of the pedicle is isolated with retraction of the thecal
sac medially using a dural retractor, and retraction of the nerve roots above and
below using brain retractors. The decancellation begins and is completed on one side
before addressing the opposite side. The center of the pedicle is removed using a high
speed 4 mm steel burr, extending the burring of bone to approximately 1 cm into the
vertebral body. A narrow rongeur or pituitary may then be used to remove the walls
of the pedicle completely (Fig. 5). The hole in the posterior cortex of the vertebral
body is widened using a Kerrison rongeur or a high speed burr. Decancellation of
the vertebral body is facilitated using angled curettes and a systematic approach
directed toward resection of a posteriorly based wedge of bone. It is important to
begin the decancellation at the posterior wall of the vertebral body, working under
the dura from the lateral cortex toward medial and distal as far as possible under
the lower nerve root. Decancellation proceeds anteriorly in the vertebral body in a
wedge shape. The superior edge of the decancellation is just under the subchondral
bone of the upper disk space. The inferior edge of the decancellation is a more

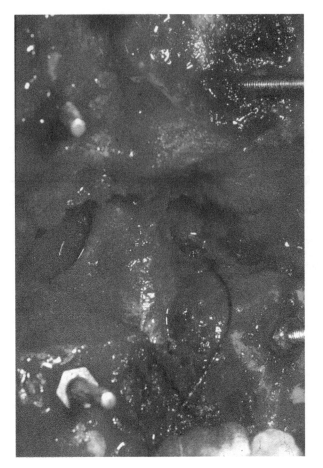

Figure 5

difficult exposure as the nerve root below the resected pedicle interferes with wide exposure of the inferior aspect of the vertebral body. Therefore, the wedge resection may not extend to the very base of the vertebral body inferiorly. Using a 10 mm osteotome, the lateral cortex of the vertebral body is cut in a wedge shape directed to the apex at a point just posterior to the anterior cortex, and in the mid-portion to the vertebral body longitudinally. Fluroscopic guidance may be helpful in visualizing the anterior cortex of the vertebral body. It is important to curette to the level of the anterior cortex in order to create a greenstick (torus type) fracture at this level. On completion of one side, thrombin-soaked gel foam is packed into the vertebral body shell, with the borders of the shell being a thin but intact posterior wall ventral to the dura, a lateral wall with a wedge resected, and an anterior cortex thinned at the apex of the wedge. The same steps are used for decancellation of the opposite side. A suction catheter may be used on the prepared side to assist with visualization of the opposite side. Bleeding is most brisk during the decancellation and slows rapidly when cortical bone is reached on each side. Using a straight curette, the anterior cortex of the vertebral body is scored in order to create a stress riser and guide the osteotomy site at the anterior vertebral body. After a complete decancellation, a reverse angle curette is used to tap the residual thinned posterior wall of the vertebral body into the decancellated space. Closure of the wedge is facilitated by reversal of the flex in the operating room table, and by compression between the pedicle screws above and below the osteotomy. During closure of the wedge resection, careful observation of the neural elements will prevent compromise of the space available. Instrumentation is placed after the wedge is closed. Additional compression of the wedge may be gained with the use of instrumentation as necessary. The fracture through the anterior cortex is a greenstick fracture (torus type) and does not involve a complete disruption of the anterior cortex. The anterior cortex serves as a hinge, and prevents translation of the spinal column. In the case of anklyosing spondylitis, special care is necessary to ensure that the anterior cortex remains a hinge and is not completely disrupted. Forceful fracture reduction should be avoided as this can lead to translation and an uncontrolled closure. Posterior compression is the key maneuver for wedge closure, and forceful maneuvers including cantilevering with a long rod may be dangerous. If the wedge is not closing easily with posterior decompression, the lateral wedges and the anterior cortex should be evaluated. A short rod may be used on one side to stabilize the spine during compression if necessary. Motor evoked and somatosensory evoked potentials are sensitive techniques for monitoring neurologic function and are followed closely during the wedge closure.

Extension of instrumentation to the pelvis using iliac screws is recommended if the osteotomy is at L4 or below, or if the patient has compromised bone stock with poor sacral fixation. The surgeon will have collected a significant amount of local bone graft from the decompression and decancellation. We harvest further autogenous bone from the iliac crest through a separate fascial incision if necessary.

RESULTS OF THE TRANSPEDICULAR WEDGE RESECTION

The efficacy of an osteotomy in correcting a sagittal and coronal deformity can be assessed by radiographic parameters and absolute correction. The clinical value of the procedure is best assessed by measurement of complications and patient satisfaction. Thomasen (33), Jaffray et al. (35), and Van Royen and Slot (13) reported significant and lasting sagittal plane correction using transpedicular wedge resection in patients with AS. Thiranont and Netrawichien (32) reported on the use of the eggshell osteotomy for the treatment of AS, demonstrating correction averaging 33°. At an average of 24 months follow-up, all cases had improvement of their general appearance, posture, and respiratory and gastrointestinal functions, and had good bony union.

In our series of 13 patients with fixed sagittal plane malalignments of various etiologies including AS, the transpedicular wedge resection osteotomy was an effective technique for radiographic improvement of fixed sagittal imbalance. Average improvement of lumbar lordosis was 30°, and a 63% improvement of global sagittal balance was observed in patients followed for a minimum of two years. Patient satisfaction with corrective osteotomy was highest in patients with AS, with all patients reporting that they were definitely satisfied with their surgery, and all would definitely repeat surgery.

ILLUSTRATIVE CASE EXAMPLE

DD is a 58-year-old male with AS that was initially diagnosed at age 28. The patient is employed as a computer systems operator and in good health. He complains of progressive difficulty standing and walking, and reports his standing tolerance is 15 minutes, and walking is limited to less than four blocks. The patient uses sulfasalazine and hydrocodone for low back pain.

1. Clinical Photos:

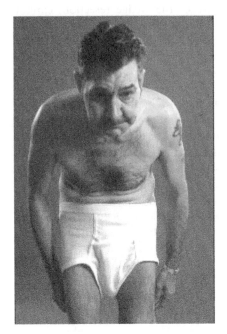
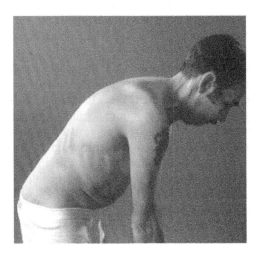

2. Radiographs: preoperative and postoperative:

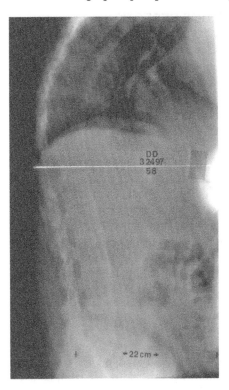
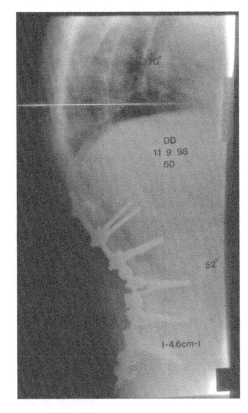

SUMMARY

Surgical correction of fixed thoracolumbar kyphosis is an important component of the spectrum of care for patients with AS. Patients with early onset of disease, and severe early involvement are most likely to develop disabling spinal deformity. The development of new disease modifying agents may improve the ability of medical management to limit progression of deformity. However, at present, there is no intervention that reliably improves the natural history of spinal deformity progression in affected patients with AS. The closing wedge osteotomy originally described by Thomasen remains the safest and most effective method for surgical correction of disabling spinal deformity in patients with AS involving the thoracolumbar spine. Patients treated with closing wedge osteotomies self-report significant improvements of pain, function, and quality of life.

REFERENCES

1. Adams JC. Techniques, dangers, and safeguards in osteotomy of the spine. J Bone Joint Surg 1952; 34B:226–232.
2. Asher MA, Lai SM, Burton DC. Further development and validation of the Scoliosis Research Society (SRS) Outcomes Instrument. Spine 2000; 25:2381–2386.
3. Bernhardt M, Bridwell KH. Segmental analysis of the sagittal plane alignment of the normal thoracic and lumbar spines and thoracolumbar junction. Spine 1989; 14:717–721.
4. Boachie-Adjei O, Bradford DS. Vertebral column resection and arthrodesis for complex spinal deformities. J Spinal Disord 1991; 4(2):193–202.
5. Booth KC, Bridwell KH, Lenke LG, Baldus CR, Blanke KM. Complications and predictive factors for the successful treatment of flatback deformity (fixed sagittal imbalance). Spine 1999; 24(16):1712–1720.
6. Bradford DS, Schumacher WL, Lonstein JE, Winter RB. Ankylosing spondylitis: experience in surgical management of 21 patients. Spine 1987; 12(3):238–243.
7. DeWald RL. Osteotomy of the thoracic/lumbar spine. In: Bradford DS, ed. Master Techniques in Orthopaedic Surgery, the Spine. Philadelphia, PA: Lippincott-Raven, 1997:229–248.
8. Jackson RP, McManus AC. Radiographic analysis of sagittal plane alignment and balance in standing volunteers and patients with low back pain matched for age, sex, and size. A prospective controlled clinical study. Spine 1994; 19:1611–1618.
9. White AA, Panjabi MM. Practical biomechanics of scoliosis and kyphosis. In: White AA, Panjabi MM, eds. Clinical Biomechanics of the Spine. Philadelphia, PA: Lippincott-Raven, 1990:127–168.
10. Glassman S, Berven S, Bridwell K, Horton W, Dimar J. Correlation of radiographic parameters and clinical symptoms in adult scoliosis. Spine 2005; 30(6):682–688.
11. Briggs H, Keats S, Schlesinger P. Wedge osteotomy of the spine with intervertebral foraminotomy. J Bone Joint Surg 1947; 29:1075–1082.
12. Smith-Peterson MN, Larson CB, Aufranc OE. Osteotomy of the spine for correction of flexion deformity in rheumatoid arthritis. J Bone Joint Surg 1945; 27:1–11.
13. Van Royen BJ, Slot GH. Closing-wedge posterior osteotomy for ankylosing spondylitis. Partila corpectomy and transpedicular fixation in 22 cases. J Bone Joint Surg 1995; 77B(1):117–121.
14. Carmargo FP, Cordeiro EN, Napoli MM. Corrective osteotomy of the spine in ankylosing spondylitis. Experience with 66 cases. Clin Orthop 1986; 208:157–167.
15. Fazl M, Bilboa JM, Hudson AR. Laceration of the aorta complicating spinal fracture in ankylosing spondylitis. Neurosurgery 1981; 8:732–734.

16. Law WA. Osteotomy of the spine. Clin Orthop 1969; 66:70–76.
17. Lichblau PO, Wilson PD. Possible mechanism of aortic rupture in orthopaedic correction of rheumatoid spondylitis. J Bone Joint Surg 1956; 38A:123.
18. McMaster MJ. Osteotomy of the spine for fixed flexion deformity. J Bone Joint Surg 1962; 44A:1206–1216.
19. Simmons EH. Kyphotic deformity of the spine in ankylosing spondylitis. Clin Orthop 1977; 128:65–77.
20. Weatherly C, Jaffray D, Terry A. Vascular complications associated with osteotomy in ankylosing spondylitis: a report of two cases. Spine 1988; 13:43.
21. LaChapelle EH. Osteotomy of the lumbar spine for correction of kyphosis in a case of ankylosing spondylo-arthritis. J Bone Joint Surg 1946; 28:851.
22. Kostuik JP, Maurais GR, Richardson WJ, Okajima Y. Combined single stage anterior and posterior osteotomy for the correction of iatrogenic lumbar kyphosis. Spine 1988; 13(3):256–266.
23. Shufflebarger HL, Clark CE. Thoracolumbar osteotomy for postsurgical sagittal imbalance. Spine 1992; 17(8S):S287–S292.
24. Kostuik J. Osteotomies. In: An HS, Riley LH, eds. An Atlas of Surgery of the Spine. Philadelphia, PA: Lippincott-Raven, 1998.
25. Michelle A, Krudger FJ. A surgical approach to the vertebral body. J Bone Joint Surgery 1949; 31A:873–878.
26. Tsuzuki N, Kostuik JP. Laminoplasty of the thoracic and lumbar spine. In: Frymoyer JW, ed. The Adult Spine: Principles and Practice. Philadelphia, PA: Lippincott-Raven, 1997:2089–2109.
27. Dawson CW. Posterior osteotomy for ankylosing arthritis of the spine. J Bone Joint Surg 1956; 38A:1393.
28. Emneus H. Wedge osteotomy of the spine in ankylosing spondylitis. Acta Orthop Scand 1968; 39:321–326.
29. Goel MK. Vertebral osteotomy for the correction of fixed flexion deformity of the spine. J Bone Joint Surg 1968; 50A:287–294.
30. Hehne HJ, Zielke K, Bohm H. Polysegmental lumbar osteotomies and transpedicled fixation for correction of long-curved kyphotic deformities in ankylosing spondylitis. Clin Orthop 1990; 258:49–55.
31. Herbert JJ. Vertebral osteotomy for kyphosis, especially in Marie-Strumpell arthritis. J Bone Joint Surg 1959; 41A:291–302.
32. Thiranont N, Netrawichien P. Transpedicular decancellation closed wedge vertebral osteotomy for treatment of fixed flexion deformity of spine in ankylosing spondylitis. Spine 1993; 18(16):2517–2522.
33. Thomasen E. Vertebral osteotomy for correction of kyphosis in ankylosing spondylitis. Clin Orthop 1985; 194:142–152.
34. Van Royen BJ, DeGast A. Lumbar osteotomy for correction of thoracolumbar kyphotic deformity in ankylosing spondylitis. A structured review of three methods of treatment. Ann Rheum Dis 1999; 58:399–406.
35. Jaffray D, Becker V, Eisenstein S. Closing wedge osteotomy with transpedicular fixation in ankylosing spondylitis. Clin Orthop 1992; 279:122–126.

19

Osteotomy of the Cervical Spine in Ankylosing Spondylitis

Hesham El Saghir and Heinrich Boehm
Department of Orthopaedics, Spinal Surgery and Paraplegiology,
Zentralklinik Bad Berka, Bad Berka, Germany

SUMMARY

Unsatisfactory results, neurological deficits, and in some instances life-threatening complications have made patients and doctors hesitant to decide for surgery in ankylosing spondylitis (AS) (1–4). However, decisive progress in surgical technique has been made toward fewer complications, less operative trauma, and better quality of life after surgery (5–7). Somatosensory evoked potential (SSEP)-monitoring allows continuous control of some functions of the spinal cord during surgery. Emphasis in this report is given to the benefits of improved instrumentation systems and better imaging studies which have made preoperative assessment and surgery of the cervical spine in ankylosing spine safer and more successful. We report on 66 AS patients (mean age: 49.4 years; male:female: 58:8) with cervical disorders treated in our institution in the period between 1994 and 2003. The material comprised subaxial disorders in the form of kyphosis in 31 patients, fractures and posttraumatic deformity in 26 patients and atlantoaxial instability and/or dislocation C1/C2 in the remaining nine patients. Surgery resulted in excellent correction of the disturbed sagittal profile with adequate stability and restoration of a horizontal axis of vision. Loosening of the screws with loss of the correction was encountered in one patient of cervicothoracic osteotomy and was successfully restored after a revision surgery. No mortalities or cord dysfunction were encountered. However, the most serious complication, partial sensory and/or motor deficit of root origin, was seen in eight patients. The C8 root was involved in six patients, followed by the C5 root in the remaining two. Remission (four patients) or substantial recovery (three patients) occurred in seven patients during the first three months after surgery.

INTRODUCTION

The role of surgery in the treatment of cervical spine disorders in AS has gained more importance and acceptance. This is attributed to several factors:

- better understanding of the disturbed biomechanics of the deformity,
- medical advances in the field of anesthesia and intensive care unit with the possibility of autotransfusion,
- spinal cord monitoring,
- development of navigation systems,
- improvement of the imaging techniques,
- availability of more reliable instrumentation systems, and
- general improvement of the surgical skills of spinal surgeons.

CERVICAL DISORDERS OF MECHANICAL ORIGIN IN AS

The cervical disorders of mechanical origin are:

- chronic neck pain,
- ankylosis and limitation of neck movements,
- cervicothoracic kyphosis,
- fractures and Anderson's lesions,
- subaxial instability,
- atlantoaxial instability, and
- craniocervical instability and/or stenosis.

Chronic Neck Pain

Chronic neck pain is a relatively common symptom in patients with AS. The pain is either inflammatory during the active stage of the disease or myogenic due to abnormal statics, which necessitate increased contractions of the extensors of the neck (Fig. 1A). However, the chronic pain may be the clue for an abnormal movement as a result of fatigue fracture or segmental instability particularly of the C1–C2 articulation (Figs. 2 and 3A,B).

Physicians should be alert regarding the different causes of neck pain AS patients. Blind treatment of chronic neck pain with analgesic anti-inflammatory drugs without proper imaging study can result in catastrophic complications.

Ankylosis and Limitation of Neck Movements

Unfortunately, the cervical spine is not immune against the inflammatory and ossifying features of AS. Usually the ankylosing process of the spine spreads in a caudocranial direction starting at the sacroiliac joint and ending at the subaxial spine or even at the craniocervical junction. According to the activity of the inflammatory process, the extent of ankylosis, and the joints affected, different degrees of limitation of the range of movements in the three planes are seen.

Cervicothoracic Kyphosis

This is the most common cervical deformity encountered in patients with AS.

Mechanisms of development of kyphosis are:

1. Kyphosis or flexion deformity at a lower level: the occurrence of thoraco-lumbar kyphosis, flattening of the lumbar lordosis and flexion deformity

(A)   (B)

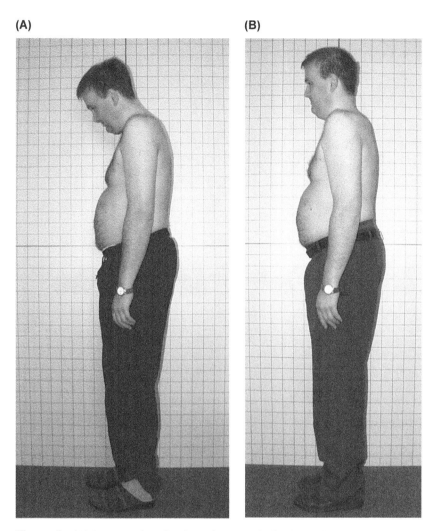

Figure 1 (A) Preoperative: fixed cervicothoracic flexion deformity of AS in a 38-year-old male. Patient in 1999 before surgery, (B) Postoperative: fixed cervicothoracic flexion deformity of AS in a 38-year-old male. Patient three months after cervicothoracic extension surgery, (C) Postoperative: whole spine X-ray of the same patient three months after cervicothoracic exten-sion surgery. Note the implants that maintain the corrected position of the head and cervical spine versus the thoracic area, (D) Postoperative: X-ray five years after cervicothoracic exten-sion surgery. Implants are still in place and no loss of correction is seen. Patient is free of pre-operative cervicothoracic pain and the marked preoperative pain at occipitocervical junction.

of the hip force the spine anterior to the plumb line. Gravity acting on the disbalanced spine then promotes further progression at a proximal level. The weight of the head and the long lever arm make the cervicothoracic junction more susceptible to the development of kyphosis. Has an angular kyphosis developed, part of the posterior neck muscles start to act as flexors rather than extensors, leading to overload of the paraspinal muscles.

2. Fractures and Anderson's lesions: in the absence of shock-absorbing inter-vertebral disks the ankylosed cervical spine is more susceptible to fractures than the mobile healthy spine. Most of these injuries can be regarded as

(C)   **(D)**

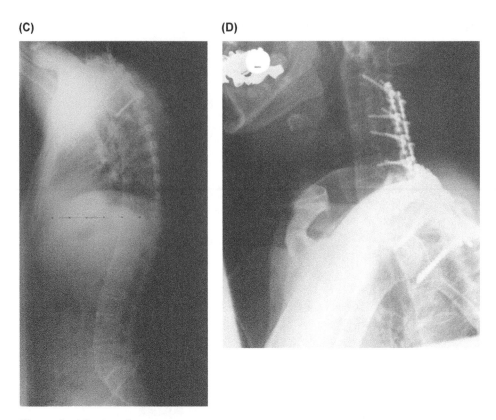

Figure 1 (*Continued*)

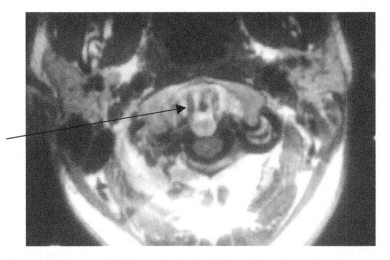

Figure 2 Details of MRI study of C1–C2 in a dislocation. Alar ligaments are orientated in the sagittal direction. Intraoperatively, the alar ligaments proved to obstruct the reduction due to ossification.

fatigue fractures occurring secondary to abnormal statics, long lever arm of the flexed head and neck, and the commonly present osteopenia and/or osteoporosis. Whatever the mechanism and cause of these injuries or lesions are, increase of the cervicothoracic kyphosis is a constant clinico-radiologic feature shared by these disorders.

3. Enthesopathy: the chronic pain resulting from the inflammatory changes is an important factor for the development of global kyphosis.

4. Weakness of the extensors of the spine is claimed to play a significant role in the development and progression of the deformity.

(A)

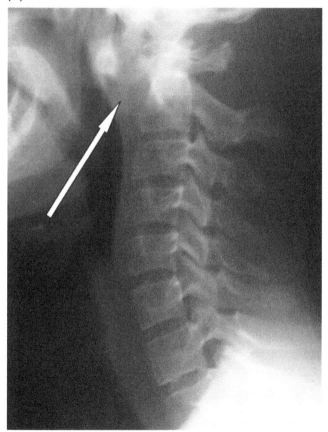

Figure 3 (A) Preoperative lateral X-ray of a 29-year-old AS patient with otherwise mainly thoracolumbar ankylosis and an onset 12 year prior. While the subaxial cervical spine had remained mobile, a rigid dislocation of the head has persisted for one year. The patient was admitted because of rapidly progressing tetraparesis. (B) Axial CT scan of the same patient: in anterior dislocation of C1 versus C2 fixed deformity. Bony bridges are hindering the reduction. Please note the malposition of the odontoid in the posterior half of the canal. (C) Post-operative lateral X-ray. The fixed atlantoaxial dislocation could be reduced by transoral and posterior osteotomy, correction and fixation by Magerl technique. Complete recovery of walking ability, partial recovery, but residual myelopathic signs in the upper extremities, and recovery of walking ability without spasticity were observed. *Abbreviations*: CT, computed tomography; AS, ankylosing spondylitis.

(B)

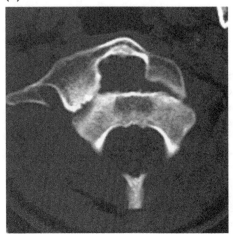 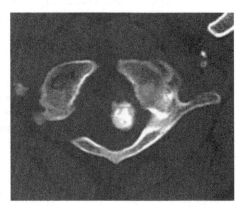

(C)

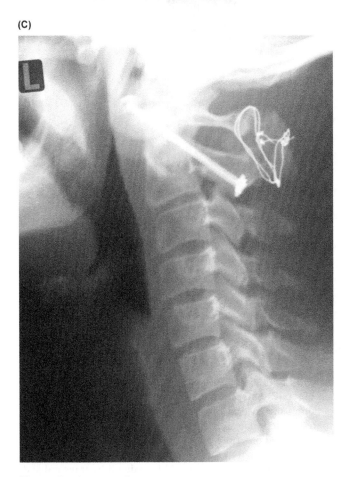

Figure 3 (*Continued*)

Sequelae of cervicothoracic kyphosis are:

1. disturbance of the axis of the field of vision,
2. susceptibility for spontaneous fractures,
3. risk of instability and stenosis at a proximal level,
4. chronic neck pain,
5. ugly deformity,
6. blocking an access to the anterior structures of the neck,
7. bad skin hygiene of the anterior part of the neck, and
8. difficult intubation and impossible access for tracheotomy if for any reason general anesthesia or emergency tracheotomy is needed.

Fractures

The abnormal statics, loss of the segmental mobility of the spine, and the osteoporotic bone make the ankylosed cervical spine more susceptible to fractures. These injuries usually follow a trivial trauma and can be easily overlooked. The trivial trauma, the already present chronic pain, and the location of the fracture at the cervicothoracic junction are responsible for the delay in diagnosis and possible occurrence of complications. Discovertebral lesions can be considered as pseudarthroses occurring on top of an overlooked fatigue fracture. Traumatic fractures in AS are completely different from fractures of the mobile spine because the ankylosed spine behaves like tubular bones. Typically in those fractures, often hyperextension injuries, the fracture line crosses the former laminar space. This can puzzle the surgeon, when in a fracture of the body of C7 he can find posterior osseous lesions at C6 or Th1. Because in plain X-rays this region cannot be visualized easily, the true extent of the trauma often needs additional imaging. The magnatic resonance imaging (MRI)—not being hampered by shoulder artifact in our experience proved to be much more helpful than the computed tomography (CT) scan. The ankylosis deprives the spine from a shock-absorbing function of the spine; this explains the high incidence of associated neurological complications.

Subaxial Instability

The progression of stiffness, ankylosis, and kyphosis imposes increased loads on the mobile segments of the cervical spine. Hypermobility at one segment can result in osteophyte formation and secondary spinal canal stenosis. Subaxial instability may also occur as a result of Anderson's lesion or an occult fracture.

Atlantoaxial Instability

Acute atlantoaxial subluxation or dislocation is a special clinicoradiologic entity not infrequently encountered in AS patients. The inflammatory process affecting the complex atlantoaxial joint and the abnormal statics are predisposing factors for the development of this disorder. A trivial trauma is sufficient to provoke the displacement. Tetraplegia due to acute neurological cord compression is a common presentation seen with this disorder. Delay in the diagnosis in cases without neurological deficits can result in chronic instability with gradual myelopathy or spontaneous fusion of the dislocated joint (Fig. 3B). Atlantoaxial instability of insidious onset and progressive course with or without myelopathy is another form seen in AS patients.

Craniocervical Instability and/or Stenosis

The craniocervical joint commonly retains a range of movement until an advanced stage of the disease. Hyperlordosis can occur as a compensatory mechanism to a global kyphosis disturbing the axis of vision. Instability with cord compression by the posterior arch of the atlas is rare but, if present, can be a source of serious high level myelopathy.

Correction of Cervicothoracic Kyphosis—General Considerations

The cervicothoracic spine is a common site for the development of kyphosis. Plain radiography can poorly image this area and MRI is very helpful in illustrating this region. The kyphotic deformity is commonly fixed. Infrequently, a mobile kyphotic deformity can be encountered particularly in those who sustained an occult fracture.

Many modifications have been done since the introduction of Urist's osteotomy (8). The osteotomy can be done under local anesthesia and a halo vest can be applied for gradual correction of the deformity. Some authors prefer to apply direct internal fixation. In our experience, osteotomy should be performed wherever bony bridges hinder a smooth and nonforceful correction of kyphosis. In the cervicothoracic junction it might be necessary posteriorly alone or in combination with previous anterior release (Fig. 4D).

Mobile Kyphosis: Technique of Correction

The surgery is done in the prone position under general anesthesia. SSEP is used for monitoring the cord function during the procedure. The spine is exposed from the midcervical region to the thoracic vertebra 3–4. A screw–rod system is used for fixation of the spine in which pedicle screws are inserted in vertebrae Th2–4. Lateral mass screws are inserted as described by Magerl in C4–C6 (9). Fluoroscopy is then done to verify the position and length of the screws. The posterior elements of C7 are removed together with part of C6 and T1 (Fig. 4D). The amount to be removed is adjusted roughly according to the amount of correction that is needed. Complete pediculotomy of Th1 is done to avoid secondary foraminal stenosis following the correction. The neck is then extended until the needed correction is obtained (Fig. 4B and C). The rods are then inserted and kept in place with the nuts. A wake-up test is then done to assure that the patient is still neurologically stable. The removed bone is then used at the osteotomy site to augment the fusion. If the anterior gap created through the correction is wide and would require a long time for spontaneous bridging, we recommend bridging it with bone graft or a cage filled with cancellous bone. This requires a second approach from the front, but usually can be performed in the same anesthesia. Due to a much more rapid bony consolidation this additional surgery usually pays very well by reducing the risk of loss of correction, and need for postoperative external support, and speeding up markedly the postoperative course.

Fixed Cervicothoracic Deformity: Technique of Correction

In this, it is preferred to start with anterior release in the form of osteotomy done at the C7–T1 disc. The patient is then turned into the prone position and the technique is completed as correction of mobile kyphosis.

(A)   **(B)**

(C)   **(D)**

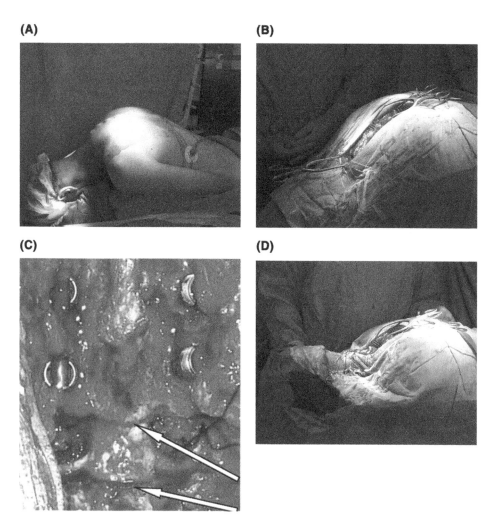

Figure 4   (**A**) Fixed cervicothoracic deformity in a 43-year-old male, 13 months after previous minor trauma. Positioning of the patient on the operative table in intubation anesthesia is shown. (**B**) Fixed cervicothoracic deformity. The same patient, with cervicothoracic spine exposed, before correction is viewed from the left side. (**C**) Details of the osteotomy site C7 before correction: laminectomy defect. The dura and both nerve roots are exposed, and both pedicles are resected. (**D**) Same patient, after posterior osteotomy and correction.

In those presenting with head on chest deformity there is no possibility to do the anterior release through an anterior approach. The anterior osteotomy is then done through a posterior approach with the aid of CT—or interventional MRI-navigation—to assure safety of the important neighboring structures.

Correction of Atlantoaxial Dislocation—General Considerations

Atlantoaxial subluxations and dislocation—though infrequently encountered—present a significant problem in AS. The mechanical overload imposed upon the relatively spared upper cervical segments in the otherwise ankylosed spine enhances the development of this complication. Significant trauma is frequently denied by these patients. Those who are lucky not to develop acute neurological manifestations are still at a high risk for the development of late myelopathy.

Atlantoaxial Dislocation, Technique of Reduction

Surgical reduction and fusion before the onset of neurological problems give excellent results as regards the correction of deformity and pain. Surgery should be considered even in neglected cases that have already developed myelopathy. Reducible C1–C2 subluxations and dislocations can be stabilized using the transarticular fixation method adopted by Magerl (9). Irreducible fixed C1–C2 dislocation with spinal canal stenosis presents a real surgical challenge. It is wise in such a situation to combine a transoral release with a posterior release, reduction, and C1–C2 transarticular fixation (Figs. 2 and 3A–C). Intraoperative spinal monitoring is an essential measure in this respect.

RESULTS

Sixty-six AS patients with cervical problems underwent corrective procedure of a deformity or instability at our institution during the period 1994–2003. Fifty-eight patients were males and eight were females reflecting the male gender predilection. The youngest patient at the time of operation was 30 years and the oldest one 78 years (mean: 49.4 years). Correction of the deformity succeeded in restoring a horizontal axis of vision in all the patients. However, due to dearrangement of posture of the lumbar and thoracic spine and fixed lordotic deformity at the craniocervical junction in 13 of these patients, the position of the head could only in 17 cases be brought optimally backward in respect to the plumb line. This is reflected in the postoperative occiput-wall distance (fleche occipitale) of 10.7 cm. Dramatic relief of pain was observed in those with preoperative painful instabilities.

Complications

No mortalities or cord injuries were encountered in this series. The most commonly encountered neurological complication was disturbed sensation or motor weakness affecting the C8 root. This was encountered in six patients and showed complete recovery in five. Temporary paresis of the C5 root occurred in two occasions. Wound infection occurred in two patients and healed after surgical debridement and re-closure of the wound. Loosening of the screws with resultant loss of correction occurred in one patient and warranted a revision surgery.

CONCLUSION

Several cervical disorders can occur in the course of the disease and can be a source of serious and life-threatening complications. Rheumatologists and orthopedic surgeons should be aware of the natural history of the disease and its complications. Proper imaging and early institution of treatment is crucial in protecting these patients from serious complications. Improvement in surgical instrumentations, advances in the tools of diagnosis and monitoring, and new options for instrumentations in this field have made surgery in ankylosing spine a real aid in improving the quality of life of these patients.

REFERENCES

1. Law WA. Osteotomy of the spine. J Bone Joint Surg Br 1959; 41:270.
2. Scudese V, Calabro JJ. Vertebral wedge osteotomy. J Am Med Assoc 1963; 186:627.
3. Smith-Peterson MN, Larson CB, Aufranc OE. Osteotomy of the spine for correction of flexion deformity in rheumatoid arthritis. J Bone Joint Surg 1945; 27:1.
4. Thomasen E. Vertebral osteotomy for correction of kyphosis in ankylosing spondylitis. Clin Orthop 1985; 194:142.
5. Boehm H, Schmelzle R, Bschorer R, eds. Zugangswege zur Wirbelsäule in Plastische und Wiederherstellungschirurgie. Unimed Verlag, 1996:638–646.
6. Boehm H. Simultaneous front and back surgery: a new technique with a thoracoscopic or retroperitoneal approach in prone position. Fourth International Meeting on Advanced Spine Techniques, Bermuda, 1997.
7. Boehm H, Hehne HJ, Zielke K. Correction of Bechterew kyphosis. Orthopade 1989; 18(2):142–154.
8. Urist MR. Osteotomy of the cervical spine: report of a case of ankylosing rheumatoid spondylitis. J Bone Joint Surg Am 1958; 41:833.
9. Magerl F, Seemann P. Stable posterior fusion of the atlas and axis by transarticular screw fixation. In: Kehr P, Weidner A, eds. Cervical Spine. New York: Springer, 1986:322–327.

20
Ankylosing Spondylitis: Complications Related to Spine Surgery

Marinus de Kleuver
Institute for Spine Surgery and Applied Research, Sint Maartenskliniek, Nijmegen, The Netherlands

INTRODUCTION

As the name suggests, ankylosing spondylitis (AS) will affect the spine in most if not all patients. Spinal surgery in these patients will generally be spinal fusions/arthrodesis, osteotomies, or spinal canal decompressions. As in all spine surgery, complications may occur, but there are certain aspects of AS which cause a specific spectrum of complications.

Biomechanic Considerations

As the disease progresses, the spine usually becomes rigid or fully ankylosed, sometimes in a kyphotic or scoliotic deformity (Fig. 1). The rigidity requires different strategies to stabilize situations of instability. The spine behaves as a long bone, and in fractures or osteotomies the proximal and distal parts of the spine act as long lever arms. Even minor movements of hips, pelvis, shoulders, or head will be directly transmitted to the fracture or osteotomy site. Therefore different (longer) instrumentation strategies are required compared to other patient categories with mobile spines. Furthermore, the spinal rigidity markedly reduces patients' ability to employ compensation mechanisms that may maintain spinal balance, and as the hips become stiffer and develop a flexion contracture, the ability to balance the trunk is compromised even further. Therefore, as the disease progresses, the patients' ability to cope with the rigid spine diminishes and postoperative malalignment is tolerated less than in other patient groups.

The spine not only becomes rigid, but often develops a kyphotic deformity. This leads to an increase in kyphotic forces in the entire spine which may induce complications such as failure of internal fixation constructions or development of junctional kyphosis above an arthrodesis, and again this has implications for the instrumentation techniques.

(A)   (B)   (C)

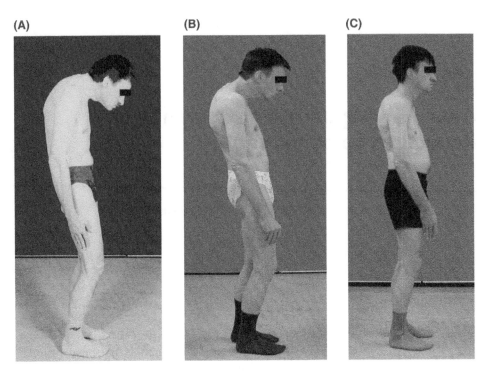

Figure 1 Patient with kyphotic deformity of the spine due to ankylosing spondylitis. (**A**) Preoperative, (**B**) after lumbar L3 closing wedge osteotomy, and (**C**) after cervical C7 osteotomy. *Note*: The eyes need to be covered, but as little as possible of the face, so that the alignment of the head can be well appreciated.

Anatomic Considerations

AS causes changes in the bone such as osteoporosis, hypertrophy of the posterior bony elements, fusion of the facet joints, and bony fusions of the intervertebral spaces (1). The ligamentum flavum ossifies, often becomes one with the posterior bony elements, and adheres to the dura mater. Intraoperative complications may result, as these bony changes may make anatomic landmarks hard to distinguish, the dural adhesions may cause dural tears during bone removal, and the osteoporosis may compromise internal fixation. If the ankylosis of the facet joints and the intervertebral disk is still at an early stage, it may be possible to treat spinal deformities in these patients with segmental corrections as in other patient categories, but mostly osteotomies will have to be performed at the facet joints to "release" the spine and allow corrections (2,3).

General Considerations

There are also certain general considerations which influence complications. AS is an autoimmune disease and is often treated with immune suppressive medication such as corticosteroids, and more recently, anti-tumor necrosis factor alpha (TNFα). This may result in wound healing problems and although there is no clear evidence available that postoperative infection rates are increased, in our own practice this does appear to be the case.

AS leads to rigidity of the chest cage, and this causes restrictive pulmonary disease resulting in increased intraoperative ventilation pressures. Postoperatively patients depend on their diaphragmatic breathing, and if they have some abdominal distension as is often the case after major spine surgery, this may easily result in pulmonary insufficiency.

A lot of AS patients often have concomitant diseases such as psoriasis or inflammatory bowel disease which can cause extra problems postoperatively.

Finally the marked kyphotic posture of the spine causes problems with positioning of the patient in the operating room and in the prevention of pressure sores.

In this chapter we will try to address the complications in spinal surgery in AS in relation to the earlier mentioned considerations, and discuss measures which may be taken to reduce the incidence of these complications.

COMPLICATIONS IN SPINE SURGERY

Complications in spinal surgery in patients with AS can be divided into three categories: intraoperative complications, postoperative complications related directly to the surgery, and postoperative general complications (Table 1), and they will be discussed in this order (4).

Intraoperative Complications

1. *Intubation problems*: due to the rigidity of the cervical thoracic spine, endotracheal intubation may be more difficult than normal. To prevent undue manipulation of the head, and possible fractures of the osteoporotic cervical spine, routine fiber-optic endotracheal intubation is advised.
2. *Patient positioning*: during most spine surgeries patients are positioned prone and due to the kyphotic spine and the flexion contracture in the hips this forms a challenge (Fig. 2).

Table 1 The Complication Classification of Spinal Corrective Surgery in Patients with AS

Intraoperative complications	Intubation problems, positioning problems, dural tears, outbreak of pedicle screws and fixation materials, incomplete reduction, profuse blood loss
Postoperative complications directly related to surgery	Wound infections: superficial and deep wound infections
	Neurological problems: SCI, nerve root dysfunction and radioculopathy
	Implant failure: loosening of nuts, rod or screw breakage and pull out
General complications	Minor general complications: urinary tract infections, pulmonary infection, disorientation, gastro-intestinal problems
	Major general complications: pulmonary embolism, blindness, gastro-intestinal perforation, death

Abbreviation: AS, ankylosing spondylitis; SCI, spinal cord and cauda injury.
Source: From Ref. 4.

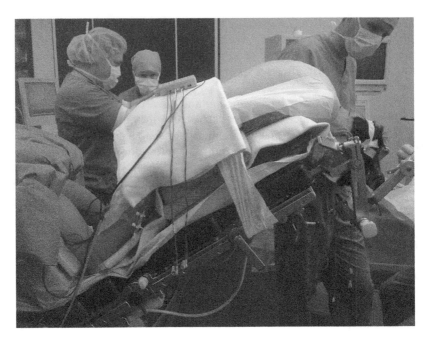

Figure 2 Problematic patient positioning due to cervico-thoracic kyphotic defromity. The head is elevated and placed in a Mayfield clamp to avoid high intraoccular pressure due to hydrostatic and contact pressures. The knees are supported to prevent the patient from slipping down the table and causing distraction of the spine or pressure sores on the chin. The arms are placed alongside the patient, as the shoulders cannot be fully elevated.

Due to the low position of the head pressure sores on face and chin may occur, and massive facial edema may form (Fig. 3). Furthermore due to the high intraocular hydrostatic pressure central optic neuropathy has been described, resulting in blindness (3–6). To keep the intraocular pressures lower, very specific care must be taken to avoid pressure on the eyeballs when the patient is prone, and the head must be kept elevated as far as possible, taking into account that the patient may then slide down the operating table.

Alternately for cervicothoracic osteotomies patients may be operated in the sitting position. Especially in patients with a chin or chest deformity this may be the only way to adequately position the patient. However, this may result in an increased rate of sometimes fatal intraoperative venous air embolism (VAE) (7).

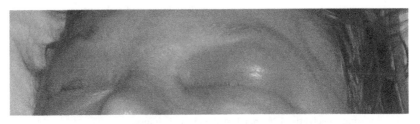

Figure 3 Facial edema after prolonged prone positioning.

3. *Lesions to dura mater*: there may be adhesions between dura mater, ligamentum flavum and bone, and intraoperatively this may easily cause lacerations and tears of the dura. Generally these can be adequately repaired with suturing, and if necessary interposition of a piece of fascia or Goretex®. Usually, if an osteotomy is performed, while extending the spine, there will be some excess dura after the correction, making closure of a laceration easier. If there is excessive correction, dural folds ("dural kinking") may develop, and this may cause neurologic compromise. Generally one would expect neurologic problems due to dural folds to occur more easily at the level of the spinal cord in the cervical spine than at cauda equina level in the lumbar spine, but in our own experience we have only once seen neorologic deficit due to dural folding in a lumbar spine osteotomy (Fig. 4).

4. *Osteoporosis and internal fixation*: due to the marked softness of the bone it is generally easier to remove bone with a rongeur than in other patients, but internal fixation poses a challenge. During correction procedures pedicle screws may easily break out. To obtain adequate fixation and to be able to use extension correction forces laminar hooks may be useful, as the laminar bony hypertrophy gives these hooks very good purchase. These hooks do not stabilize adequately against translation or rotation, and must be supplemented with pedicle screw constructs. At the lower end of a lumbar construct pedicle screws in S1 generally have very good grip, as the quality of bone in the sacrum is good due to the sacroiliitis, and pull through of these screws is seldom (if ever) seen.

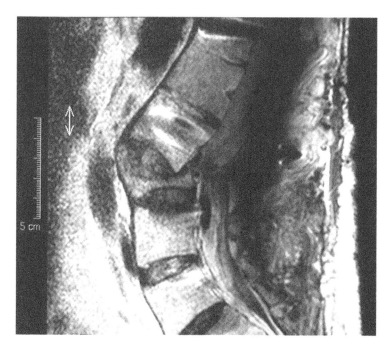

Figure 4   Direct postoperative MRI after L3 closing wedge ostetomy. The patient has almost complete quadriceps muscle paralysis, with intact motor functions in the lower legs and intact sensations. There is anterior translation and marked "dural kinking" resulting in compression of the lumbar cauda equina. *Abbreviation*: MRI, magnetic resonance imaging.

5. Profuse blood loss can be a problem encountered during osteotomy surgery, often from the osteoporotic bone and the epidural veins. It may partly be caused by high intra-abdominal pressures due to difficulties in adequately positioning these often very stooped patients. Adequate blood management must of course be applied. Intraoperatively routine surgical measures can be taken, using bipolar electrocautery, gelfoam, and other clotting agents, but in extreme cases it may be necessary to pack the wound and delay further surgery to a second stage at a later date.

Postoperative Complications Directly Related to the Surgery

1. *Infections*: in our own experience we have had a high rate of deep wound infections after osteotomy surgery in patients with AS. Before 1998 we had 11.7% deep wound infections. There may be several explanations for this. Patients have an autoimmune disease, and use medication that is often immune suppressive. This combination makes them more susceptible to deep wound infections. Furthermore blood loss is generally large, and blood transfusions may have an autoimmune suppressive effect. Finally patients were originally treated postoperatively with a plaster of Paris thoracolumbo sacral orthosis (TLSO) which was applied directly postoperatively with the patient still under anesthesia. Although this is common practice in other fields of orthopedic surgery, such as foot and ankle surgery, the significant postoperative wound drainage into the cast of these patients may have created a favorable environment for bacterial growth resulting in an increased infection rate. Since 1998 we are employing a rigid blood management protocol and immune suppressive autologous blood transfusions have become very rare. Due to more extensive internal fixation direct postoperative immobilization in a plaster of Paris cast is no longer necessary. With this new postoperative regimen the infection rate has been reduced to 2.6%. Perioperatively patients should receive adequate antibiotics, based on the bacteria most frequently found in the hospital's area. In our clinic patients currently receive an intravenous second generation cephalosporine at induction of anesthesia and during the first 24 hours postoperative. An extra dose of antibiotics is given after 2 L of blood loss or two hours of surgery. It is questionable whether longer postoperative antibiotics can prevent infections, and they may possibly have a detrimental effect by causing infections with resistant bacteria.

2. *Neurologic complications*: in our series of osteotomy patients we have had a relatively high rate of neurologic complications (15%) (4). Half of these patients have recovered fully, but ultimately 9 of 115 patients have had permanent neurologic deficit varying from radiculopathy to partial spinal cord injuries. However all patients in our series have remained community ambulators. There are several causes for neurologic injuries. The dural folding has been mentioned earlier. During closure of closing wedge osteotomies nerve roots may get entrapped in the foramen if inadequate bone resection has been performed. Furthermore, if inadequate removal of lamina bone has been performed during closure of a closing wedge osteotomy (pedicle substraction osteotomy) the lamina may impinge on the dura and the spinal cord. Finally, during correction of an osteotomy

inadvertent translation of the two vertebral bodies may occur, causing severe spinal stenosis (Fig. 5). Almost all neurologic injuries in these patients are due to mechanical compromise of the neurostructures. For this reason all surgery must be performed under adequate neuromonitoring, preferably including motoring evoked potentials. If reduction of signals

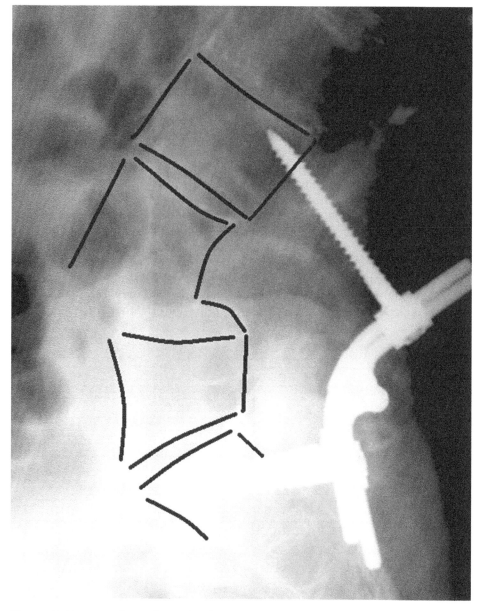

Figure 5 Postoperative radiograph after unsuccessful L4 closing wedge osteotomy in a 58-year-old man, weighing 120 kg. The L3 and L4 vertebrae have translated anterior, with resultant pull-out of the L3 pedicle screws. The patient had a cauda equina syndrome that recovered partially after re-intervention.

is seen, then the first step must be to ensure adequate hemodynamic perfusion with a mean arterial pressure above 60 mmHg. If there is no quick recovery, the correction must be reduced and this may often give marked recovery of signals (Fig. 6). Then further bony resection can be performed, so that further correction can again be attempted.

As nerve roots may be entrapped in the foramina, selective intraoperative electromyography (EMG) monitoring of several peripheral muscle groups (e.g., quadriceps, anterior tibial and gastrocnemius muscles) can help demonstrate nerve root entrapment, much more specifically than somato sensory evoked potentials (SSEPs), and for this reason multimuscle motor evoked potential monitoring is recommended (8).

If despite normal neuromonitoring and intraoperative findings there is a postoperative nerve root problem, further postoperative diagnostics are required such as a computed tomography (CT)-scan and a magnetic resonance imaging (MRI). However in our experience very frequently radiculopathy will recover with time. A direct postoperative MRI-scan is very difficult to interpret due to the implants (titanium), edema, hematoma, and marked changes in anatomy due to the osteotomy. The images are often alarming. Radiculopathy or single nerve root dysfunction should generally not be treated immediately, but several days to weeks may be waited before possible surgical re-exploration is attempted.

3. *Failure of internal fixation*: postoperative failure of internal fixation of fractures or osteotomies may occur due to failure of the implant bone interface (breakout of hooks and screws) or failures of the implants themselves. With older thin threaded rod implants up to 20% failures of the implants has been described; with current pedicle screw–solid rod constructs implant failures should rarely occur (4). By employing sufficient internal fixation at least three levels above and three levels below an osteotomy or fracture it is

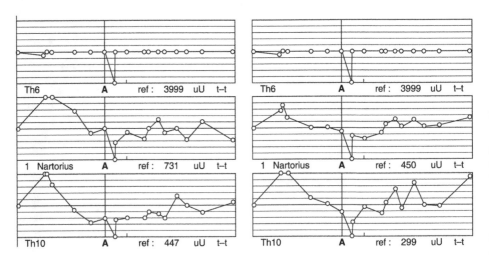

Figure 6 Intraoperative motor evoked potential responses. At point "A" during a cervical osteotomy procedure the head position is corrected to lordosis, and the response amplitude is reduced in all six muscle groups measured. After diminishing the correction, the responses recover fully. The patient had no postoperative deficits.

generally sufficient to prevent failures of fixation. In the cervical thoracic spine we prefer six lateral mass screws (three left, three right) in the cervical spine above the osteotomy or fracture, and four to six pedicle screws in the high thoracic spine, supplemented by a laminar hook at the lower end of the construct to prevent pull out. In the lumbar spine we prefer six pedicle screws in the lower spine including S1 due to the good fixation in the sclerotic sacrum, and four to six pedicle screws and two laminar hooks at the top of the construct, again to prevent the pull out due to the kyphotic forces.

4. *Postoperative fractures*: due to the marked kyphotic deformity there are huge kyphogenic forces on the spine. When an osteotomy is performed on the lumbar or cervical spine, this will markedly improve posture, but the thoracic hyperkyphosis is not addressed. If spinal balance is inadequately restored the kyphogenic forces may cause a junctional kyphosis or fractures (Fig. 7). This may require another operation and further internal fixation. Fractures have a tendency to heal poorly due to the long lever arms of the rigid spine, and the osteoporotic bone. The situation that

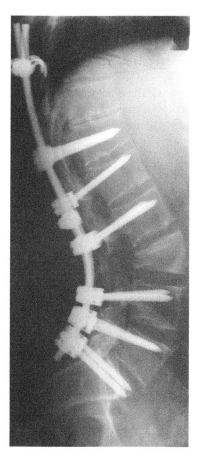
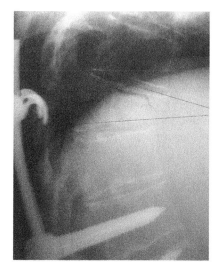

Figure 7 A 46-year-old male patient, three months after L3 closing wedge osteotomy. The osteotomy has consolidated. There is a spontaneous fracture at the top of the instrumented part of the spine. This may be due to the fact that the instrumentation ended at the apex of the thoracic kyphosis.

develops is similar to the pseudarthrosis that develops after spontaneous "discitis" also known as an Andersson lesion (9,10). Extension of the instrumentation, and sometimes combined anterior and posterior procedures are necessary to treat these lesions.

To prevent these fractures and junctional kyphosis above a fusion mass, long instrumentations should be used, and the instrumentation should never end at the apex of a kyphosis. This may mean that even for a lumbar osteotomy the instrumentation may have to be continued up high into the thoracic spine.

General Postoperative Complications

In our experience around 10% of the AS patients have serious complications after major spine surgery, such as pulmonary embolism, gastrointestinal complications, cerebral hemorrhage, acute respiratory distress syndrome, multiple organ failure, and one case of bacterial meningitis after a dural leak. We have had two deaths (out of 115 patients operated), one due to cardiac arrest and one due to a cerebral hemorrhage. Many of these major catastrophes are difficult to prevent, but they illustrate that these patients are prone to complications. Of course it implies that adequate care must be taken of these patients, including routine anticoagulation therapy, adequate pulmonary exercises (especially considering the rigid chest pulmonary infections are frequent), and attention to the gastrointestinal system (especially considering the frequent concomitant colitis and the occurrence of a paralytic postoperative ileus after spine surgery). In our series we saw a very high rate of major complications in patients who underwent combined anterior and posterior spine surgery, and for this reason we do our utmost to prevent combined surgery in this patient category.

CONCLUSIONS

Spine surgery, and especially osteotomy surgery in patients with AS is associated with a high complication rate that appears to be higher than other adult spinal deformity surgery (11). Patients must be made aware of this, and preoperative information should be adapted to these patients. Despite these complications, patients are often severely restricted in their daily life, and will often accept these risks. It cannot be shown from any data, but common sense suggests that complications occur more frequently during difficult surgery and major corrections. Therefore it may be wise to offer surgery to these patients at a relatively early stage of deformity, and not to wait until they are so kyphotic that the required corrections are enormous and neurologic injury and instrumentation failures are more likely.

Some complications seem to be specifically related to the AS (intraoperative positioning, screw pull out, deep wound infections, and comorbidity). Therefore as the underlying disease seems to contribute so much to the type and incidence of complications, these surgeries should be performed by a team experienced in treating patients with AS and not just an experienced spine team. A team that is aware of the possible complications can to a certain extent prevent them by adequate intraoperative positioning, blood management, neuro-monitoring, adequate surgical decompressions, and adapted instrumentation techniques, and can adequately address the complications if they do occur.

REFERENCES

1. Stafford L, Youssef PP. Spondyloarthropathies: an overview. Intern Med J 2002; 32(1–2):40–46.
2. Puschel J, Zielke K. Corrective surgery for kyphosis in Bekhterev's disease—indication, technique, results. Z Orthop Ihre Grenzgeb 1982; 120(3):338–342.
3. Van Royen BJ, de Kleuver M, Slot GH. Polysegmental lumbar posterior wedge osteotomies for correction of kyphosis in ankylosing spondylitis. Eur Spine J 1998; 7(2): 104–110.
4. Willems KF, Slot GH, Anderson PG, Pavlov PW, de Kleuver M. Spinal osteotomy in patients with ankylosing spondylitis: complications during first postoperative year. Spine 2005; 30(1):101–107.
5. Luken MG III, Patel DV, Ellman MH. Symptomatic spinal stenosis associated with ankylosing spondylitis. Neurosurgery 1982; 11(5):703–705.
6. Simmons EH. The surgical correction of flexion deformity of the cervical spine in ankylosing spondylitis. Clin Orthop 1972; 86:132–143.
7. Schmitt HJ, Hemmerling TM. Venous air emboli occur during release of positive end-expiratory pressure and repositioning after sitting position surgery. Anesth Analg 2002; 94(2):400–403.
8. Langeloo DD, Lelivelt A, Louis JH, Slappendel R, de Kleuver M. Transcranial electrical motor-evoked potential monitoring during surgery for spinal deformity: a study of 145 patients. Spine 2003; 28(10):1043–1050.
9. Andersson A. Röntgenbilden vid spondylarthritis ankylopoetica. Nord Med Tidskr 1937; 14:200.
10. Obradov M, Schonfeld DH, Franssen MJ, de Rooy DJ. Andersson lesion in ankylosing spondylitis. JBR-BTR 2001; 84(2):71.
11. Bridwell KH, Lewis SJ, Lenke LG, Baldus C, Blanke K. Pedicle subtraction osteotomy for the treatment of fixed sagittal imbalance. J Bone Joint Surg Am 2003; 85-A(3): 454–463.

21

Atlantoaxial Subluxation in Ankylosing Spondylitis

Cesar Ramos-Remus, Antonio Barrera-Cruz, and Francisco J. Aceves-Avila
Department of Rheumatology, Centro Médico Nacional de Occidente,
IMSS, Guadalajara, Mexico

Miguel A. Macias-Islas
Department of Neurology, Centro Médico Nacional de Occidente, IMSS,
Guadalajara, Mexico

INTRODUCTION

Several textbooks and reviews have underscored the importance of atlantoaxial subluxation (AAS) in ankylosing spondylitis (AS). It has been considered as a rare feature of classical AS, yet several studies reveal that the frequency of spontaneous AAS may be as high as 21% and can cause intense pain, a myriad of neurological symptoms, and even death. In this chapter we present some anatomic considerations of the craniovertebral junction, definitions, and pertinent data on the frequency, clinical implications, and potential risk factors for AAS in primary AS patients.

ANATOMIC CONSIDERATIONS AND DEFINITIONS

Most of the clinical and radiological manifestations of AS are explained by alterations in synovial and cartilaginous joints and in sites of tendon and ligament attachment to bone, named enthesitis.

Four synovial articulations occur between the atlas and axis: two lateral atlantoaxial joints, one on each side, between the inferior facet of the lateral mass of the atlas and the superior facet of the axis; and two median synovial joints, one minor between the anterior arch of the atlas and the odontoid process of the axis and a second and larger lies between the cartilage-covered anterior surface of the transverse ligament of the atlas and the grooved posterior surface of the odontoid process. In addition to these synovial articulations, syndesmoses between the atlas and axis include continuations of the anterior longitudinal ligament anteriorly and the ligamenta flava posteriorly (1). The joints are stabilized by a large number of ligaments, including the transverse ligament, the alar ligament, and the accessory atlantoaxial ligaments (2).

Atlantoaxial subluxation has been classified as congenital, traumatic, or spontaneous. Spontaneous AAS usually occurs in association with an infectious or inflammatory process. Spontaneous AAS is described as a complication of various rheumatic conditions, including rheumatoid arthritis, rheumatic fever, systemic lupus erythematosus, mixed connective tissue disease, psoriatic arthritis, reactive arthritis, inflammatory bowel disease, Behcet's syndrome, osteoarthritis, ossification of the posterior longitudinal ligament, diffuse idiopathic skeletal hyperostosis (DISH) Marfan syndrome, and Lesch–Nyhan syndrome (3–19).

Atlantoaxial subluxation can occur anteriorly, posteriorly, vertically, laterally, and/or rotationally. Anterior AAS is characterized by an increase in the atlas–dens interval on a plain radiograph taken in the neutral position or with the neck flexed (Fig. 1). There is no agreement on the definition of the minimal distance required to diagnose anterior AAS. Early reports suggested that the distance between the anterior aspect of the odontoid and the posterior aspect of the anterior arch of the atlas never exceeded 2 mm or 2.5 mm in lateral films taken in flexion and extension in normal adults (8,20). Others determined that the normal distance in adults is 1.238 − (0.0074 × age in years), ±0.90 mm in women, and 2.052 − (0.0192 × age in years), ±1.00 mm in men (21). A subsequent study of 1292 healthy adults found that 99.4% had a distance of 3 mm or less, 0.5% a distance between 3.1 and 3.5 mm, 0.08% between 3.6 and 4 mm, and 0.8% between 4.1 and 4.5 mm; none had a distance > 4.5 mm. The authors concluded that a distance of more than 3 mm after the age of 44 and more than 4 mm in younger people should be considered abnormal (4). Yet we have used ≥4 mm to define anterior AAS in research to avoid borderline cases

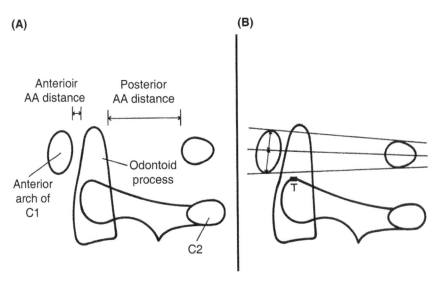

Figure 1 (A) Anterior atlantoaxial interval is the distance between the anterior aspect of the odontoid and the posterior aspect of the anterior arch of the atlas. Posterior atlantoaxial interval is the distance between the posterior margin of the odontoid and the anterior rim of the posterior arch of C1. (B) The Sakaguchi–Kauppi method to assess vertical atlantoaxial subluxation. In normal situation (grade I), the tips of the facets of the axis are situated under a line drawn from the lower part of the posterior atlas arch to the lowest part of the anterior atlas arch (the lower atlas arch line). Vertical subluxation is diagnosed when the atlas falls around the axis; it is categorized into grades II, III, or IV.

(22,23). However, Boden et al. found that the distance between the posterior margin of the odontoid and the anterior rim of the posterior arch of C1 (posterior atlas–odontoid interval) (Fig. 1) showed stronger correlation with the risk of neurological compromise than the atlas–odontoid interval. All of their rheumatoid arthritis patients whose posterior atlas–odontoid interval was <14 mm had neurological abnormalities (24). If other studies confirm these findings, measuring the posterior atlas–odontoid interval may be used for surgical decisions.

Superior migration of the odontoid process, or vertical AAS, is better assessed in lateral films taken in neutral position. Several measurements have been used to determine it, including Chamberlain's line, McRae's line, McGregor's line, Rana-wat's method, Redlund's method, and Sakaguchi–Kauppi method (reviewed in Ref. 25). McRae's and McGregor's lines may be both less sensitive if the apex of the odontoid is eroded. If the apex of the odontoid cannot be identified, these methods cannot be used. Ranawat's method has not gained wide acceptance because the radiological landmarks are difficult to define. Redlund's method is based on measurements of the distance from the endplate of the axis to the McGregor's line. These landmarks are easy to find, and this is a good method for follow-up of vertical AAS. Unfortunately it is not satisfactory for screening because results depend on the height of the axis which has a wide distribution in healthy individuals (26). For screening purposes we use the Sakaguchi–Kauppi method; vertical AAS is diagnosed when the atlas falls around the axis; it is categorized into grades II, III, or IV (Fig. 1) (25).

Lateral AAS has been rarely reported in AS. In this situation, C1 is displaced laterally, resulting in abnormal head posture, and indicates unilateral or asymmetric involvement of the lateral atlantoaxial joint. Loss of all the cartilage and of no more than 1 mm of subchondral bone on the lateral mass of C1 or articular process of C2 allows a 2.5 mm lateral shift of C1. The upwardly directed superior articular process of C2 prevents further slippage. When more than 1 mm of bone is lost, the displacement can reach 5 mm and is limited by contact between the lateral mass of C1 and the odontoid. At the same time, the lateral mass of C1 touches C2, so that C1 is not only shifted laterally but also tilted. The diagnosis is provided by an anteroposterior open-mouth radiograph, which shows involvement of one or both C1–C2 joints with a >2 mm shift of C1 on C2 and tilting of C1 on C2. The degree of tilting reflects the extent of the damage to the lateral mass of C2 (27). The lateral view shows no evidence of lateral AAS.

Rotatory AAS has also been reported in AS patients. Rotatory AAS results from unilateral C1–C2 joint damage with disruption of the transverse ligament. The best incidence for demonstrating the dislocation by plain radiography is the open-mouth incidence, which shows lateral displacement of the odontoid, asymmetry of the C1 lateral masses with respect to the odontoid, and abnormal lateral mass geometry (the anteriorly displaced mass seems larger and closer to the odontoid, whereas the other mass seems smaller and farther from the odontoid). Persistence of these abnormalities when the neck is rotated confirms the diagnosis. Computerized tomography (CT) is currently the investigation of choice because it shows rotation of C1 on C2. CT images in maximum inverse rotation are particularly useful (27).

Posterior AAS is when the anterior arch of C1 moves upward and the posterior arch tilts downward until it lodges in front of the spinous process of C2. On imaging studies, the posterior margin of the anterior arch of C1 lies posterior to the anterior edge of the C2 vertebral body.

MECHANISMS EXPLAINING AAS

To the best of our knowledge, there are no reports on the mechanism explaining AAS in AS patients. In one experimental study on traumatisms De la Caffinière et al. (28) established that C1 cannot slip anteriorly over C2 unless the transverse ligament is disrupted. The maximum displacement is 5 mm when the other ligaments are intact but reaches 6.5–10 mm and 7 mm when the alar or accessory atlantoaxial ligaments are disrupted also, respectively, and 12 mm when all three ligaments are disrupted.

The advocated mechanisms to produce AAS in AS patients are similar to those reported in rheumatoid arthritis: the odontoid forms a synovial bursa with the anterior arch of the atlas and the transverse ligament; thus, chronic inflammation and pannus formation of the synovial tissue might cause odontoid erosions and AAS. Yet other mechanisms are worth considering. The basic problem in AS is inflammation at sites of tendon and ligament attachments, described as enthesitis. The transverse ligament, the alar ligament and the accessory atlantoaxial ligaments form multiple entheses. It is well known that enthesitis may produce bone erosions in AS patients, and thus, explain the reported erosions in odontoid. Enthesitis, with or without bone erosions, may produce ligament laxity, thus AAS. Indeed, ligaments and entheses involvement have also been reported in rheumatoid arthritis and systemic lupus erythematosus, among others (9,29).

PREVALENCE OF AAS IN AS

Patients with advanced AS are prone to fractures of the lower cervical spine following minor injuries, and their occurrence is 3.5 times greater than in the normal population (30–32). Sixty-six percent of the fracture subluxations of the ankylosed spine are associated with injury to the spinal cord, and the mortality rate is 40%; most of the AS patients are injured by falls (33,34). Despite the higher risk of cervical fractures in AS, there are few case reports in the literature of traumatic AAS in AS. For instance, Liang et al. (35) report on a 46-year-old man who sustained injury in a traffic accident. He developed quadriplegia and spontaneous eye opening, and deep coma later on. He had a 20-year history of AS. Radiographs showed advanced AS changes and atlantoaxial fracture dislocation with complete dissociation of the atlantoaxial junction. The patient died on the seventh day after admission.

On the other hand, the literature reveals several case reports or case series, five cross-sectional studies, and one follow-up report of spontaneous AAS since 1933 (4,5,22,23,36–58). Altogether we identified 106 cases of AAS in patients with primary AS-77% had anterior AAS, 10% vertical, 8.5% rotatory, and 4% mixed forms. For instance, Sharp and Purser (4) described a case series of 18 patients with AS with anterior AAS ($\geq$3 mm). Disease duration in this series ranged from 3 to 31 years and the atlantoaxial distance ranged from 4 to 16 mm. Six of 18 patients (33%) had some degree of neurological manifestations. In a study by Martel (5), 31 patients with AS were assessed because of persistent neck discomfort and/or severe, progressive disease. In this selected group anterior AAS was diagnosed at $\geq$3 mm and was observed in four patients (13%). The disease duration ranged from 15 to 25 years and the atlantoaxial distance from 3 to 5 mm. In another study, where no selection criteria or definition of anterior AAS were described, five of 73 (6.8%) patients with AS were reported to have anterior AAS, with a disease duration of 1 to 32 years and atlantoaxial distance between 4 and 16 mm (57). In a case series of AAS in six patients with AS,

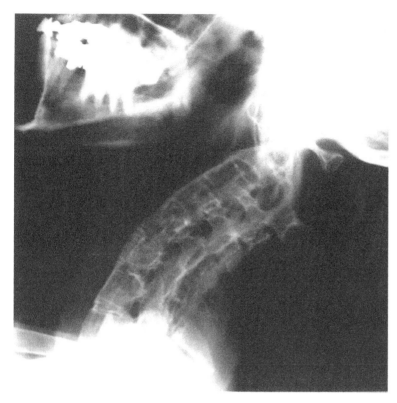

Figure 2 In a 52-year-old man with a 25-year history of ankylosing spondylitis, a lateral position plain film of the cervical spine reveals anterior atlantoaxial subluxation, apophyseal joint ankylosis, and syndesmophytosis.

Halla et al. (37) described two anterior AAS (>3 mm), one vertical AAS, six lateral AAS, and four rotative AAS. The range of disease duration was 8 to 18 years. Suarez-Almazor and Russell (56) reported an association between AAS and peripheral arthritis: six of 17 patients with diverse seronegative spondyloarthropathies (SpA) and peripheral arthritis had anterior AAS, compared to none of 21 patients with SpA without peripheral arthritis. We studied 103 patients with AS consecutively recruited from two secondary care outpatient rheumatology clinics within a six month period, all of them having primary AS, and were not selected on the basis of cervical involvement. The mean age was 35 years, 74% were male, and the mean disease duration was 10 years (SD ±7.9). We found that 22 patients (21%) (confidence interval from 13% to 29%) had anterior AAS using a distance ≥4 mm as a criterion; 17 patients (16%) had a distance between 4 and 6 mm, four patients (4%) between 6.5 and 9.0 mm and one patient (1%)≥9.5 mm. Two patients with anterior AAS also had vertical AAS (Figs. 2 and 3) (22). Lee et al. (58) reported that 13.8% of their 181 AS patients had AAS; this point prevalence is similar to the confidence interval we had reported.

CLINICAL CONSIDERATIONS AND FOLLOW-UP

Atlantoaxial subluxation may be developed at any time during the course of AS. There are at least eight case reports in the literature where AAS was diagnosed

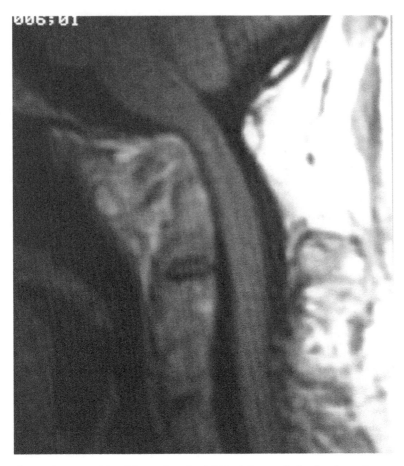

Figure 3   T1-weighted fast-spin echo MRI of the cervical spine from the same patient shows anterior atlantoaxial subluxation, a poorly defined odontoid process, and integrity of spinal cord.

before or shortly after clinically apparent AS; some of them were in juvenile AS. However, one cross-sectional study did not find significant association between the age at onset or the age at diagnosis and the presence of AAS (22). The reported association between peripheral arthritis and anterior AAS in patients with diverse SpA was not found in a study of patients with primary AS (22,56). Yet it was found that anterior AAS was associated with the presence of posterior longitudinal ligament ossification at cervical level, and the mean anterior atlantoaxial distance increased with sacroiliitis grade, reaching statistical significance for grade IV sacroiliitis (22). It is also reported that condylar erosions in temporomandibular joints were associated with anterior AAS (59).

In most of the published case reports, spontaneous AAS was diagnosed after clinical symptoms and the reported follow-up was related to the results of therapeutic interventions; the overall short-term outcome in these cases was good in 46 of 48 patients, where this information was available. Twenty-nine (60%) of these patients underwent surgery, 18 (38%) were handled with traction, cervical collar and/or plaster, and one with no intervention. The main reported indication for surgery was neck pain.

Although the information is scanty regarding the course of spontaneous AAS in those patients where the diagnosis was made for screening purposes, it seems that at least in one-third of AS patients the anterior AAS will increase in the following two years. In the case series of Sharp and Purser (4), 13 of the 18 patients with AS had radiographs of the cervical spine taken at some time before the diagnosis of AAS (mean 2.3 years, range one month to six years). Progression of anterior AAS was observed in 11 (85%) patients and the magnitude of the progression, calculated as percentage progression from the first film, ranged from 20% to 800%; in some cases, notable progression occurred in <2 years.

However, magnification factors may represent a source of error that precludes accurate linear measurements. Magnification error is governed by the subject-to-cassette and tube-to-cassette distances. Although standardized techniques are used in radiology departments, small variations in these distances may produce magnification error in bone measurements (60,61). The effect that magnification creates on different structures (e.g., C1–odontoid distance or the thickness of the cervical prevertebral soft tissues) is controversial (62,63). In one study assessing the progression of anterior and vertical AAS in AS patients, magnification issues were present in eight of 16 available paired films, and its presence affected differences by no more than 0.8 mm (23). In this study, anterior AAS was detected in 22 patients at baseline examination, and two of them also had vertical AAS. At two years follow-up, one patient had died of acquired immunodeficiency syndrome, three could not be reached, and the two who had undergone surgical fusion due to severe myelopathy, now showed complete neurological recovery. Of the remaining 16 patients, seven (32%) showed progression and nine (41%) showed no change in the C1–odontoid distance; the progression ranged from 0% to 120%. Vertical AAS developed in one patient. Three additional patients had surgical fusion because of notable progression of AAS, despite absence of neurological signs. No variable registered at baseline, including age at onset, AS characteristics, neurological findings and radiological features, was identified as a predictor of AAS progression (23). Long-term follow-up studies are necessary to determine whether apophyseal fusion and/or ossification of the longitudinal ligaments can arrest, at least in some, the progression of anterior and/or vertical AAS.

On the contrary, AAS may be a feature of a subgroup of patients with AS with more severe axial enthesopathy, considering that it may be present early in the course of AS, and its association with ossification of the posterior longitudinal ligament, condylar erosions in temporomandibular joints, and grade IV radiological sacroiliitis (22).

SYMPTOMS AND SIGNS OF AAS

The clinical picture of severe AAS is characteristic and easily recognized. In less severe degrees of displacement when the diagnosis is not too obvious, symptoms including those due to neurological changes may remain unexplained unless this complication is considered. The clinical expression and severity depends on three factors: the individual variation between the spinal cord volume and space available in the bony canal, and the swiftness and type of AAS. These factors may explain that there is no clear relationship between the radiological features and the neurological signs (Figs. 2 and 3) (2).

It has been reported that AAS in AS patients may produce a myriad of neurological and vascular symptoms, including severe neck pain, myelopathy, multiple cerebellar infarction due to vertebral artery obstruction and bulbar symptoms,

Table 1 Suggested Strategies for Clinical and Radiological Screening and Follow-Up of Atlantoaxial Subluxation in Ankylosing Spondylitis

At baseline obtain radiographs of the cervical spine: anteroposterior open-mouth and lateral in neutral position and flexion

	Clinical condition	Follow-up	Scenarios	Follow-up
No AAS is observed	Patient has sacroiliitis grade ≤III	Obtain the same cervical radiographs every 5 years	Development of AAS	Same as in AAS is observed
	Patient has sacroiliitis grade IV, and/or OPLL, and/or TMJ dysfunction	Obtain the same cervical radiographs every 2 years		
	If anterior odontoid–atlas interval ≤6 mm and/or posterior odontoid–atlas interval ≥15 mm	Obtain the same cervical radiographs every year	AAS progression or new development of vertical AAS	Perform full neurological assessment and extensive imaging studies; discussion by rheumatologist and surgeon of the need for fusion
AAS is observed	If anterior odontoid–atlas interval ≥6 mm and/or posterior odontoid–atlas interval ≤15 mm, and/or vertical AAS	Perform full neurological assessment and extensive imaging studies; discussion by rheumatologist and surgeon of the need for fusion		
Patient undergoing any kind of surgical procedures involving intubation		Obtain the same cervical radiographs before surgery; discussion by surgeon and anesthesiology of risks of intubation		
Patient having at any time vascular or neurological symptoms		Perform full neurological assessment and extensive imaging studies		

Abbreviations: AAS, atlantoaxial subluxation; OPLL, ossification of the posterior longitudinal ligament; TMJ, temporomandibular joint.

and vertebrobasilar insufficiency, but its real frequency is difficult to assess. A number of factors can be concurrent in patients with AS and produce vascular and neurological symptoms or signs, such as a specific type of myelopathy, myopathy, disuse muscle atrophy, ossification of the posterior longitudinal ligament, and nonspecific alterations in somatosensory evoked potentials (22,64–69). Furthermore, subtle neurological and vascular manifestations of AAS, such as tinnitus or autonomic dysfunction, have not been properly assessed.

SUGGESTED STRATEGIES FOR CLINICAL AND RADIOLOGICAL FOLLOW-UP OF AAS IN AS

There are no established guidelines for the management of spontaneous AAS in patients with AS. In most instances, the management has been similar to that suggested for patients with rheumatoid arthritis. Surgical stabilization has been recommended when displacement is >5 mm, severe pain cannot be controlled by a collar, displacement of the sagittal diameter of the spinal canal is 30% or greater, or there are neurological symptoms or signs (36,44,45). Three of our reported patients had surgical fusion even in the absence of myelopathy or pain, because of craniocervical instability and a high risk of sudden death (22,23). Indeed, Agarwal et al. (70) recommended early C1–C2 fusion in patients with rheumatoid AAS before basilar invagination develops, to reduce the risk of future progression of cervical spine instability and its associated complications. Matsunaga et al. found better survival rates in their rheumatoid arthritis patients after surgical fusion when compared with nonsurgical treatment (71). Yet there are reports in patients with AS of reduction of the C1–odontoid distance after either a period of continuous halo traction, use of a collar, or spontaneous fixation of the atlantoaxial joint occurring during spontaneous apophyseal fusion (4,38,53).

Even though there are several unanswered questions regarding the clinical impact, screening procedures, management, and prognosis of AAS in AS patients, we may say that this complication is not uncommon and may produce significant morbidity and risk of death. Meanwhile we use the strategies in Table 1 for screening and follow-up of AAS in our AS patients.

REFERENCES

1. Resnick D, Niwayama G. Anatomy of individual joints. In: Resnick D, ed. Diagnosis of Bone and Joint Disorders. Philadelphia, PA: Saunders, 1995:672–768.
2. Bland J, Boushey D. Anatomy and physiology of the cervical spine. Semin Arthritis Rheum 1990; 20:1–20.
3. Bland JH. Rheumatoid subluxation of the cervical spine. J Rheumatol 1990; 17:134–137.
4. Sharp J, Purser DW. Spontaneous atlanto-axial dislocation in ankylosing spondylitis and rheumatoid arthritis. Ann Rheum Dis 1961; 20:47–77.
5. Martel W. The occipito–atlanto-axial joints in rheumatoid arthritis and ankylosing spondylitis. Am J Roentgenol 1961; 86:223–240.
6. Castro S, Verstraete K, Mielants H, Vanderstraeten G, de Reuck J, Veys EM. Cervical spine involvement in rheumatoid arthritis: a clinical, neurological and radiological evaluation. Clin Exp Rheumatol 1994; 12:369–374.
7. Komusi T, Munro T, Harth M. Radiologic review: the rheumatoid cervical spine. Semin Arthritis Rheum 1985; 14:187–105.

8. Coutts MB. Atlanto-epistropheal subluxation. Arch Surg 1934; 29:297–311.

9. Babini SM, Maldonado-Cocco JA, Babini JC, de la Sota M, Arturi A, Marcos JC. Atlantoaxial subluxation in systemic lupus erythematosus: further evidence of tendinous alterations. J Rheumatol 1990; 17:173–177.

10. Stuart RA, Maddison PJ. Atlantoaxial subluxation in a patient with mixed connective tissue disease. J Rheumatol 1991; 18:1617–1620.

11. Laiho K, Kauppi M. The cervical spine in patients with psoriatic arthritis. Ann Rheum Dis 2002; 61:650–652.

12. Fox B, Sahuquillo J, Poca MA, Huguet P, Lience E. Reactive arthritis with a severe lesion of the cervical spine. Br J Rheumatol 1997; 36:126–129.

13. Jordan JM, Obeid LM, Allen NB. Isolated atlantoaxial subluxation as the presenting manifestation of inflammatory bowel disease. Am J Med 1986; 80:517–520.

14. Koss JC, Dalinka MK. Atlantoaxial subluxation in Behcet's syndrome. Am J Roentgenol 1980; 134:392–393.

15. Daumen-Legre V, Lafforgue P, Champsaur P, et al. Anteroposterior atlantoaxial subluxation in cervical spine osteoarthritis: case reports and review of the literature. J Rheumatol 1999; 26:687–691.

16. Takasita M, Matsumoto H, Uchinou S, Tsumura H, Torisu T. Atlantoaxial subluxation associated with ossification of posterior longitudinal ligament of the cervical spine. Spine 2000; 25(16):2133–2136.

17. Verdone F. Anterior atlantoaxial subluxation in a patient with DISH. J Rheumatol 1999; 26:1639–1640.

18. Herzka A, Sponseller PD, Pyeritz RE. Atlantoaxial rotatory subluxation in patients with Marfan syndrome. A report of three cases. Spine 2000; 25:524–526.

19. Shewell PC, Thompson AG. Atlantoaxial instability in Lesch–Nyhan syndrome. Spine 1996; 21:757–762.

20. Jackson H. The diagnosis of minimal atlanto-axial subluxation. Br J Radiol 1950; 26:672–674.

21. Hinkck VS, Hopkins CE. Measurement of the atlanto-dental interval in the adult. Am J Roentgenol 1960; 84:945–947.

22. Ramos-Remus C, Gomez-Vargas A, Guzman-Guzman JL, et al. Frequency of atlantoaxial subluxation and neurologic involvement in patients with ankylosing spondylitis. J Rheumatol 1995; 22:2120–2125.

23. Ramos-Remus C, Gomez-Vargas A, Hernandez-Chavez A, Gamez-Nava JI, Gonzalez-Lopez L, Russell AS. Two year followup of anterior and vertical atlantoaxial subluxation in ankylosing spondylitis. J Rheumatol 1997; 24:507–510.

24. Boden S, Dodge L, Bohlmann H, Rechtine G. Rheumatoid arthritis of the cervical spine. J Bone Joint Surg 1993; 75A:1282–1297.

25. Kauppi M, Sakaguchi M, Konttinen YT, Hämäläinen M. A new method of screening for vertical atlantoaxial dislocation. J Rheumatol 1990; 17:167–172.

26. Eulderich F, Meijers KAE. Pathology of the cervical spine in rheumatoid arthritis. J Pathol 1976; 120:91–108.

27. Bouchaud-Chabot A, Lioté F. Cervical spine involvement in rheumatoid arthritis. A review. J Bone Spine 2002; 69:141–154.

28. De la Caffinière JY, Seringe R, Roy-Camille R, Saillant G. Étude physiopathologiques des lésions ligamentaries graves dans les traumatismes de la charnière occipito-rachidienne. Rev Chir Orthop Reparatrice Appar Mot 1972; 58:11–19.

29. Ball J. Enthesopathy of rheumatoid and ankylosing spondylitis. Ann Rheum Dis 1971; 30:213–223.

30. Hunter T, Forster B, Dvorak M. Ankylosed spines are prone to fracture. Can Fam Physician 1995; 41:1213–1216.

31. Salathe M, Johr M. Unsuspected cervical fractures a common problem in ankylosing spondylitis. Anesthesiology 1989; 70:869–870.

32. Olerud C, Frost A, Brin J. Spinal fractures in patients with ankylosing spondylitis. Eur Spine J 1996; 5:51–55.
33. Kewalramani LS, Taylor RG, Albrand OW. Cervical spine injury in patients with ankylosing spondylitis. J Trauma 1975; 15:931–934.
34. Rowed DW. Management of cervical spinal cord injury in ankylosing spondylitis: the intervertebral disc as a cause of cord compression. J Neurosurg 1992; 77:241–246.
35. Liang Ch-L, Lu K, Lee T-Ch, Lin Y-Ch, Chen H-J. Dissociation of atlantoaxial junction in ankylosing spondylitis. J Trauma 2002; 53:1173–1175.
36. Sorin S, Askari A, Moskowitz RW. Atlantoaxial subluxation as a complication of early ankylosing spondylitis. Two case reports and review of the literature. Arthritis Rheum 1979; 22:273–276.
37. Halla JT, Fallahi S, Hardin JG. Nonreducible rotational head tilt and atlantoaxial lateral mass collapse. Arch Intern Med 1983; 143:471–474.
38. Santavirta S, Slätis P, Sandelin J, Lindqvist C, Konttinen YT. Atlanto-axial subluxation in patients with seronegative spondylarthritis. Rheumatol Int 1987; 7:43–46.
39. Leventhal MR, Maguire JK, Christian CA. Atlantoaxial rotary subluxation in ankylosing spondylitis. Spine 1990; 15:1374–1376.
40. Thompson GH, Khan MA, Bilenker RM. Spontaneous atlantoaxial subluxation as a presenting manifestation of juvenile ankylosing spondylitis. Spine 1982; 7:78–79.
41. Hamilton MG, MacRae ME. Atlantoaxial dislocation as the presenting symptom of ankylosing spondylitis. Spine 1993; 18:2344–2346.
42. Reid GD, Hill RH. Atlantoaxial subluxation in juvenile ankylosing spondylitis. J Pediatr 1978; 93:531–532.
43. Kernodle GW, Allen NB, Kredich D. Atlantoaxial subluxation in juvenile ankylosing spondylitis. Arthritis Rheum 1987; 20:837–838.
44. Stammers FAR, Frazer P. Spontaneous dislocation of the atlas. Lancet 1933; 2: 1203–1205.
45. Kornblum D, Clayton ML, Nash HH. Nontraumatic cervical dislocations in rheumatoid spondylitis. J Am Med Assoc 1952; 149:431–435.
46. Margulies ME, Katz I, Rosenberg M. Spontaneous dislocation of the atlanto-axial joint in rheumatoid spondylitis. Neurology 1955; 5:290–294.
47. Wilkinson M, Bywaters EGL. Clinical features and course of ankylosing spondylitis. Ann Rheum Dis 1958; 17:209–228.
48. Martel W, Page JW. Cervical vertebral erosions and subluxations in rheumatoid arthritis and ankylosing spondylitis. Arthritis Rheum 1960; 3:546–556.
49. Lourie H, Stewart WA. Spontaneous atlantoaxial dislocation. A complication of rheumatoid disease. N Engl J Med 1961; 265:677–681.
50. Cruckshank B. Pathology of ankylosing spondylitis. Clin Orthop 1971; 74:43–58.
51. Little H, Swinson DR, Cruckshank B. Upward subluxation of the axis in ankylosing spondylitis. Am J Med 1976; 60:279–285.
52. Wainstein PR, Karpman RR, Gall EP, Pitt M. Spinal cord injury, spinal fracture, and spinal stenosis in ankylosing spondylitis. J Neurosurg 1982; 57:609–616.
53. Hunter T. The spinal complications of ankylosing spondylitis. Semin Arthritis Rheum 1989; 19:172–182.
54. Elia M, Mazzara JT, Fielding JW. Onlay technique for occipitocervical fusion. Clin Orthop 1992; 280:170–174.
55. Fox MW, Onofrio BM, Kilgore JE. Neurological complications of ankylosing spondylitis. J Neurosurg 1993; 78:871–878.
56. Suarez-Almazor ME, Russell AS. Anterior atlantoaxial subluxation in patients with spondyloarthropathies: association with peripheral disease. J Rheumatol 1988; 15:973–975.
57. Meijers KAE, Heerman van Voss SFC, Francois RJ. Radiological changes in the cervical spine in ankylosing spondylitis. Ann Rheum Dis 1968; 27:333–338.

58. Lee HS, Kim TH, Yun HR, et al. Radiologic changes of cervical spine in ankylosing spondylitis. Clin Rheumatol 2001; 20:262–266.
59. Ramos-Remus C, Major P, Gomez-Vargas A, et al. Temporomandibular joint osseous morphology in a consecutive sample of ankylosing spondylitis patients. Ann Rheum Dis 1997; 56:103–107.
60. Stevens PM. Radiographic distortion of bones: a marker study. Orthopedics 1989; 12:1457–1463.
61. Heller JG, Viroslav S, Hudson T. Jefferson fractures: the role of magnification artifacts in assessing transverse ligament integrity. J Spinal Disord 1993; 6:392–396.
62. Sistrom CL, Southall EP, Peddada SD, Shaffer HA. Factors affecting the thickness of the cervical prevertebral soft tissues. Skeletal Radiol 1993; 22:167–171.
63. Locke GR, Gardner JI, Van Epps EF. Atlas-dens interval (ADD) in children. A survey based on 200 normal cervical spines. Am J Radiol 1966; 97:135–140.
64. Shim SC, Yoo DH, Lee JK, et al. Multiple cerebellar infarction due to vertebral artery obstruction and bulbar symptoms associated with vertical subluxation and atlanto-occipital subluxation in ankylosing spondylitis. J Rheumatol 1998; 25:2464–2468.
65. Dolan AL, Gibson T. Intrinsic spinal cord lesions in 2 patients with ankylosing spondylitis. J Rheumatol 1994; 21:1160–1161.
66. Simmons EH, Graziano GP, Heffner R Jr. Muscle disease as a cause of kyphotic deformity in ankylosing spondylitis. Spine 1991; 16(suppl):S351–S360.
67. Ho EK, Leong JC. Traumatic tetraparesis: a rare neurologic complication in ankylosing spondylitis with ossification of posterior longitudinal ligament of the cervical spine. A case report. Spine 1987; 12:403–405.
68. Ramos-Remus C, Russell AS, Gomez-Vargas A, et al. Ossification of the posterior longitudinal ligament (opll) in 3 geographically and genetically different populations of ankylosing spondylitis and other spondyloarthropathies. Ann Rheum Dis 1998; 57:429–433.
69. Pillay N, Hunter T. Delayed evoked potentials in patients with ankylosing spondylitis. J Rheumatol 1986; 13:137–141.
70. Agarwal AK, Peppelman WC, Kraus DR, et al. Recurrence of cervical spine instability in rheumatoid arthritis following previous fusion. Can disease progression be prevented by early surgery? J Rheumatol 1992; 19:1364–1370.
71. Matsunaga S, Sakou T, Onishi T, et al. Prognosis of patients with upper cervical lesions caused by rheumatoid arthritis: comparison of occipitocervical fusion between C1 laminectomy and nonsurgical management. Spine 2003; 28:1581–1587.

22

Management of Cervical Spinal Fractures in Ankylosing Spondylitis

David M. Hasan and Vincent C. Traynelis
Department of Neurosurgery, University Hospitals, Iowa City, Iowa, U.S.A.

INTRODUCTION

The first reported case of cervical spine injury in a patient with ankylosing spondylitis (AS) appeared in 1933 (1). Subsequently, numerous publications have shown the incidence of traumatic cervical injury in patients with AS to be appreciably higher than the general population without AS (2,3). There are several major reasons for this discrepancy. Patients with AS are more prone to fall because of the compromised balance which accompanies the disease. Additionally, the lack of spinal mobility coupled with the frequent comorbidity of osteoporosis increases the risk of fracture to such an extent that cervical spinal injuries occur regularly following even trivial falls (2,4–11). Frequently all the spinal elements across the anterior–posterior (AP) plane are disrupted, resulting in complete three-column instability. Cervical spinal fractures in the presence of AS are particularly serious, and the mortality ranges from 35% to 50% depending on the series (6,7,12,13). Although reports by several groups have implicated hyperextension as the most frequent mechanism of injury to the cervical spine, forces in any vector can result in fractures. Flexion injuries, in particular, may lead to vertebral body fractures (7,10,13–18).

The cervical spine may be altered by AS in a number of ways. The disease often results in osteoporosis, which has a predilection for affecting the vertebral bodies. Stress fractures may develop in patients with advanced osteopenia (19,20). The facet joints undergo progressive destructive changes, leading to eventual ossification, joint narrowing, and ankylosis (11). The intervertebral disks and their annuli may become calcified. Calcification of the annulus fibrosis reduces the movement and elasticity of the intervertebral disk, and frequently this point is the site of least resistance when the spine is subjected to trauma (2). Any or all of the cervical spinal ligaments may become calcified. Overall, the more pronounced these effects are, the more brittle the cervical spine becomes (2,20). The multiple fused vertebral segments cause the fractured ankylotic spine to resemble a long-bone fracture (2). These patients are also more prone to formation of epidural hematomas with cervical fractures as compared to the general population without AS (21).

The cervical spine is divided into three segments based on both anatomical and biomechanical considerations. The upper cervical region, also termed the craniovertebral junction (CVJ), consists of the occipital–cervical articulation, the atlas, and the axis. The subaxial cervical spine includes the bony vertebrae from C3 through C6 and their associated disks and articulations. The cervicothoracic junction is the third segment. This is comprised of the transitional C7 vertebra and its articulation with T1. In this chapter, cervical spine fractures in AS patients will be discussed for each of these regions.

THE UPPER CERVICAL SPINE

The occipital-atlanto-axial segment can be divided into two components: bony structures and the discoligamentous elements.

On the lateral sides of the foramen magnum, the oval and convex occipital condyles articulate with the superior facets of the atlas. The condyloid fossae located dorsal to the occipital condyles receive the posterior portions of the superior articular processes of the atlas when the head is extended. The external occipital crest, a ridge which extends from the opisthion to the inion, serves as the attachment site for the ligamentum nuchae.

The atlas is an irregular ring and contains two separate lateral masses. Two-fifths of the circumference of the ring is made up of the lateral masses. The anterior arch forms one-fifth and the posterior arch forms the remainder of the atlas (22). Within the ring a pair of tubercles is present slightly anterior to the AP midline of the atlas. These serve as attachment points for the transverse portion of the cruciate ligament. The superior and inferior surfaces of the lateral masses constitute the articular facets. Each atlantal facet is uniquely shaped to accommodate the occipital condyles and superior facets of the axis. The transverse processes of the atlas extend more laterally than those of the subaxial cervical vertebrae. A groove containing the vertebral artery lies within the posterior arch of the atlas. The fovea dentis is an indentation of the posterior surface of the anterior arch and is the site for anterior odontoid articulation (22).

The anterior portion of the axis is comprised of a vertebral body with a cephalad-projecting extension named the odontoid process or dens. A transverse groove lies across the dorsal aspect of the dens. The transverse ligament passes over this groove. The laminae of the posterior arch of C2 are thick and stout. The atlas has a relatively large and long pars interarticularis. This structure serves to transition the facet articulation from the relatively anterior position of the occipital condyle and C1 to the more dorsal location of the lateral masses of the subaxial cervical spine. Fractures of the pars interarticularis of the atlas are termed hangman's fractures because of their constant appearance following judicial hangings. The large, bifid spinous process provides an anchor point for many strong tendons and ligaments.

The ligaments that maintain the craniocervical articulation can be divided into two groups. The first set attaches the skull to the atlas and includes the articular capsule ligaments, the anterior and posterior atlanto-occipital ligaments, and two lateral atlanto-occipital ligaments. The anterior atlanto-occipital ligament is a continuation of the anterior longitudinal ligament, and the posterior atlanto-occipital ligament spans between the posterior border of the foramen magnum and the posterior atlantal arch. The cruciate ligament (the horizontal member of which is the important transverse ligament) also contributes to the stability of this articulation.

A second set of ligaments secures the cranium to the axis, and it is this group that provides the primary source of stability across the CVJ. These ligaments include the apical dental ligament, the alar ligaments, the tectorial membrane, and the ligamentum nuchae (23,24). The alar ligaments are paired structures, each of which contains a duo of ligaments: the atlantal alar and the occipital alar. These ligaments connect the tip of the odontoid to the occipital condyles and the lateral masses of the atlas, respectively (25). The alar ligaments are the main restraints for axial rotation, which occurs mostly across the C1–C2 articulation. They also are important in preventing AP translation and lateral flexion (23). The tectorial membrane is a continuation of the posterior longitudinal ligament. It reaches from the dorsal surface of the odontoid to insert on the ventral surface of the foramen magnum (26,27). The tectorial membrane resists hyperextension (23). If the tectorial membrane is incompetent, contact between the posterior arches of the atlas and the occiput will limit hyperextension (27). Flexion is restricted by contact of the odontoid process with the anterior foramen magnum (23). The apical dental ligament and the ligamentum nuchae contribute only slightly to the stability of the CVJ.

The brittle spine and ossified ligaments in AS patients make them more susceptible to atlanto-axial subluxation/dislocation than the general population because of transverse ligamentous injury, odontoid process fractures, and hangman's fractures (28). Significant neck pain after minor trauma or the presence of symptoms and/or clinical signs of myelopathy warrants a full imaging evaluation with plain radiographs and thin-cut computerized tomography (CT). Two-dimensional reconstructions of the CT images are often very useful for accurate delineation of fractures in patients with AS. Magnetic resonance (MR) scans are optimal for the evaluation of spinal cord impingement or contusions and hematomas.

Anterior or posterior subluxation of C1 on C2 secondary to a transverse ligament rupture or an odontoid process fracture may be initially managed via closed reduction with gentle cervical traction to correct the alignment. The vector of the traction should be anterior and superior to the axis of the spine to re-establish the pre-injury alignment, and the weight should not exceed five pounds (2). Careful and frequent radiographic monitoring of the CVJ is essential during the application of traction. If the malalignment is successfully reduced, then application of a halo crown and vest or operative fusion with internal fixation are both management options. If external immobilization is utilized, the halo should be worn for a minimum of three months. Careful inspection for skin breakdown while wearing the halo vest is paramount, as AS patients are more prone to decubiti because of the marked cervicothoracic kyphosis. Follow-up CT scanning of the cervical spine may be required to verify bony healing.

Failure to achieve closed reduction coupled with progressive neurologic deterioration is an absolute indication for early surgical intervention. Surgery is also indicated if the transverse ligament is disrupted, if the external orthosis cannot hold the fractured elements adequately, or if the patient has failed to heal after an appropriate period of halo immobilization. Surgery is often an attractive alternative to prolonged halo immobilization. Even if a nonoperative strategy is chosen, open fusion and internal stabilization may be necessary if these patients develop moderate to severe erosive skin ulcers, pin site infection, or skull penetration by halo pins.

Several surgical techniques have been used to achieve C1–C2 fusion. Brooks and Jenkins (29) described a technique compressing an iliac crest wedge graft between the laminae utilizing C1 and C2 sublaminar wires or cables. The interspinous technique achieves fixation via a C1 sublaminar cable which wraps around the spinous process of C2. An autograft is compressed between the C1 and C2 dorsal elements (30,31). Biomechanically, interlaminar clamp fixation behaves in a manner similar to the Brooks fusion technique although the clinical success rate may be less (32–34). The successful fusion rate for these procedures markedly varies throughout the literature (35).

Magerl and Seemann (32) proposed a transarticular screw technique, which is superior in terms of minimizing axial rotation and AP transition. Optimally, this method is combined with posterior wiring, which results in a fusion rate from 87% to 100% (31,34–39). Transarticular screw fixation across the C1–C2 joint is a demanding procedure. The risk of vertebral artery injury can be minimized by careful preoperative radiographic evaluation and normalization of CVJ alignment. Image guidance may improve the safety of this procedure. Patients with AS frequently have an exaggerated cervicothoracic kyphosis which may preclude transarticular screw fixation.

Placement of polyaxial screws in the C1 lateral masses and C2 pars interarticularis and fixing these bone anchors on each side with longitudinal rods affords the surgeon the opportunity to achieve an excellent fusion rate (40,41). Furthermore, it is possible to perform this technique when anatomical constraints, such as severe cervicothoracic kyphosis or the location of the vertebral artery within the C2 pars interarticularis, preclude transarticular screw fixation. Similar to C1–C2 transarticular screw fixation, a dorsal cable and graft construct should augment the rigid fixation.

Ideally, patients treated with nonrigid fixation should be immobilized with a halo in the postoperative period. When screws or screw/rod implants are employed, a collar is sufficient.

THE SUBAXIAL CERVICAL SPINE

The subaxial cervical spine consists of the C3 through C6 vertebrae, their intervertebral disks and annuli, and the supporting discoligamentous complex, which includes the anterior and posterior longitudinal ligaments, ligamentum flavum, and interspinous ligaments. Throughout this region the bony and soft tissue anatomy of the cervical spine is fairly consistent. Distortion of the bony structures and obliteration of the pliable ligaments are hallmarks of AS.

Subaxial cervical spinal fractures in patients with AS are almost always injuries which completely disrupt all of the spinal elements across the affected horizontal plane. Such complete segmental lesions coupled with the long stiff portions of the spine above and below the traumatic level increase the risk of neurological injury occurring at the time of impact. The radiographic workup is similar to that of the CVJ, with two-dimensional CT reconstructions playing a valuable role.

Realignment of displaced subaxial cervical spinal fractures in the setting of AS is difficult and treacherous. Generally, fractures behave mechanically as midshaft long bone fractures, with two extended lever arms confounding the realignment process. The treatment options include traction or repositioning by adjusting a halo immobilization device. The patient's overall alignment and presumed pretrauma alignment should be considered as traction is instituted. Generally, a force exerted by the cervical traction coursing anterior and superior to this vector is most likely to promote restoration of the usual pre-injury cervical alignment in patients with AS (2). The applied force should not be excessive, and successful closed reduction with weights less than 10 pounds has been reported (2). Alternatively, the patient may be placed in a halo vest orthosis and serial adjustments made until acceptable alignment is achieved. In some cases, it may be difficult or impossible to maintain alignment in a halo. For that reason, the adjustments should be made with the patient in the supine position, and only after the fractured fragments are reapproximated should the patient begin the mobilization process.

Patients who are adequately reduced with either traction or positioning are candidates for treatment with a halo vest orthosis. In such cases, the patient should be slowly mobilized with frequent radiographic assessments. The halo vest is employed for an average duration of three months. Persistent motion across the fractured level while in the halo is an indication for surgery. Many AS patients have a significant thoracic kyphosis which increases the risk of skin breakdown while in a halo. Surgical intervention should be considered for these individuals.

If the neural elements cannot be decompressed by a closed reduction, surgical intervention is indicated. Failure to maintain stable and proper alignment or intolerance of the halo vest are also indications for an operative intervention. Likewise, treatment of a symptomatic intraspinal hematoma requires prompt surgical attention. Surgical reduction and stabilization with internal fixation will eliminate compression of the neural elements and provide the optimal environment for bony healing.

Patients with incompetence of the anterior column require an anterior approach. While destruction of the anterior load-bearing column can occur acutely, AS patients are prone to have undetected fractures that slowly lead to significant bone erosion and subsequent deformity and instability. The surgical positioning and exposure for an anterior decompression and stabilization is safe and simple. The damaged spinal elements are removed and a graft is inserted. Great forces may be exerted across the treated level; therefore, solid fixation is necessary. Anterior instrumentation can and should be extended to achieve fixation at least two segments above and below the injury. As significant AS usually produces a completely fused spine, this will not result in further loss of motion. A long plate should be firmly secured at each end initially. Screws are then placed in the segments rostral and caudal to the injury. Simultaneously tightening the two screws at each segment will minimize stripping of the screws within the vertebral bodies and maximize the ability of the instrumentation to achieve reduction when it is necessary. The traction should be released before this maneuver is performed. The bone in patients with AS is often osteoporotic; therefore, bicortical fixation is preferable. Once the instrumentation is secured, the construct can be tested for stability by having the anesthesiologist try to gently flex the neck under continuous fluoroscopic monitoring. It should be remembered at this time that the spine is rigid and the head only needs to be lifted a short distance to detect abnormal motion. If there are any concerns about the strength of the construct, the patient should be immobilized postoperatively in a halo vest or a posterior fixation procedure performed (Fig. 1).

Posterior surgery alone may be considered when the anterior column is capable of bearing an axial load. This is often the case if an acute linear fracture is present. Posterior instrumentation can also be used to augment anterior column reconstruction, as mentioned previously. Decompression of the neural elements in AS patients with a cervical fracture is often achieved by restoration of proper alignment; therefore, bony decompression is not usually necessary. Treatment of an intraspinal hematoma will require removal of the laminae, but barring this entity, the dorsal bony structures are usually not removed. Anatomically, all of the posterior elements can be used in stabilization of the cervical spine, including the spinous processes, laminae, facets, and lateral masses. Exposure of the subaxial cervical spine should be sufficient to perform the procedure safely; however, the muscular

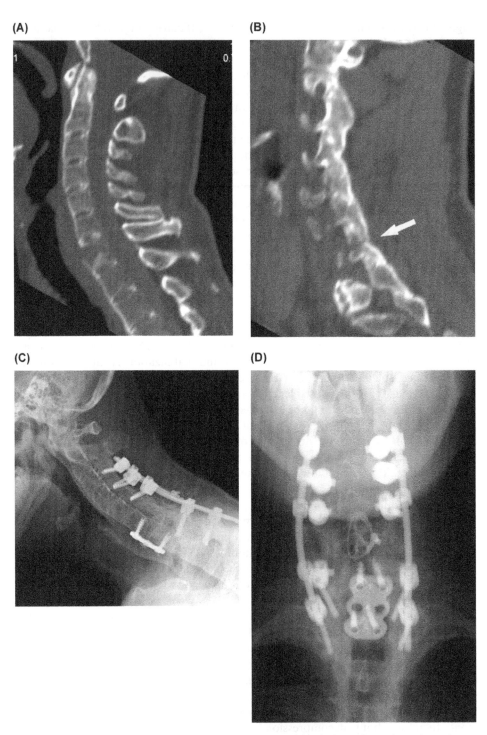

Figure 1 (**A**) CT demonstrating a subaxial fracture resulting in loss of anterior column integrity. (**B**) The fracture extended through the posterior structures bilaterally. (**C**) Lateral radiograph demonstrating reconstruction of the anterior column and posterior stabilization. (**D**) AP radiograph demonstrating reconstruction of the anterior column and posterior stabilization. *Abbreviations*: CT, computerized tomography; AP, anterior–posterior.

and ligamentous attachments to the large C2 spinous process should be left intact whenever possible (42).

There are several techniques available to achieve posterior subaxial cervical fusion. The choice of the method of stabilization must be based on the individual patient, the injury, and the surgeon's experience. These techniques include: simple spinous process wiring, Bohlman's triple wire technique, and rigid rod and screw fixation (43–46). Sublaminar wiring does not offer a biomechanical advantage over spinous process fixation and is associated with an increased risk of spinal cord injury (43). Furthermore, it may be very difficult to perform in the patient with AS as the disease process often results in obliteration of the interlaminar space secondary to the development of dorsal ossifications. One should keep in mind the prevalence of distortion of the bony anatomy in both the injured and uninjured segments. Reapproximation of the fractured spine will result in bony healing; therefore, no grafts are necessary (although they are frequently added).

It is our preference to perform both spinous process wiring and lateral mass fixation whenever possible. This is especially important if fixation is achieved solely from the posterior route. The spinous processes are connected to each other with cables extending at least two segments above and below the fracture line. Alternatively, securing an autologous rib graft to the spinous processes with cables may increase the stiffness of the construct (Fig. 2) (47). Extending the levels of fixation rarely results in lengthening the fusion as the entire subaxial cervical spine is almost always completely ankylosed from the primary disease.

Screw fixation of the lateral masses can be challenging in patients with AS. The primary problem in such individuals is the loss of bone and facet joint landmarks which are necessary for safe screw insertion. Optimally, surgeons choosing to employ lateral mass fixation in patients with AS should be well experienced in placing articular pillar screws in situations where the anatomy is more straightforward. Unicortical fixation over multiple segments can provide adequate stability and yet minimize the risk of nerve root or vertebral artery injury (46). The development of rigid systems which allow the surgeon to place each screw precisely represents an advance over the earlier nonrigid screw/plate devices. The bony anchors of the rigid systems are secured to longitudinal members which may be cross-linked for further stability (43,44,48–50).

THE CERVICOTHORACIC JUNCTION

The transition from the relatively flexible cervical spine to the more rigid thoracic spine makes the cervicothoracic junction anatomically and biomechanically complex (51–57). Independent biomechanical studies have shown that the lower cervical spine is more flexible in extension than the mid-cervical spine (58) and that motion segments of the thoracic spine are more flexible in flexion than extension (59). Moving caudally from the lower cervical spine into the upper thoracic region, the lateral masses decrease in size while the pedicles become larger (60). The transitional nature of C7 makes both lateral mass and pedicle fixation relatively more difficult (61,62). In the subaxial cervical spine, screws may be placed in the lateral masses or in the pedicles; however, at C7, T1, and T2, the lateral masses are much smaller and the transverse processes become large. Hence, the anatomy of the cervicothoracic junction necessitates the use of pedicle screws for C7–T2 (61) or C7 lateral mass and T1–T2 pedicle screws. The change from the lordotic cervical spine to the kyphotic

(A)

(B)

(C)

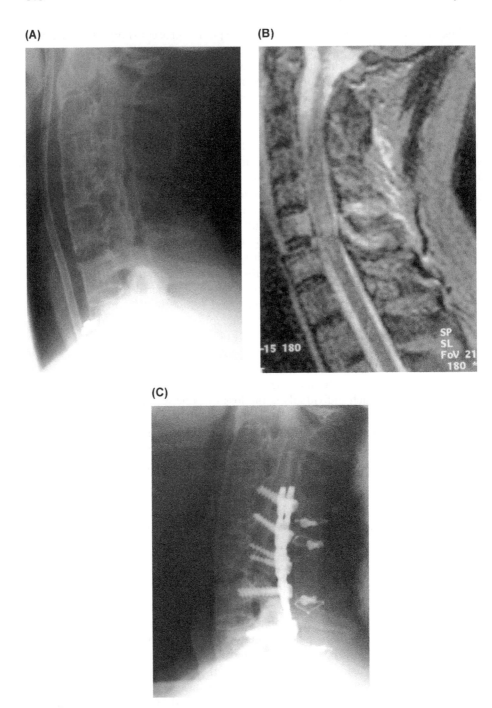

Figure 2 (**A**) Lateral radiograph demonstrating a subaxial fracture with preserved anterior column integrity. (**B**) T2-weighted MRI of the same patient. (**C**) Postoperative radiograph showing fixation of the lateral masses and the spinous processes. *Abbreviation*: MRI, magnetic resonance imaging.

thoracic spine is frequently more marked in AS, a situation which increases the difficulty of contouring the plates or rods (63).

The radiographic workup is similar to that of the subaxial region except that it is exceptionally difficult to image this region with lateral radiographs.

It is very difficult to safely treat cervicothoracic fractures with traction in patients with AS, and generally this management strategy is not recommended. Likewise, it is difficult to immobilize the lower cervical spine, specifically the cervicothoracic segment, with external orthoses, even with a halo vest and crown. This, combined with the other negative effects of halo immobilization, renders this management strategy generally suboptimal; therefore, acute restoration of spinal alignment and stability of the cervicothoracic junction is usually achieved surgically.

Whenever possible, anterior grafting and instrumentation should be used to treat cervicothoracic instability in patients with AS. This is because positioning is safest with an anterior approach, and internal fixation can be achieved prior to turning for a posterior instrumentation if it is necessary. Anterior approaches are not always possible, however, because these patients frequently have exaggeration of the upper thoracic kyphosis that always confounds the exposure and frequently makes it impossible. Furthermore, intraoperative radiographic assessment of the anterior cervicothoracic junction exposure is very difficult.

Bilateral multisegment rigid fixation is recommended to achieve adequate stabilization. Spinous process wiring alone or with a bone graft cannot be trusted to provide enough support, and this technique should be reserved for augmenting the screw/plate or screw/rod construct. Lateral mass screws are adequate bone anchors in the cervical region, and pedicle screws provide solid fixation in T1, T2, and T3. The thoracic pedicles decrease in size over the next several segments, making pedicle screw fixation more difficult and less secure. Placement of a laminar hook at the most caudal level of pedicle fixation can markedly decrease the risk of screw pull-out without adding an additional level to the fusion.

CONCLUSION

The management of cervical fractures in patients with AS is complex and difficult. Nonoperative treatment of these patients with cervical traction and immobilization with a halo crown and vest does not provide sufficient immobilization in many cases and carries a high risk of decubitus ulcer. Frequently, surgical stabilization with rigid fixation is necessary.

REFERENCES

1. Stiasny H. Fraktur der halswirbelsaule bei spondylarthritis ankylopoetica (Bechterew). Zentralbl Chir 1933; 60:998–1001.
2. Detwiler KN, Loftus CM, Godersky JC, Menezes AH. Management of cervical spine injuries in patients with ankylosing spondylitis. J Neurosurg 1990; 72:210–215.
3. Grisolia A, Bell RL, Peltier LF. Fractures and dislocations of the spine complicating ankylosing spondylitis. A report of six cases. J Bone Joint Surg 1967; 49A:339–344.
4. Bohlman HH. Acute fractures and dislocations of the cervical spine. An analysis of three hundred hospitalized patients and review of the literature. J Bone Joint Surg 1979; 61A: 1119–1142.

5. Guttman L. Traumatic paraplegia and tetraplegia in ankylosing spondylitis. Paraplegia 1966; 4:188–203.
6. Murray GC, Persellin RH. Cervical fracture complicating ankylosing spondylitis: a report of eight cases and review of the literature. Am J Med 1981; 70:1033–1041.
7. Woodruff FP, DeWing SB. Fracture of the cervical spine in patients with ankylosing spondylitis. Radiology 1963; 80:17–21.
8. Fast A, Parikh S, Marin EL. Spine fractures in ankylosing spondylitis. Arch Phys Med Rehabil 1986; 67:595–597.
9. Foo D, Bignami A, Rossier AB. Two spinal cord lesions in a patient with ankylosing spondylitis and cervical spine injury. Neurology 1983; 33:245–249.
10. Osgood CP, Abbasy M, Mathews T. Multiple spine fractures in ankylosing spondylitis. J Trauma Inj Infect Crit Care 1975; 15:163–166.
11. Weinstein PR, Karpman RR, Gall EP, Pitt M. Spinal cord injury, spinal fracture, and spinal stenosis in ankylosing spondylitis. J Neurosurg 1982; 57:609–616.
12. Hansen ST Jr, Taylor TK, Honet JC, Lewis FR. Fracture-dislocations of the ankylosed thoracic spine in rheumatoid spondylitis. Ankylosing spondylitis, Marie–Strumpell disease. J Trauma Inj Infect Crit Care 1967; 7:827–837.
13. Kewalramani LS, Taylor RG, Albrand OW. Cervical spine injury in patients with ankylosing spondylitis. J Trauma Inj Infect Crit Care 1975; 15:931–934.
14. Rand RW, Stern WE. Cervical fractures of the ankylosed rheumatoid spine. Neurochirurgia 1961; 4:137–148.
15. Burke DC. Hyperextension injuries of the spine. J Bone Joint Surg 1971; 53B:3–12.
16. Cheshire DJ. The stability of the cervical spine following the conservative treatment of fractures and fracture-dislocations. Paraplegia 1969; 7:193–203.
17. Symonds C. The interrelation of trauma and cervical spondylosis in compression of the cervical cord. Lancet 1953; 1:451–454.
18. Taylor AR. Mechanism and treatment of spinal-cord disorders associated with cervical spondylosis. Lancet 1953; 1:717–720.
19. Yau ACMC, Chan RNW. Stress fracture of the fused lumbo-dorsal spine in ankylosing spondylitis. A report of three cases. J Bone Joint Surg 1974; 56B:681–687.
20. Cruickshank B. Histopathology of diarthrodial joints in ankylosing spondylitis. Ann Rheum Dis 1951; 10:393–404.
21. Farhat SM, Schneider RC, Gray JM. Traumatic spinal extradural hematoma associated with cervical fractures in rheumatoid spondylitis. J Trauma Inj Infect Crit Care 1973; 13:591–599.
22. VanGilder JC, Menezes AH, Dolan KD. Anatomy of the craniovertebral junction. The Craniovertebral Junction and Its Abnormalities. Mount Kisco, NY: Futura, 1987:9–27.
23. Werne S. Studies in spontaneous atlas dislocation. Acta Orthop Scand Suppl 1957; 23:1–150.
24. White AA III, Panjabi MM. The clinical biomechanics of the occipitoatlantoaxial complex. Orthop Clin North Am 1978; 9:867–878.
25. Exner G, Botel U, Kluger P, Richter M, Eggers C, Ruidisch M. Treatment of fracture and complication of cervical spine with ankylosing spondylitis. Spinal Cord 1998; 36:377–379.
26. Wiesel S, Kraus D, Rothman RH. Atlanto-occipital hypermobility. Orthop Clin North Am 1978; 9:969–972.
27. Wiesel SW, Rothman RH. Occipitoatlantal hypermobility. Spine 1979; 4:187–191.
28. Toussirot E, Benmansour A, Bonneville JF, Wendling D. Atlantoaxial subluxation in an ankylosing spondylitis patient with cervical spine ossification. Br J Rheumatol 1997; 36:293–295.
29. Brooks AL, Jenkins EB. Atlanto-axial arthrodesis by the wedge compression method. J Bone Joint Surg 1978; 60A:279–284.
30. Dickman CA, Sonntag VKH, Papadopoulos SM, Hadley MN. The interspinous method of posterior atlantoaxial arthrodesis. J Neurosurg 1991; 74:190–198.

31. Farey ID, Nadkarni S, Smith N. Modified Gallie technique versus transarticular screw fixation in C1–C2 fusion. Clin Orthop 1999; 359:126–135.

32. Magerl F, Seemann PS. Stable posterior fusion of the atlas and axis by transarticular screw fixation. In: Kehr P, Weidner A, eds. Cervical Spine I. Vienna: Springer-Verlag, 1987:322–327.

33. Moskovich R, Crockard HA. Atlantoaxial arthrodesis using interlaminar clamps. An improved technique. Spine 1992; 17:261–267.

34. Grob D, Crisco JJ, Panjabi MM, Wang P, Dvorak J. Biomechanical evaluation of four different posterior atlantoaxial fixation techniques. Spine 1992; 17:480–490.

35. Taggard DA, Kraut MA, Clark CR, Traynelis VC. Case–control study comparing the efficacy of surgical techniques for C1–C2 arthrodesis. J Spinal Disord Tech 2004; 17:189–194.

36. Dickman CA, Sonntag VKH. Posterior C1–C2 transarticular screw fixation for atlantoaxial arthrodesis. Neurosurgery 1998; 43:275–281.

37. Grob D, Jeanneret B, Aebi M, Markwalder TM. Atlanto-axial fusion with transarticular screw fixation. J Bone Joint Surg 1991; 73B:972–976.

38. Haid RW Jr, Subach BR, McLaughlin MR, Rodts GE Jr, Wahlig JB Jr. C1–C2 transarticular screw fixation for atlantoaxial instability: a 6-year experience. Neurosurgery 2001; 49:65–70.

39. Stillerman CB, Wilson JA. Atlanto-axial stabilization with posterior transarticular screw fixation: technical description and report of 22 cases. Neurosurgery 1993; 32:948–955.

40. Fiore AJ, Haid RW, Rodts GE, et al. Atlantal lateral mass screws for posterior spinal reconstruction: technical note and case series. Neurosurg Focus 2002; 12(1):1–6.

41. Harms J, Melcher RP. Posterior C1–C2 fusion with polyaxial screw and rod fixation. Spine 2001; 26:2467–2471.

42. Stauffer ES. Wiring techniques of the posterior cervical spine for the treatment of trauma. Orthopedics 1988; 11:1543–1548.

43. Coe JD, Warden KE, Sutterlin CE III, McAfee PC. Biomechanical evaluation of cervical spine stabilization methods in a human cadaveric model. Spine 1989; 14:1122–1131.

44. Sutterlin CE III, McAfee PC, Warden KE, R'ey RM Jr, Farey ID. A biomechanical evaluation of cervical spinal stabilization methods in a bovine model. Static and cyclical loading. Spine 1988; 13:795–802.

45. Taggard DA, Traynelis VC. Management of cervical spinal fractures in ankylosing spondylitis with posterior fixation. Spine 2000; 25:2035–2039.

46. Wellman BJ, Follett KA, Traynelis VC. Complications of posterior articular mass plate fixation of the subaxial cervical spine in 43 consecutive patients. Spine 1998; 23:193–200.

47. Sawin PD, Traynelis VC, Menezes AH. A comparative analysis of fusion rates and donor-site morbidity for autogeneic rib and iliac crest bone grafts in posterior cervical fusions. J Neurosurg 1998; 88:255–265.

48. Gill K, Paschal S, Corin J, Ashman R, Bucholz RW. Posterior plating of the cervical spine. A biomechanical comparison of different posterior fusion techniques. Spine 1988; 13:813–816.

49. Montesano PX, Juach EC, Anderson PA, Benson DR, Hanson PB. Biomechanics of cervical spine internal fixation. Spine 1991; 16(suppl 3):S10–S16.

50. Mummaneni PV, Haid RW, Traynelis VC, et al. Posterior cervical fixation using a new polyaxial screw and rod system: technique and surgical results. Neurosurg Focus 2002; 12(1):1–5.

51. An HS, Vaccaro A, Cotler JM, Lin S. Spinal disorders at the cervicothoracic junction. Spine 1994; 19:2557–2564.

52. Anderson PA, Henley MB, Grady MS, Montesano PX, Winn HR. Posterior cervical arthrodesis with AO reconstruction plates and bone graft. Spine 1991; 16(suppl 3): S72–S79.

53. Chapman JR, Anderson PA, Pepin C, Toomey S, Newell DW, Grady MS. Posterior instrumentation of the unstable cervicothoracic spine. J Neurosurg 1996; 84:552–558.

54. Evans DK. Dislocation at the cervicothoracic junction. J Bone Joint Surg 1983; 65B: 124–127.
55. Miller MD, Gehweiler JA, Martinez S, Charlton OP, Daffner RH. Significant new observations on cervical spine trauma. AJR Am J Roentgenol 1978; 130:659–663.
56. Nichols CG, Young DH, Schiller WR. Evaluation of cervicothoracic junction injury. Ann Emerg Med 1987; 16:640–642.
57. Vaccaro R, Conant RF, Hilibrand AS, Albert TJ. A plate-rod device for treatment of cervicothoracic disorders: comparison of mechanical testing with established cervical spine in vitro load testing data. J Spinal Disord 2000; 13:350–355.
58. Shea M, Edwards WT, White AA, Hayes WC. Variations of stiffness and strength along the human cervical spine. J Biomech 1991; 24:95–107.
59. Panjabi MM, Brand RA Jr, White AA III. Three-dimensional flexibility and stiffness properties of the human thoracic spine. J Biomech 1976; 9:185–192.
60. Bailey AS, Stanescu S, Yeasting RA, Ebraheim NA, Jackson WT. Anatomic relationships of the cervicothoracic junction. Spine 1995; 20:1431–1439.
61. An HS, Gordin R, Renner K. Anatomic considerations for plate-screw fixation of the cervical spine. Spine 1991; 16(suppl 10):S548–S551.
62. Panjabi MM, Duranceau J, Goel V, Oxland T, Takata K. Cervical human vertebrae. Quantitative three-dimensional anatomy of the middle and lower regions. Spine 1991; 16:861–869.
63. Kreshak JL, Kim DH, Lindsey DP, Kam AC, Panjabi MM, Yerby SA. Posterior stabilization at the cervicothoracic junction: a biomechanical study. Spine 2002; 27:2763–2770.

23

Management of Thoracolumbar Spinal Fractures in Ankylosing Spondylitis

Aaron M. From and Patrick W. Hitchon
Department of Neurosurgery, University Hospitals, Iowa City, Iowa, U.S.A.

FRACTURES OF THE ANKYLOSED SPINE

Owing to stiffness and osteoporosis, spinal fractures are four times more likely in ankylosing spondylitis (AS) than they are in age-matched controls (1–5). Due to the kyphotic deformity of the spine, falls often result in extension fractures. Minor trauma in AS such as simple falls can result in spinal fractures with serious neurological deficit in at least half of the patients (3,6,7). An earlier review at the University of Iowa revealed that minor injuries were responsible for thoracolumbar fractures in 7 of 12 patients with AS (3,7). Therefore, in the avoidance of these fractures and associated neurological deficit, prevention of minor injuries in AS is of utmost importance (2–14). Both cervical and thoracic fractures can occur simultaneously mandating radiological studies of the entire spine in any AS patient presenting with possible fracture (7,11,15–17).

The chronic inflammation and calcification of ligaments and joints that occurs in AS results in a spine that is brittle and fused. Thus when a fracture occurs it is more often than not unstable involving all three columns: the anterior column consisting of the anterior half of the bodies and intervening disk space, the middle column including the posterior half of the bodies and the disk space between, and the posterior column comprising the neural arches, facet joints and ligaments (17). For the delineation of the extent of fractures, plain films, supplemented with computerized axial tomography (CT), and three-dimensional reconstructions are often helpful and necessary. As a result of this focal area of spinal thypermobility or instability, cord compression, dural laceration, or epidural hematoma can occur at the site of fracture (9–11,18–22). For the extent of soft tissue injury and neural compression, magnetic resonance imaging (MRI) is indicated.

NONOPERATIVE MANAGEMENT OF THORACIC AND LUMBAR FRACTURES OF THE ANKYLOSED SPINE

In the absence of three-column injury and dislocation, with minimal or no neurological deficit, nonoperative management may be all that is needed in some patients (3,8,7,23). Patients with AS often have associated systemic problems with increased morbidity and mortality as a result of surgery (3,5). Furthermore it has been suggested that bony growth occurs at an accelerated rate in AS patients because of the underlying inflammatory process, hastening the fusion of fractures (10). In general, for thoracic and lumbar fractures in AS that are associated with minimal or no neurological deficit, and in the absence of instability, bed rest until pain relief is achieved is instituted. Generally this period of time is in the order of a few days to one week, followed by ambulation with bracing in a Jewett brace for thoracic fractures, or thoracolumbosacral orthosis (TLSO) clam-shell orthosis for thoracolumbar fractures. Orthoses are generally worn for three to five months depending on the angulation and loss in height. Any progression or complication may require operative management (5,15,24,25).

At times patients with AS present with back pain, and are found on subsequent diagnostic study to have a fracture, but cannot report a specific traumatic event. These are most likely pseudarthroses or nondisplaced stress fractures. Such fractures can occur anywhere along the spine (body or disk space). A trial of nonsurgical treatment is always undertaken, though increasing pain may entail eventual surgery (2,5,6,8,9,25,26).

(A)

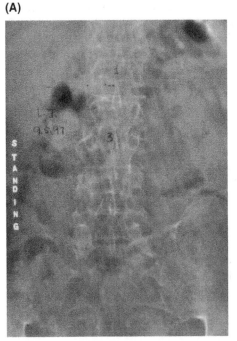

(B)

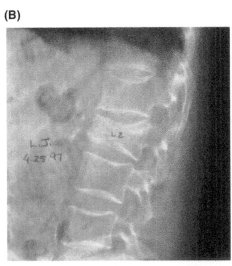

Figure 1   (**A**) Antero-posterior and (**B**) lateral plain radiograph of a 61-year-old male with an L2 compression fracture complicating AS after a lifting injury. The patient had no neurological deficit at presentation and was treated conservatively with stable neurological function at latest follow-up. *Abbreviation*: AS, ankylosing spondylitis.

(A)

(B)

Figure 2   (A) Antero-posterior and (B) lateral plain radiograph of a 57-year-old male with T9–T10 pseudoarthrosis four weeks after falling from a step ladder. He presented with pain only and no neurological deficit. He was treated conservatively with stable neurological function at latest follow-up.

Three of the 12 AS patients with thoracolumbar fractures reported earlier were treated nonsurgically (3). All three had fractures involving the anterior two columns without dislocation. Two of these three patients, a 61-year-old intact male with an L2 compression fracture (Fig. 1), and a 57-year-old male with pseudoarthrosis at T9–T10 (Fig. 2), presented with pain only without neurological deficit. A third patient, a 74-year-old male with a superior end-plate fracture of L5, presented with paraparesis. His other medical problems included cirrhosis, obesity, anticoagulation for pulmonary embolism, and obstructive pulmonary disease. This patient did, however, improve and was ambulating at latest follow-up. All three were treated with recumbency for up to one week, followed by gradual mobilization in thoracolumbar orthoses for at least three months.

OPERATIVE MANAGEMENT OF THORACIC AND LUMBAR FRACTURES OF THE ANKYLOSED SPINE

Operative management is indicated for unstable three-column injuries (5–7). Where cord or cauda equina compression exists, decompression generally by laminectomy is indicated (5–8,18) as was performed in four of nine patients (3). Instrumentation consists of rods and pedicle screws where possible (Fig. 3), or hooks if difficulty is encountered with screw insertion (Fig. 4). Laminar hooks may at times be difficult to insert because of calcification of the ligamentum flavum. Instrumentation is always supplemented with posterolateral bony fusion. Patients are always braced

(A)

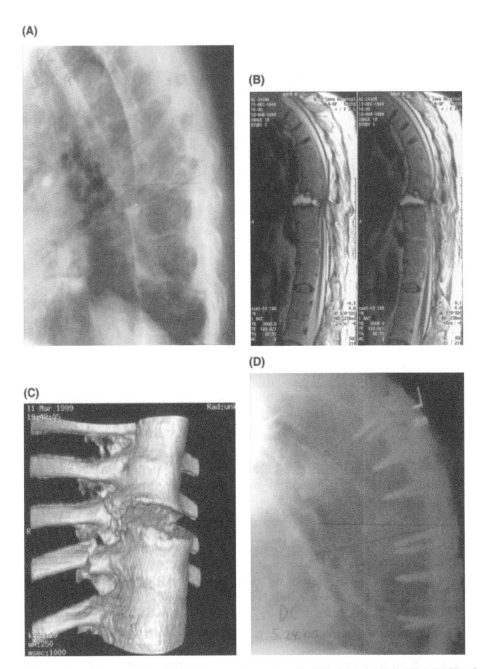

(B)

(D)

(C)

Figure 3 (**A**) Preoperative lateral plain radiograph, (**B**) T2-weighted MRI, (**C**) 3-D CT of a T7–T8 extension fracture in a 49-year-old male which occurred while being moved in a Hoyer lift, and (**D**) Postoperative lateral radiograph after posterior fusion with rods and screws. *Abbreviations*: MRI, magnetic resonance imaging; CT, computerized axial tomography.

postoperatively for up to five months in thoracolumbar clam-shells, or corsettes in the case of lumbar fractures (15,24).

Of the 12 patients reviewed at the University of Iowa nine underwent surgery for spinal stabilization with hardware and bony fusion. Instrumentation included

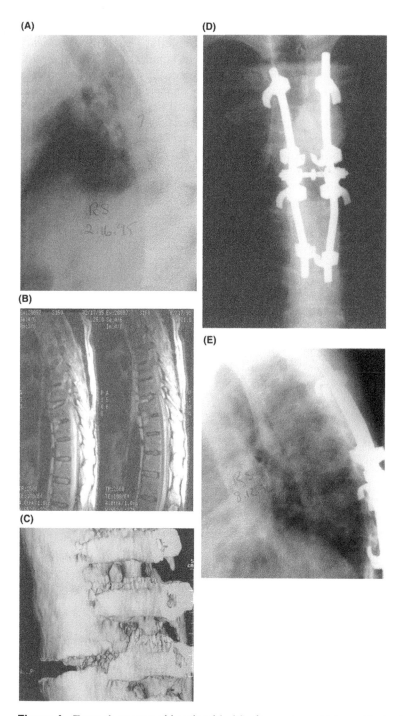

Figure 4 Forty-three-year-old male with AS after motor vehicle accident with an extension fracture through the T7–T8 disk space as shown on (**A**) lateral plain radiograph, (**B**) T2-weighted MRI and (**C**) 3-D CT reconstruction. Posterior hooks and rods were used in the stabilization of this fracture as seen on postoperative, (**D**) antero-posterior and (**E**) lateral plain radiograph. The patient presented initially with no neurological deficit and was clinically unchanged at latest follow-up. *Abbreviations*: AS, ankylosing spondylitis; MRI, magnetic resonance imaging; CT, computerized axial tomography.

either hooks (in three patients) or pedicle screws (in six patients) to secure rods or plates. Two patients underwent both posterior and anterior fusion. Four patients diagnosed with posterior cord compression underwent laminectomy (3,7).

Based on Frankel scores at admission and subsequent follow-up, four of the nine surgical patients did not suffer motor or sensory damage as a result of fracture. Of the five patients who had a postinjury neurological deficit, two demonstrated neurological improvement after treatment, whereas three showed no change in Frankel score. Spinal deformity was corrected as a result of surgery in seven of the nine operative patients by $12 \pm 10°$ (mean $\pm$ standard deviation) (3,7).

In conclusion, because of osteoporosis and rigidity, the spine in AS is prone to fracture, at times secondary to minor injuries only. Half of these fractures are associated with neurological deficit, and the majority require surgical stabilization.

REFERENCES

1. Mitra D, Elvins DM, Speden DJ, Collins AJ. The prevalence of vertebral fractures in mild ankylosing spondylitis and their relationship to bone mineral density. Rheumatology 2000; 39:85–89.
2. Hanson JA, Mirza S. Predisposition for spinal fracture in ankylosing spondylitis. AJR Am J Roentgenol 2000; 174:150.
3. Hitchon P, From A, Brenton M, Glaser J, Torner J. Fractures of the thoracolumbar spine complicating ankylosing spondylitis. J Neurosurg 2002; 97(suppl 2):218–222.
4. Cooper C, Carbone L, Michet CJ, Atkinson EJ, O'Fallon WM, Melton J. Fracture risk in patients with ankylosing spondylitis: a population based study. J Rheumatol 1994; 21(10):1877–1882.
5. Fox M, Onofrio B. Ankylosing spondylitis. In: Menezes AH, Sonntag VH, eds. Principles of Spinal Surgery. Section 4. Chapter 47. New York: McGraw-Hill, 1996:735–750.
6. Fox MW, Onofrio BM, Kilgore JE. Neurological complications of ankylosing spondylitis. J Neurosurg 1993; 78(6):871–878.
7. From AM, Hitchon PW, Peloso PM, Brenton M. Ankylosing spondylitis and spinal complications. In: Lewandrowski et al., eds. Advances in Spinal Fusion-Molecular Science, Biomechanics and Clinical Management. Chapter 13. New York: Marcel Dekker, 2003.
8. Weinstein P, Karpman R, Gall E, Pitt M. Spinal cord injury, spinal fracture and spinal stenosis in ankylosing spondylitis. J Neurosurg 1982; 67:609–616.
9. Graham GP, Evans PD. Spinal fractures in patients with ankylosing spondylitis. Injury 1991; 22(5):426–427.
10. Hunter T, Dubo HI. Spinal fractures complicating ankylosing spondylitis. A long-term follow-up study. Arthritis Rheum 1983; 26(6):751–759.
11. Foo D, Bignami A, Rossier AB. Two spinal cord lesions in a patient with ankylosing spondylitis and cervical spine injury. Neurology 1983; 33(2):245–249.
12. Graham B, Van Peteghem PK. Fractures of the spine in ankylosing spondylitis. Diagnosis, treatment, and complications. Spine 1989; 14(8):803–807.
13. Alaranta H, Luoto S, Konttinen YT. Traumatic spinal cord injury as a complication to ankylosing spondylitis. An extended report. Clin Exp Rheumatol 2002; 20:66–68.
14. Kauppi M, Belt EA, Soini I. "Bamboo spine" starts to bend—something is wrong. Clin Exp Rheumatol 2000; 18:513–514.
15. Osgood CP, Abbasy M, Mathews T. Multiple spine fractures in ankylosing spondylitis. J Trauma Inj Infect Crit Care 1975; 15(2):163–166.
16. Finkelstein JA, Chapman JR, Mirza S. Occult vertebral fractures in ankylosing spondylitis. Spinal Cord 1999; 37:444–447.

17. Denis F. The three column spine and its significance in the classification of acute thoracolumbar spinal injuries. Spine 1983; 8(8):817–831.
18. Grisolia A, Bell RL, Peltier LF. Fractures and dislocations of the spine complicating ankylosing spondylitis. A report of six cases. J Bone Joint Surg 1967; 49(2):339–344.
19. Kewalramani LS, Taylor RG, Albrand OW. Cervical spine injury in patients with ankylosing spondylitis. J Trauma 1975; 15(10):931–934.
20. Donnelly S, Doyle DV, Denton A, Rolfe I, McCloskey EV, Spector TD. Bone mineral density and vertebral compression fracture rates in ankylosing spondylitis. Ann Rheum Dis 1994; 53:117–121.
21. Foo D, Rossier AB. Post-traumatic spinal epidural hematoma. Neurosurgery 1982; 11(1 pt 1): 25–32.
22. Rowed DW. Management of cervical spinal cord injury in ankylosing spondylitis: the intervertebral disc as a cause of cord compression. J Neurosurg 1992; 77(2):241–246.
23. Hansen ST, Taylor TKF, Honet JC, Lewis FR. Fracture-dislocations of the ankylosed thoracic spine in rheumatoid spondylitis. J Trauma 1967; 7(6):827–837.
24. Apple DF Jr, Anson C. Spinal cord injury occurring in patients with ankylosing spondylitis: a multicenter study. Orthopedics 1995; 18(10):1005–1011.
25. Thorngren KG, Lidberg E, Aspelin P. Fractures of the thoracic and lumbar spine in ankylosing spondylitis. Arch Orthop Trauma Surg 1981; 98:101–107.
26. Detwiler KN, Loftus CM, Godersky JC, Menezes AH. Management of cervical spine injuries in patients with ankylosing spondylitis. J Neurosurg 1990; 72:210–215.

24

Total Hip Replacement in Ankylosing Spondylitis

David H. Sochart
The Manchester Arthroplasty Unit, North Manchester General Hospital, Crumpsall, Manchester, U.K.

INTRODUCTION

The hallmark of ankylosing spondylitis (AS) is involvement of the axial skeleton, but up to 25% of patients will actually first present with pain involving the peripheral joints, particularly the hip (1). Up to 50% of patients with AS will eventually develop symptomatic arthritis of the hip and in the majority of these patients both hips will be involved (2–4).

There tend to be two distinct types of hip involvement. First, a relatively pain-free form with rapid progression to fibrous or bony ankylosis, and second, a more painful and typically inflammatory process with supervening changes of osteoarthritis (Fig. 1).

For patients with fixed kyphotic spinal deformities the hip involvement and subsequent development of flexion contractures may be the most prominent symptom and complaint. This limits their ability to walk and further compromises their posture leaving them unable to look above the horizon, becoming the major source of their disability.

The main indications for total hip arthroplasty in patients with AS are pain, stiffness, and compromised posture. The aims of surgery are pain relief, eradication of flexion contractures, increased range of motion of the hip joint, improved mobility, and correction of posture.

Unlike the majority of the inflammatory arthropathies, AS tends to affect young males who are otherwise economically, socially, and physically active. A further aim of surgery is therefore to enable these patients to continue or return to working, while sexual and family issues are also of great concern. These young, high-demand patients are not willing to accept the inferior results of arthrodesis or osteotomy, which in any case would rarely be indicated in AS, and demand the more predictable and rapid results of joint replacement.

The typical patient with AS is therefore very different from those with other inflammatory arthropathies, being relatively young, predominantly male, with sparing of the upper limbs and a greater potential to return to a high level of activity after

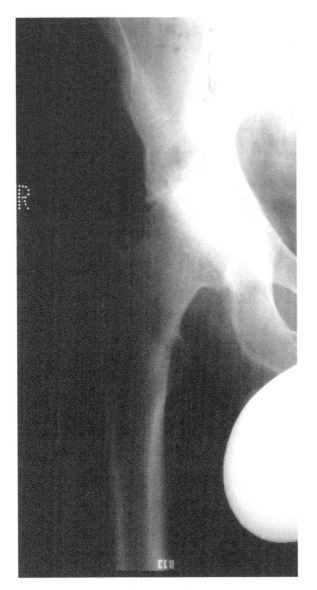

Figure 1 Osteoarthritic pattern in 27-year-old male with AS. *Abbreviation*: AS, ankylosing spondylitis.

surgery. Another major concern is therefore the longevity of the joint replacement and the long-term stability of fixation in young, active patients, particularly with the additional stresses imposed by concomitant fixed spinal deformities.

In early series reporting the results of hip replacement in patients with AS, reliable and rapid pain relief was reported. Concerns were however, raised over the relatively high rates of complication, such as infection, dislocation, and heterotopic ossification, as well as the development of radiological appearances indicative of mechanical failure of the implant in the short to mid-term. Failure of the implant would then lead to the requirement for more technically demanding revision surgery and the law of diminishing returns would apply.

There is however a lack of quality literature on the subject, with many of the early series grouping patients with AS together with those suffering from other inflammatory arthropathies, in an attempt to boost the low numbers in the study. Follow-up was often incomplete and of short duration, with a variety of implants and surgical approaches being included in a single study. The methods used to report clinical results and radiological findings were often different and incompatible and it was very difficult to extract meaningful data to aid in the selection of implants and the appropriate preoperative counseling of patients.

Only within the last five years papers have been published determining the long-term results of total hip arthroplasty in well defined patient groups, using standardized reporting techniques and including survivorship analysis (4–8). The most encouraging results have been obtained with the use of conventional cemented implants such as the Charnley low-friction arthroplasty, but other designs such as uncemented components and resurfacing arthroplasty are also showing promising early results (8,9).

TECHNICAL CONSIDERATIONS

Meticulous preoperative planning of the surgical procedure is essential and there are technical considerations for both anesthetists and surgeons.

From the anesthetic perspective, neck stiffness and temporomandibular and cricoarytenoid joint disease may make intubation difficult, while lumbar spine disease associated with ossified ligaments may make spinal or epidural anesthesia impossible. Thoracic involvement reduces chest expansion and vital capacity and there may also be cardiac involvement. The long-term use of anti-inflammatory analgesics can predispose to increased bleeding, while long-term steroid use can lead to osteoporosis, poor wound healing, and an increased risk of infection.

Positioning of the patient requires great care particularly in the presence of spinal deformity and contractures of one or both hips. Unrecognized and uncorrected pelvic obliquity may lead to malposition of the acetabular component and subsequent dislocation, while involvement of the knee can make the assistants' task and positioning of the femoral component more difficult.

The choice of surgical approach is also crucial, with trochanteric osteotomy having been associated with an increased risk of heterotopic ossification. Previous surgical procedures may have been performed, with old incisions being awkwardly placed as well as the perils of removing antiquated and unfamiliar plates or implants. More extensive soft tissue releases are usually required as well as more extensive capsulotomies or capsulectomies.

The introduction of aseptic techniques, with disposable impermeable drapes, antibiotic prophylaxis, and laminar airflow theaters has minimized the risk of infection. Gentle and precise surgical technique is crucial to reduce the risks of heterotopic ossification or femoral shaft fracture. In the ankylosed hip it will be necessary to section the femoral neck in situ, but in cases with protrusio or marked stiffness this would also be a sensible move.

Correct orientation of the components is essential, but there are many factors that can compromise this, leading to dislocation or early mechanical failure because of aseptic loosening. The effects of pelvic obliquity, spinal deformity, and other joint contractures must be remembered as well as the effects of any previous surgical procedures leading to an alteration in the anatomy. To optimize the longevity of the implant the center of rotation of the prosthetic joint should ideally be reconstructed at the correct anatomical level. It can, however, be very difficult to establish the true inferior and medial margins of the acetabulum in the presence of an ankylosed hip, and the use of radiology with intra-operative image intensifiers may be required. There may be protrusio acetabulae leading to the risk of acetabular perforation with injudicious reaming or the requirement for bone grafting. The femoral intramedullary canal is often narrowed or may be deformed or partially obliterated following a previous surgical procedure, particularly an osteotomy.

In the majority of cases hip involvement is bilateral and there may also be involvement of the knees with joint contractures. In these cases it is important to replace the other joints soon after the initial hip replacement in order to facilitate rehabilitation, optimizing the gains in motion and preventing the recurrence of soft tissue contractures through lack of use. As part of the preoperative assessment these coexisting problems must be identified and the patient counseled and advised that they may be required to undergo several joint replacements in relatively quick succession. There are various arguments as to whether multiple joint replacements should be performed in one sitting, or staged, but other factors must be considered such as general health and comorbidities, the ease of anesthesia, patient and surgeon preferences, and rehabilitative requirements.

In summary, the relatively high rates of infection, dislocation, fracture, and early loosening reported in the early series have been reduced as surgical techniques and awareness have improved. But despite these facts there are no grounds for complacency because these cases remain technically and emotionally challenging, with careful planning and precise surgical technique as essential prerequisites for a successful outcome.

RESULTS OF TOTAL HIP REPLACEMENT

In the Lancet paper of 1961 entitled "Arthroplasty of the Hip. A New Operation" (10), Charnley stated that the objectives of total hip replacement must be reasonable and that "neither surgeons nor engineers will ever make an artificial hip joint which will last 30 years and at some time in this period enable the patient to play football."

As previously mentioned the typical patient with AS is relatively young, active, and male, which means that he will place high demands on the implant and is likely to disregard any advice that he feels unfairly limits his lifestyle. The aims of surgery must, however, be realistic. First, pain must be relieved, contractures eradicated and range of motion improved, leading to improvements in function, mobility, and posture.

Clinical Results

It has been reported that up to 25% of patients with AS first present because of pain in the hip. In the majority of these cases hip joint involvement is bilateral, and in many cases the pain arising from the hip can overshadow the other symptoms.

In the majority of series from 89% to 100% of patients reported experiencing little or no pain arising from the replaced hip (11–17). This pain relief was well maintained in the long-term and 86% to 91% were rated good or excellent at latest follow-up (Table 1).

Several authors originally suggested that the gains in range of motion following total hip arthroplasty for AS would be relatively modest. This was the result of the presence of joint contractures, very restricted movements, and ankylosis prior to

Table 1 Previous Studies of Total Hip Replacement in AS

	Hips	Patients	Follow-up (yr)	Age	Implants[a]
Baldurson	18	10	3.8 (1–6)	32 (18–61)	2
Bhan	19	12	3.8 (3–5)	25 (19–40)	1
Bisla	34	23	4 (1–6)	41 (20–75)	4
Brinker	20	12	6.2 (2–10)	35 (23–53)	4
Finsterbush	35	23	7.5 (4–9)	N/S (21–44)	N/S
Gualtieri	73	39	7.5 (6–9)	50 (32–64)	2
Joshi[b]	181	103	10 (2–27)	47 (17–77)	1
Kilgus	53	31	6.3 (2–18)	43 (18–65)	6
Lehtimaki[b]	76	54	N/S (8–28)	40 (16–67)	1
Resnick	21	11	3 (1/12–6)	49 (24–73)	3
Shanahan	16	12	7.4 (0.5–12)	43 (17–76)	1
Shih	74	46	8.3 (3–14)	36 (20–75)	6
Sochart '97[b]	43	24	22.7 (2–30)	29 (19–70)	1
Sochart '01[b]	95	58	17 (2–30)	40 (19–70)	1
Sundaram	98	66	N/S (>1)	N/S	1
Tang[b]	95	58	11.3 (2–28)	39 (19–79)	3
Toni	28	22	N/S (2–14)	N/S (21–68)	5
Walker	29	19	4.8 (2–6)	53 (2–74)	7
Welch	33	20	2.6 (1–6)	43 (N/S)	1
Williams	86	53	3 (0.5–10)	42 (18–67)	2

Note: N/S, not specified in the study.
[a]Number of different designs of implant included in the study.
[b]Survivorship analysis performed.
Abbreviation: AS, ankylosing spondylitis.

operation. Bhan and Malhotra (2) reported an average preoperative flexion contracture of 43° in a series of 19 hips, Bisla et al. (12) an average of 38° in 34 hips, Kilgus et al. (18) an average of 33° in 53 hips, and Brinker et al. (9) an average of 20° in 20 hips. Preoperative ankylosis was reported in 6 of 18 hips (33%) by Baldursson et al. (11), 42 of 181 hips (23%) by Joshi et al. (5), 12 of 33 hips (36%) by Kilgus et al. (18), 26 of 74 hips (35%) by Shih et al. (15), and 10 of 95 hips (11%) by Sochart and Porter (7). It was also suggested that there would be a significant risk of developing heterotopic ossification or re-ankylosis following surgery (19,20).

When the results were analyzed there was an almost universally significant increase in the range of movement of the artificial joint, which was maintained in the long-term thereafter, with few cases of significant heterotopic ossification or re-ankylosis (see section "Heterotopic Ossification"). Range of movement was expressed either as an arc of flexion (FL) or a total cumulative range (Table 2). Postoperative arcs of flexion of 86–90° were reported and total cumulative ranges of 148–194° (2,6,7,9,11,12,15–18,21).

Scores for overall function following total hip replacement were originally designed to assess the results in patients undergoing surgery for monoarticular osteoarthritis. Clearly these will be affected by other factors such as polyarticular disease and medical comorbidities. Despite this, such systems can provide a useful guide to the early results following surgery. In a series of 95 Charnley low-friction arthroplasties, reported by Sochart and Porter in 2001 (7), it was noted that the functional score, using the six-point scale of Merle d'Aubigne and Postel (22), increased from an average of 2.7 points preoperatively (range 1–5 points) to an average of

Table 2 Clinical Results Following Total Hip Replacement in AS

	Heterotopic ossification[a] (%)	Class 3 and 4[b] (%)	Range of movement	No pain (%)
Baldurson	28	0	90 FL	94
Bhan	0	0	194	92
Bisla	62	26	148	91
Brinker	35	0	187	90
Finsterbush	17	N/S	86 FL	N/S
Gualtieri	N/S	21	N/S	89
Joshi[c]	12	0	N/S	96
Kilgus	45	11	176	N/S
Resnick	57	43	N/S	N/S
Shanahan	100	36	N/S	94
Shih	65	8	190	97
Sochart '97[c]	14	0	185	100
Sochart '01[c]	25	2	185	100
Sundaram	40	11	N/S	N/S
Tang[c]	74	21	N/S	94
Toni	50	21	N/S	N/S
Walker	77	23	168	97
Welch	N/S	N/S	160	100
Williams	55	11	N/S	B73

Note: N/S, not specified in the study.
[a]Heterotopic ossification of any degree.
[b]Heterotopic ossification of Brooker Class 3 or 4.
[c]Survivorship analysis performed.
Abbreviations: AS, ankylosing spondylitis; FL, arc of flexion.

5.4 points (range 2–6 points) 12 months postoperatively. This represented an improvement from only being able to walk with sticks to being able to walk long distances without sticks, but with a slight limp.

Following total hip replacement, patients therefore achieved rapid and reliable pain relief, a significantly increased range of hip movement, and a marked improvement in their overall walking ability. These clinical results have been shown to be well maintained in the long term.

Radiographic Results and Survival Analysis

Only five studies have reported the long-term results of total hip arthroplasty performed in patients with AS with more than 10 years average duration of follow-up and survivorship analysis using the Kaplan–Meier technique (23). Four of these studies looked at the results of a single design of implant, the Charnley low-friction arthroplasty (4–7), which is a cemented total hip arthroplasty, with the final study analyzing the results of both cemented and uncemented implants (8).

In a paper, published in 1997, Sochart and Porter (6) specifically looked at the long-term results in young patients with AS, aged less than 40 at the time of surgery. The results of 43 Charnley low-friction arthroplasties performed on 24 patients, with an average age of 29 (19–39 years) and an average duration of follow-up of 23 years, were analyzed. Using revision as the end point, survivorship of both of the original components was 92% at 10 years, 72% at 20 years and 70% at 30 years. Femoral component survivorship was similar at 10 years (93% vs. 91%), but at 20 years (91% vs. 72%) and 25 years (83% vs. 72%) femoral component survivorship was significantly higher. Aseptic loosening had occurred in a total of 33% of the acetabular components and in 10% of the femoral components. It was noted that failed implants had a significantly higher average annual wear rate of the polyethylene acetabular component than surviving implants.

In a paper published in 2001, Lehtimaki et al. (4) analyzed the results of 76 Charnley low-friction arthroplasties performed on 54 patients, with a follow-up of between 8 and 28 years, and an average age of 40 years (16–67 years). Survivorship of both of the original components was 80% at 10 years, 66% at 15 years and 62% at 20 years. Survivorship was similar for both acetabular and femoral components at all time intervals, with 20-year femoral survivorship being 77% and acetabular survivorship being 73%. No wear measurements or radiological analysis were reported.

In a paper published in 2002, Joshi et al. (5) analyzed the results of 181 Charnley low-friction arthroplasties performed on 103 patients, with an average follow-up of 10 years (range: 2–27 years), and an average age of 47 years (17–77 years). Survivorship of both of the original components was 87% at 10 years, 81% at 15 years and 72% at 27 years. It was once again demonstrated that long-term femoral component survivorship was superior to that of the acetabulum, with the 27-year femoral survivorship being 85% and the survivorship of the acetabulum being 74%. No wear measurements or detailed radiological analysis of surviving implants had been performed.

In 2001 Sochart and Porter (7) published the results of 95 Charnley low-friction arthroplasties performed on 58 patients with an average age of 40 years (19–70 years) and an average duration of follow-up of 17 years (2–30 years). Survivorship of both of the original components was 92% at 10 years, 83% at 15 years and 71% at 25 years. The total rate of aseptic loosening of the acetabulum was 21% and for the femur was 16%. The main factor determining the outcome for each implant was the average annual wear rate of the acetabular component and the average rate for the entire series was 0.1 mm per year. The average wear rate for failed implants was 0.19 mm per year as opposed to an average of 0.09 mm per year for surviving implants, which was highly statistically significant.

The fact that the average annual wear rate was the single most important factor in determining the long-term outcome of total hip arthroplasty was first established and quantified in a paper analyzing the long-term results of total hip arthroplasty performed on young patients, which was published in 1999 (24), with three subsequent papers reaching similar conclusions. As the average annual wear rate increases, the risk of acetabular and femoral loosening and revision have been shown to increase significantly, with implants which have an average annual wear rate of >0.2 mm per year being at particularly high risk of early failure. This is because the polyethylene wear debris produced by the implant stimulates the host's, immune response mechanism leading to macrophage and osteoclast stimulation resulting in the development of peri-prosthetic osteolysis, bone loss, and implant loosening.

In 2000, Tang and Chiu (8) analyzed the results of 95 arthroplasties performed on 57 patients, with an average age of 39 years (19–79 years) and an average duration of follow-up of 11 years (2–28 years). Six different implants were used in the series, three cemented and three uncemented, which clearly weakened the study. The probabilities of survival of the original implants were 98.5%, 96.8%, and 66.3% at 5, 10, and 15 years, respectively, when the results for the entire series were included. The probabilities of survival of the cemented prostheses were 100% at 5 years and

97.7% at 10 years, with the results for the uncemented prostheses being 95.5% at both five and 10 years. It was however noted that the survivorship for the uncemented components fell sharply at 11 years to only 66%, with the cemented component survivorship only falling to similar levels at 16 years. This is the only paper to date that presents the long-term survivorship of uncemented components, but the series was relatively small, multiple implant designs were grouped together, no wear results were provided, and no detailed radiological analysis was reported.

HETEROTOPIC OSSIFICATION

Heterotopic ossification is the formation of bone outside the skeleton and has been reported to occur in the soft tissues adjacent to the hip following surgical intervention. The precise activating factors of the condition are not known, but it is believed that ectopic bone formation is the result of the inappropriate differentiation of pluripotential mesenchymal cells within the connective tissues into osteoblastic stem cells. Contamination of the operative field with bone fragments is also thought to be a factor and, as always, meticulous surgical technique is essential.

Several conditions have been associated with an increased risk of ectopic bone formation following total hip replacement (Table 3), and there were several early reports implicating AS as a major risk factor. The reported incidences did however vary widely, with most authors reporting rates of between 12% and 62% in patients with AS (5,9,11,12,14,21,25,26).

The most widely used classification is that of Brooker et al. (27) published in 1973. The authors discovered ectopic bone formation in 21% of a consecutive series of 100 cases. They described four classes of ectopic bone formation of increasing severity. In Class 1 there were islands of bone within the soft tissues, and in Class 2 there were bony spurs extending from the pelvis or proximal femur, leaving more than 1 cm between opposing bone surfaces. In Class 3 cases the gap between the opposing surfaces was <1 cm, and in Class 4 there was complete bony ankylosis (Fig. 2).

Although heterotopic ossification was frequently observed radiologically, it was seldom of clinical importance, with only Class 3 or 4 changes potentially leading to any compromise of range of movement or function. In practice, only the Class 4

Table 3 Conditions Associated with the Development of Heterotopic Ossification

Male, prolonged operating time, advanced age (>65 years), increased blood loss
Heterotopic ossification following previous surgery or hip replacement on the same or
  opposite hip
Ankylosed or stiff hip preoperatively
Trochanteric bursitis
Hypertrophic osteoarthritis with large osteophytes
Post-traumatic arthritis
Postoperative infection
Surgical approaches: trochanteric osteotomy or anterolateral rather than posterior
DISH: disseminated idiopathic skeletal hyperostosis
Paget's disease
AS

Abbreviation: AS, ankylosing spondylitis.

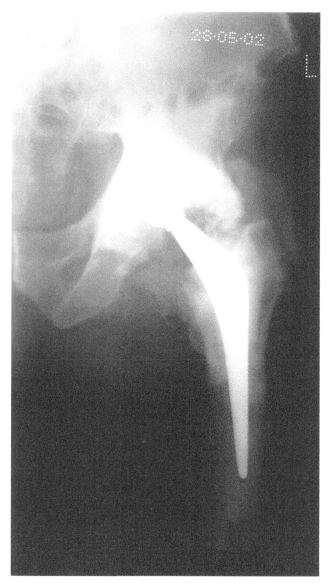

Figure 2 Class 4 heterotopic ossification with reankylosis.

cases demonstrated any significant clinical problems. In the larger series reporting the results of total hip replacement for AS, Class 3 or 4 changes have been reported in 2% to 43% of hips (Table 3), but complete ankylosis occurred in only 1% to 7% of hips in some series (8,12,15,18,26), with many series reporting no cases with Class 4 changes (2,5–7,9,11,14,17).

Because of the relatively high risk in patients with AS, routine prophylaxis against heterotopic bone formation has been advocated. The most commonly used methods are nonsteroidal anti-inflammatory agents and localized radiotherapy (28–31), but these also have potential side effects and morbidities. It has been suggested that there is a greater risk of ectopic bone formation when several risk factors coexist (32–34)

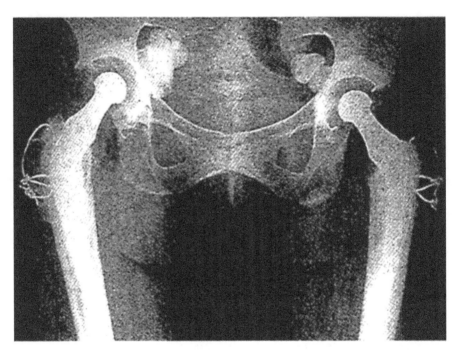

Figure 3 One year postoperative radiograph showing bilateral Charnley low-friction arthro-plasties in 1967. *Source:* From **JBJS** paper; Fig. 1B.

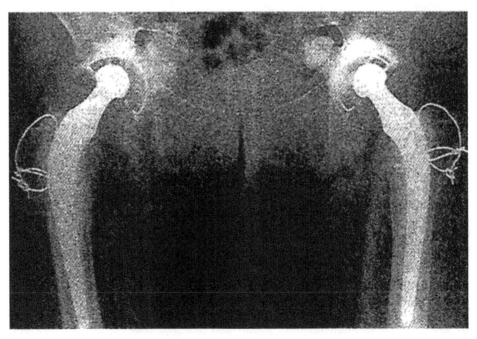

Figure 4 Thirty year postoperative radiograph taken in 1996, showing no evidence of loosening and acceptable rate of wear.

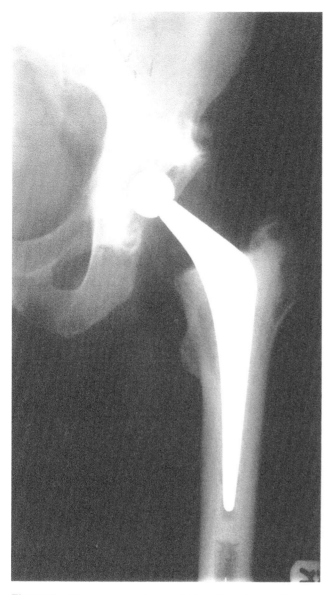

Figure 5 Modern cemented total hip arthroplasty using a polished tapered stem.

and it is likely that targeted prophylaxis in high-risk patients with multiple risk factors would be more appropriate than routine prophylaxis in all cases.

CONCLUSIONS

Total hip replacement has now been shown to provide rapid and reliable pain relief in patients with AS. Range of movement and function are significantly increased and all of the benefits are well maintained in the long term. The re-ankylosis rate is low and could be improved further with the use of targeted prophylaxis against heterotopic ossification in high-risk cases. Component survivorship

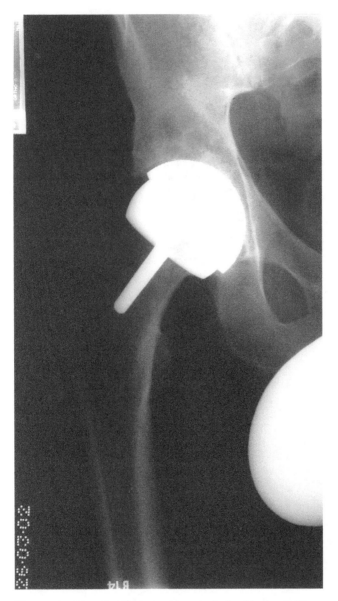

Figure 6 Resurfacing arthroplasty of the hip in a 27-year-old male patient with AS. *Abbreviation*: AS, ankylosing spondylitis.

has been shown to be comparable with other patient groups when using a tried and tested implant (35). However, dealing with these young, active, and highly motivated patients is often both emotionally demanding and technically challenging and such cases should only be operated upon by experienced hip surgeons (Figs. 3 and 4).

There remains a relative paucity of long-term studies, with only cemented total hip arthroplasties having been thoroughly assessed (Fig. 5), and the Charnley low-friction arthroplasty remaining the benchmark (4–7). The major factor determining the long-term outcome of total hip arthroplasty, particularly in young patients, is wear of the polyethylene acetabular component and alternative bearing surfaces and other technologies, such as uncemented implants and resurfacing arthroplasty, are being studied (Fig. 6).

REFERENCES

1. Dwosh I, Resnick D, Becker M. Hip involvement in ankylosing spondylitis. Arthritis Rheum 1976; 19:683–692.
2. Bhan S, Malhotra R. Bipolar hip arthroplasty in ankylosing spondylitis. Arch Orthop Trauma Surg 1996; 115:94–99.
3. Forouzesh S, Bluestone R. The clinical spectrum of ankylosing spondylitis. Clin Orthop Relat Res 1979; 143:53–58.
4. Lehtimaki M, Lehto M, Kautiainen H, Lehtinen K, Hamalainen M. Charnley total hip arthroplasty in ankylosing spondylitis. Acta Orthop Scand 2001; 72:233–236.
5. Joshi A, Markovic L, Hardinge K, Murphy J. Total hip arthroplasty in ankylosing spondylitis. J Arthroplasty 2002; 17:427–433.
6. Sochart DH, Porter ML. Long-term results of total hip replacement in young patients who had ankylosing spondylitis. J Bone Joint Surg 1997; 79A:1181–1189.
7. Sochart D, Porter M. Long-term results of Charnley low friction arthroplasty for ankylosing spondylitis. Hip Int 2001; 11:59–70.
8. Tang W, Chiu K. Primary total hip arthroplasty in patients with ankylosing spondylitis. J Arthroplasty 2000; 15:52–58.
9. Brinker M, Rosenberg A, Kull L, Cox D. Primary non-cemented total hip arthroplasty in patients with ankylosing spondylitis. J Arthroplasty 1996; 11:802–812.
10. Charnley J. Arthroplasty of the hip. A new operation. Lancet 1961; 1(7187):1129–1132.
11. Baldursson H, Brattstrom H, Olsson T. Total hip replacement in ankylosing spondylitis. Acta Orthop Scand 1977; 48:499–507.
12. Bisla R, Ranawat C, Inglis A. Total hip replacement in patients with ankylosing spondylitis with involvement of the hip. J Bone Joint Surg 1976; 58A:233–238.
13. Gualtieri G, Gualtieri I, Hendriks M, Gagliardi S. Comparison of cemented ceramic and metal–polyethylene coupling hip prostheses in ankylosing spondylitis. Clin Orthop Relat Res 1992; 282:81–85.
14. Shanahan W, Kaprove R, Major P, Hunter T, Baragar F. Assessment of long-term benefit of THR in patients with ankylosing spondylitis. J Rheumatol 1982; 9:101–104.
15. Shih L, Chen T, Lo W, Yang D. Total hip arthroplasty in patients with ankylosing spondylitis: long-term follow-up. J Rheumatol 1995; 22:1704–1709.
16. Walker LG, Sledge CB. Total hip arthroplasty in ankylosing spondylitis. Clin Orthop Relat Res 1991; 262:198–204.
17. Welch RB, Charnley J. Low friction arthroplasty in rheumatoid arthritis and ankylosing spondylitis. Clin Orthop Relat Res 1970; 72:22–32.
18. Kilgus D, Namba R, Gorek J, Cracchiolo A, Amstutz H. Total hip replacement for patients who have ankylosing spondylitis. J Bone Joint Surg 1990; 72A:834–839.
19. Resnick D, Dwosh I, Goergen T, Shapiro R, D'Ambrosia R. Clinical and radiographic 'reankylosis' following hip surgery in ankylosing spondylitis. AJR Am J Roentgenol 1976; 126:1181–1188.
20. Wilde A, Collins H, MacKenzie A. Reankylosis of the hip joint in ankylosing spondylitis after total hip replacement. Arthritis Rheum 1972; 15:493–496.
21. Finsterbush A, Amir D, Vatashki E, Husseini N. Joint surgery in severe ankylosing spondylitis. Acta Orthop Scand 1988; 59:491–496.
22. Merle d'Aubigne R, Postel M. Functional results of hip arthroplasty with acrylic prosthesis. J Bone Joint Surg 1954; 36A:451–475.
23. Kaplan EL, Meier P. Nonparametric observation from incomplete observations. J Am Stat Assoc 1958; 53:457–481.

24. Sochart D. Relationship of acetabular wear to osteolysis and loosening in total hip arthroplasty. Clin Orthop Relat Res 1999; 363:135–150.
25. Toni A, Baldini N, Sudanese A, Tigani D, Giunti A. Total hip arthroplasty in patients with ankylosing spondylitis with a more than two year follow-up. Acta Orthop Belg 1987; 53:63–66.
26. Williams E, Taylor A, Arden G, Edwards D. Arthroplasty of the hip in ankylosing spondylitis. J Bone Joint Surg 1977; 59B:393–397.
27. Brooker A, Bowerman J, Robinson R, Riley L. Ectopic ossification following total hip-replacement. J Bone Joint Surg 1973; 55A:1629–1632.
28. Lima D, Venn-Watson E, Tripuraneni P, Colwell C. Indomethacin versus radiation therapy for heterotopic ossification after hip arthroplasty. Orthopaedics 2001; 24:1139–1143.
29. Neal B, Rogers A, Dunn L, Fransen M. Non-steroidal anti-inflammatory drugs for preventing heterotopic bone formation after hip arthroplasty. The Cochrane Library Issue 2, 2003.
30. Seegensschmeidt M, Makoski H, Micke O. Radiation prophylaxis of heterotopic ossification about the hip joint—a multicentre study. Int J Radiat Oncol Biol Phys 2001; 51:756–765.
31. Vielpeau C, Joubert J, Hulet C. Naproxen in the prevention of heterotopic ossification after total hip replacement. Clin Orthop Relat Res 1999; 369:279–288.
32. Iorio R, Healy W. Heterotopic ossification after hip and knee arthroplasty. J Am Acad Orthop Surg 2002; 10:409–416.
33. Lewallen D. Heterotopic ossification following total hip arthroplasty. Instr Course Lect 1995; 44:287–292.
34. Pai V. Heterotopic ossification in total hip arthroplasty. J Arthroplasty 1994; 9:199–202.
35. Sochart DH, Porter ML. The long-term results of Charnley low-friction arthroplasty in young patients who have congenital dislocation, degenerative arthrosis or rheumatoid arthritis. J Bone Joint Surg 1997; 79A:1599–1617.

25

Total Knee Arthroplasty for Patients with Ankylosing Spondylitis

John Minnich and Javad Parvizi

Department of Orthopaedics, Rothman Institute, Philadelphia, Pennsylvania, U.S.A.

INTRODUCTION

Although ankylosing spondylitis (AS) is more commonly associated with amphi-arthrodial joints, it has been reported to affect peripheral diarthrodial joints, like the knee, in up to 70% of the patients (1–3). The rapid progression to ankylosis of the joints, in patients with AS, may lead to severe stiffness and immobility. Joint pain may be due to "coxitis," i.e., the inflammatory process affecting the joint or in the advanced stage of the disease due to development of severe degenerative joint disease. Treatment options for arthritis of the knee in AS patients are similar to other patients with osteoarthritis. The management strategy includes institution of non-operative treatments such as weight loss, activity modification, anti-inflammatory medication, corticosteroid injections, and even viscosupplementation injections whenever indicated. Because of the potential failure of nonoperative treatment for the degenerative joint disease, some of these patients will seek treatment from the orthopedic surgeon for their end-stage joint disease.

Although total knee arthroplasty (TKA) is known to have a durable and excellent outcome for patients with osteoarthritis, rheumatoid arthritis, or avascular necrosis, its results in patients with AS is largely unknown (4–8). In some series, a few total knee arthroplasties in patients with AS have been reported. Based on the information from those reports, it is difficult to ascertain the clinical outcome in this patient subgroup, as the results are reported together, with a much greater number of total knee arthroplasties performed in patients with osteoarthritis and rheumatoid arthritis. Fintersbush et al. (9) reported on the result of joint surgery in 35 patients with AS. They noted excellent pain relief following knee arthroplasty in six of the patients in their series. The functional result of TKA was, however, less predictable and noted to deteriorate with time in all of the six patients who underwent TKA.

The result of TKA for patients with AS is likely to be compromised for various reasons. First, patients with AS are often young and moderately active patients both of which adversely affect the survivorship of TKA (7,10). Second, patients with AS may have involvement of other joints which could in turn influence the mechanics of gait and the long-term outcome of the arthroplasty. Finally, patients with AS are known to be predisposed to stiffness which could also compromise the outcome of TKA (11). In fact, some of the major reasons cited as the cause of inferior outcome for TKA for patients with AS are postoperative stiffness and the development of heterotopic ossification (11,12). Both of the latter result in limited motion of the knee following TKA and adversely affect the functional outcome.

INSTITUTIONAL EXPERIENCE

A retrospective review of 23 patients (34 arthroplasties) with AS undergoing TKA at Mayo Clinic over a 15-year period was conducted. During the study period 13,821 had undergone TKA at our institution. It is therefore apparent that only a small portion of the joint arthroplasty population is comprised of patients with AS. All patients included in this study were examined by a rheumatologist and met the New York criteria for AS (13). Human leukocyte antigen (HLA)-B27 assay was positive in 16 patients (25 knees). Chest expansion was tested and found to be limited to < 2.5 cm as measured at the fourth intercostal space in all the patients in this study. Extraskeletal manifestation of AS was also present in the form of iritis in three patients, apical fibrosis in one patient, and aortitis in one patient. In addition, 17 patients admitted to some degree of fatigue, weight loss, and anorexia. The characteristic radiographic changes of subchondral sclerosis with complete amelioration of the sacroiliac joint and squaring of the anterior vertebral borders were present in all patients. Ossification of the anterior longitudinal ligaments leading to bamboo spine was also seen in 18 patients who were radiographed. Six patients underwent surgery on other joints for deformity and pain. This included ipsilateral total hip arthroplasty in three patients, contralateral total hip arthroplasty in two patients, and shoulder arthroplasty in one patient.

There were 17 males and 3 females with a mean age of 55 years (range 28–67 years) at the time of surgery. The mean weight of the patients was 76.4 kg (range 50–105 kg) and the mean height for the patients in the study was 166.6 cm (range 150–179 cm). All patients had a cemented condylar prosthesis. Ten of the patients had bilateral knee replacements of which five were simultaneous and five were staged bilateral arthroplasties. All patients had their patella resurfaced with a cemented all-polyethylene button. Five knees had been operated on before the knee arthroplasty: two knees had medial meniscectomy, one knee upper tibial osteotomy, one knee synovectomy, and one knee arthroscopic debridement. The average duration of AS prior to surgery was 25 years (range 1–57 years) and the average duration of symptomatic knee involvement prior to surgery was 12 years (range 3–29 years).

Clinical and radiographic data were collected preoperatively and at two months, one year, two years, and every five years postoperatively. Knee scores were calculated using the Knee Society knee scoring system consisting of a score for pain and a score for function, each with a maximum of 100 points (14). Knee scores were assessed before surgery, at two-years, and at latest follow-up examination. Surveillance averaged 11.2 years (range 3–24 years) for clinical and 8.6 years (range 2–22 years) for radiographic follow-up.

Preoperatively, the Knee Society scores averaged 14 (range 0–37) for pain and 16.3 (range 0–40) for function. The average scores improved to 87.5 (range 75–100) for pain and 80 (range 30–90) for function at two-year follow-up and then declined to 76.3 (range 45–100) for pain and 58.7 (range 0–85) for function at the latest follow-up.

At two year follow-up three knees had extensor lag ≥10°. The range of motion had deteriorated over the years with the number of knees with extensor lag ≥10° being present in 10 knees.

(A)

(B)

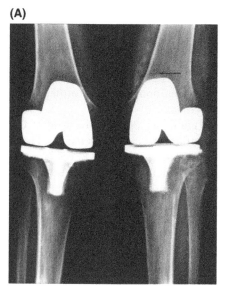
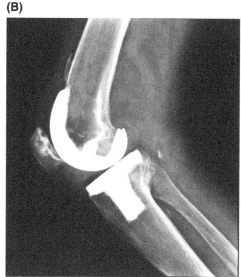

Figure 1 Radiograph of the knee of a 51-year-old man with AS. (**A**) Anteroposterior and (**B**) lateral postoperative radiograph at four years confirms presence of heterotopic ossification. There was a significant decline in the range of motion of this patient over the ensuing years. *Abbreviation*: AS, ankylosing spondylitis.

Preoperatively, there were two patients who could not walk secondary to their knee pathology, 6 patients (10 knees) who required a walker, and 12 patients (18 knees) who required a cane or crutches full time. At two years postoperatively, all patients could walk without assistance. At the latest follow-up, only three patients (five knees) were able to walk without any aids, two patients could not walk, and 15 patients (23 knees) needed some help from an assistance to ambulate.

Three patients required manipulation under anesthesia postoperatively in an attempt to improve their poor range of motion. One knee was revised at 10 years postoperatively for aseptic loosening of the patellar component (the tibial and femoral components were stable).

Heterotopic ossification was found on the latest follow-up radiographs of six knees (Fig. 1). Only one of the patients had moderate symptoms of pain. Three of the six knees had prior surgery on the affected knee and two of the knees had a postoperative manipulation. Sub-analysis was performed to evaluate the mean arc of motion for the six knees (four patients) with heterotopic ossification. This was found to be 73° (range 25–90°) preoperatively improving only slightly to 76° (range 30–95°) at the latest follow-up. The mean arc of motion for patients with heterotopic ossification was significantly less than the remaining patients without heterotopic ossification, both preoperatively ($p < 0.05$) and at the latest follow-up ($p < 0.007$).

There was no significant difference in the erythrocyte sedimentation rate in patients with and without evidence of heterotopic ossification.

DISCUSSION

In spite of the retrospective nature of the study, with its innate limitations, and the relatively small number of patients, we were able to make some conclusive deductions. We observed that TKA provided an excellent and predictable outcome with regard to pain relief in patients with AS. Although ambulation potential and functional ability also improved in these patients, the gain in range of motion was less optimal. The reason for inferior range of motion in these patients, we believe, was related to three important factors: the nature of the disease in causing soft tissue and joint ankylosis, the poor preoperative range of motion, and the formation of heterotopic ossification following TKA in these patients.

Because of the inherent nature of AS, as the name suggests, involvement of the soft tissues and joint ankylosis results in deterioration in motion over time. There were three patients in our series who required manipulation of their knees because of poor postoperative range of motion. The rate of manipulation of the knee following TKA is usually <2%. The postoperative knee manipulation rate in patients with AS is therefore undeniably high when compared to patients with underlying diagnosis of osteoarthritis or rheumatoid arthritis.

Although the main indication for TKA in this group of patients was pain, unresponsive to conservative treatment, 98% of the patients also complained of severe stiffness and inability to bend or straighten their knees. In addition, the majority of the patients in this series had considerable degrees of flexion contracture preoperatively. Severe, fixed flexion contracture associated with end-stage arthritis of the knee is one of the more technically challenging situations encountered in TKA (15,16). Technical difficulties in achieving satisfactory correction of the contracture and deformity were encountered in over 75% of the total knee arthroplasties in this study. Additional distal femur resection, up to the point of insertion of the collateral ligament, was felt to be necessary in eight knees for correction of the flexion contracture. It is clear that poor preoperative range of motion with coexistent flexion contracture and deformity adversely affected the functional outcome in these patients.

Another reason for deterioration in motion over time could be explained by the higher rate of development of heterotopic ossification in patients with AS. The prevalence of heterotopic ossification in our patients with AS is similar to what has been reported in patients who have undergone total hip arthroplasty. (Almost one-third of the patients in this study developed some degree of heterotopic ossification over the ensuing years following the TKA.) Although heterotopic ossification was responsible for functional disability in only one of our patients, it seems intuitive that development of heterotopic ossification would undoubtedly have some deleterious effect on the range of motion in the remainder of patients who developed some degree of heterotopic ossification.

The reason for a higher preponderance of patients with AS for development of heterotopic ossification remains unknown. Previous studies evaluating the results of total hip arthroplasty in patients with AS have also observed a higher incidence of heterotopic ossification formation in these patients (1,11,12,17–19). Heterotopic ossification developed in as high as 76% of the patients in some of these studies but was functionally disabling in only 9% of the patients. We observed that the incidence of heterotopic ossification was higher in previously operated knees and heterotopic ossification was more likely to develop in a knee with heterotopic ossification on the contralateral knee. Incidentally, heterotopic ossification developed following manipulation in two knees. It is difficult to ascertain whether the poor range of motion, with tendency for ankylosis, in these two patients requiring manipulation was the cause or consequence of heterotopic ossification formation. It is, however, plausible that manipulation may be another predisposing factor for development of heterotopic ossification. There were four patients in our study who received ibuprofen preoperatively. None of these patients developed heterotopic ossification, despite the fact that one of these patients had developed severe heterotopic ossification in the hip. Based on these results it would be difficult to advocate routine administration of heterotopic ossification prophylaxis for patients with AS undergoing knee arthroplasty, but any patient with a history of previous knee surgery, and those with evidence of heterotopic ossification in the contralateral joint as well as patients with severe preoperative knee stiffness should be considered for heterotopic ossification prophylaxis. In agreement with a previous study we also found that the level of erythrocyte sedimentation rate did not have any effect on the incidence of heterotopic ossification formation (19).

The incidence of other complications, following TKA, in patients with AS was not found to be any higher, despite the systemic nature of the disease. Patients with AS, because of the involvement of costovertebral joints, are known to have a compromised lung vital capacity. One might expect these patients to be at a greater risk of developing intraoperative or postoperative pulmonary complications. We were surprised to discover the low incidence of pulmonary complications in our patients with AS. There were only two patients who developed postoperative atelactasis that resolved with minimal intervention. No other intraoperative or postoperative pulmonary complications were observed. It is important to note that the awareness for potentially higher complication rates for patients with AS may have encouraged the use of specific measures to minimize the risk of these complications. For example, because of severe cervical spine ankylosis, fiber-optic intubations were used in seven patients. Also most patients required higher mean airway pressures than the general population for adequate ventilation during anesthesia.

CONCLUSIONS

Total knee arthroplasty is a viable treatment option for AS patients who have significant and debilitating degenerative arthritis in the knees. Patients can expect excellent pain relief, although functional outcomes are more variable. Therefore, medical management should be exhausted and patients should be counseled about the unique risks involved in the procedure. In particular, postoperative care should be aimed at maximizing range of motion and surgeons should consider prophylaxis against heterotopic ossification in high-risk patients. Lastly, surgeons should avoid performing bilateral total knee replacements in AS patients because of the increased morbidity, difficult rehabilitation, and less predictable outcome.

REFERENCES

1. Brinker MR, Rosenberg AG, Kull L, Cox DD. Primary noncemented total hip arthroplasty in patients with ankylosing spondylitis: clinical and radiographic results at an average follow-up period of 6 years. J Arthroplasty 1996; 11:802–812.
2. Forouzesh S, Bluestone R. The clinical spectrum of ankylosing spondylitis. Clin Orthop 1979; 43:53–58.
3. Resnick D. Patterns of peripheral joint disease in ankylosing spondylitis. Radiology 1976; 110:523–532.
4. Ito J, Koshino T, Okamoto R, Saito T. 15-year follow-up study of total knee arthroplasty in patients with rheumatoid arthritis. J Arthroplasty 2003; 18(8):984–992.

5. Seldes RM, Tan V, Duffy G, Rand JA, Lotke PA. Total knee arthroplasty for steroid-induced osteonecrosis. J Arthroplasty 1999; 14(5):533–537.
6. Lachiewicz PF, Soileau ES. The rates of osteolysis and loosening associated with a modular posterior stabilized knee replacement. Results at five to fourteen years. J Bone Joint Surg Am 2004; 86-A(3):525–530.
7. Kelly MA, Clarke HD. Long-term results of posterior cruciate-substituting total knee arthroplasty. Clin Orthop 2002; 404:51–57.
8. Gill GS, Joshi AB, Mills DM. Total condylar knee arthroplasty. 16- to 21-year results. Clin Orthop 1999; 367:210–215.
9. Fintersbush A, Amir D, Vatashki E, Husseini N. Joint surgery in severe ankylosing spondylitis. Acta Orthop Scand 1988; 59:491–496.
10. Duffy GP, Trousdale RT, Stuart MJ. Total knee arthroplasty in patients 55 years old or younger. 10- to 17-year results. Clin Orthop 1998; 356:22–27.
11. Kilgus DJ, Namba RS, Gorek JE, Cracchiolo A, Amstutz HC. Total hip replacement for patients who have ankylosing spondylitis. J Bone Joint Surg 1990; 72A:834–839.
12. Shih L-Y, Chen T-H, Lo W-H, Yang D-J. Total hip arthroplasty in patients with ankylosing spondylitis: long-term follow-up. J Rheum 1995; 22:1704–1709.
13. Moll JM, Wright V. New York clinical criteria for ankylosing spondylitis: a statistical evaluation. Ann Rheum Dis 1973; 324:354–363.
14. Insall JN, Dorr LD, Scott RD, Scott, RN. Rationale of the Knee Society clinical rating system. Clin Orthop 1989; 248:13–14.
15. Lu H-S, Mow CS, Lin J-H. Total knee arthroplasty in the presence of severe flexion contracture. J Arthroplasty 1999; 14:775–780.
16. Naranja RJ Jr, Lotke PA, Pagnano MW, Hanssen AD. Total knee arthroplasty in a previously ankylosed or arthrodesed knee. Clin Orthop 1996; 331:234–237.
17. Baldursson H, Brattstrom H, Olsson TH. Total hip replacement in ankylosing spondylitis. Acta Orthop Scand 1977; 48:499–507.
18. Bisla RS, Ranawat CS, Inglis AE. Total hip replacement in patients with ankylosing spondylitis with involvement of the hip. J Bone Joint Surg 1976; 58A:233–238.
19. Sundram NA, Murphy JCM. Heterotopic bone formation following total hip arthroplasty in ankylosing spondylitis. Clin Orthop 1986; 207:223–226.

26

Ankylosing Spondylitis in 2015

Debby Vosse and Sjef van der Linden
Division of Rheumatology, Department of Internal Medicine, University Maastricht, Maastricht, The Netherlands

Although nowadays ankylosing spondylitis (AS), also known as Morbus Bechterew or Bechterew's disease, is a well-recognized entity, it should be noted that this disease for a long time (up to the early 1960s) had been regarded as a variant of rheumatoid arthritis (RA) (1,2). The disease was often referred to as rheumatoid spondylitis. At that time Wright and Moll had proposed the unifying concept of the spondyloarthropathies or spondylarthritides (SpA) (3). With the advent of classification criteria and improved epidemiological tools, and also due to thorough clinical research, and the important contribution of human leukocyte antigen (HLA)-typing it became quite clear that AS is in fact the prototype of this group of related diseases (4). The modified New York criteria, in which the presence of radiographic sacroiliitis was made a conditio sine qua non for the diagnosis of AS have had widespread acceptance for standardization of surveys of the disease among populations (5). In daily practice, however, occasionally clinical cases of AS without radiographic sacroiliitis may occur (6). It is now known that magnetic resonance imaging (MRI) techniques are more sensitive in detecting inflammation of the sacroiliac joints among symptomatic people than conventional radiographs or computer tomographic imaging of these joints (7–9). The idea, therefore, is that conventional radiography may lack sensitivity to detect these occasional patients who otherwise may show all usual signs and symptoms of AS. It should also be noted that dealing with sacroiliitis there is considerable intra- and inter-observer variation in the interpretation of conventional radiographs of the sacroiliac joints (10).

In this chapter we will briefly review some major features regarding the etiology, diagnosis, classification, prognosis, treatment, and outcome assessment of AS. We will do so concentrating on such questions as what do we currently know of these features, what do we not yet know, and what will we probably know one decade from now, that means by the year 2015? The assumption is that a large number of these questions will be put on the agenda of researchers and that relevant answers will be found within the next decade or so. Our questions are intended to be clinically important and are largely related to the following clinical case.

CASE DESCRIPTION

A male person, aged 39 years, having an administrative job, has had inflammatory low back pain of insidious onset for more than 10 years. At physical examination considerable loss of motion of the lumbar and thoracic spine and an increased occiput-to-wall distance were noted. Conventional radiographs of the spine and the pelvis demonstrated clear-cut sacroiliitis grade 2 bilaterally and one small syndesmophyte at the lumbar spine, but were otherwise completely normal. In addition, there was mild inflammation of both knee joints. Psoriasis was absent. There was a questionable history of chronic inflammatory bowel disease and he had experienced one attack of acute anterior uveitis. The family history is negative for AS. He is HLA-B27 positive. The diagnosis of AS was established 10 years after the onset of symptoms. His Bath AS Functional Index (BASFI) score indicated considerably reduced physical capacity.

Questions That Might Come Up from This Case

The questions are grouped under etiology, diagnosis, prognosis, and treatment. Regarding prognosis one should preferably distinguish between prognosis given the "natural history of the disease" and changes in prognosis due to the effects of or responses to one or more interventions (pharmaceutical or nonpharmaceutical). In fact, the observed outcome is the end result of the natural history of the disease and any superimposed effects of pharmaceutical and nonpharmaceutical interventions.

Questions on Etiology and Pathogenesis

- What is the cause of the disease?
- What anatomical substrate causes the extensive limitation of spinal mobility in this patient in the absence of syndesmophytes? Might advanced imaging techniques show extensive fibrosis without calcification and new bone formation?

Questions on Diagnosis and Classification

- How can we effectively shorten the diagnostic delay, i.e., the time interval between first complaints and establishing the clinical diagnosis? What is in this respect the role of education and whom should we educate? What are effective modes of education to reach the goal of early diagnosis?

Questions on Prognosis and Prevention

- Can the prognosis due to the natural history of the disease for a particular patient be estimated at—or shortly after—establishing the diagnosis of AS for that patient? The aim is to differentiate those with a bad prognosis from those with a good prognosis.
- Can attacks of anterior uveitis be prevented by biologicals? Do the several anti-tumor necrosis factor (TNF)-α blockers differ in efficacy in preventing such events?
- Is HLA-B27 a prognostic factor or primarily associated with susceptibility for AS?
- What is the exact relationship between radiological outcome and clinical outcome? In particular, how does physical function relate to damage?
- Can bad spinal posture be predicted and prevented?

- What is the relationship between bad posture and physical functioning?
- Can radiographic damage (osteoporosis, syndesmophytosis) be predicted and prevented (at the group and at the individual level)?
- Will patients such as the one provided in our case description eventually after long follow-up develop extensive syndesmophytosis?
- How can, at an early stage of the disease, the development of syndesmophytes be predicted for individual patients?
- Does disease activity overtime really predict outcomes relevant for patients and society?

Questions on Treatment

- Does *early* treatment improve radiographic and clinical outcome? Is there a therapeutic window of opportunity?
- To what degree can physical functioning be improved (or can functional decline be prevented) by nonpharmacological interventions such as regular exercises, physiotherapy, or spa treatment? Can the efficacy of such interventions be increased and, if so, how should this be done and by what mechanisms are these effects brought about?
- How much can dissemination and broad implementation of those interventions that are currently already known to be effective, but that are not yet generally applied in daily practice, contribute to promote improvement of outcome of current AS patients?
- Does pharmacological treatment with nonsteroidal anti-inflammatory drugs (NSAIDs) or biologicals improve outcome in terms of preventing structural damage (including syndesmophytes and osteoporosis) and associated decline in physical functioning?
- How can we soon after establishing the diagnosis predict response to therapy (in particular treatment with biologicals)? Are those patients who would have a worse outcome by natural history of disease equally responsive to disease-modifying interventions as those patients who might expect a more favorable course of disease by natural history?
- Would early treatment with biologicals prevent the particular type of loss of spinal mobility as observed in the case presented? Radiological damage of the spine is almost lacking in this patient.
- Does treatment with biologicals make physiotherapeutic modalities such as daily exercises or spa therapy unnecessary or should these interventions still be continued on a regular basis during pharmacological treatment?

Questions on Outcome Assessment

- How valid is the current assessment of patient outcome?
- Is outcome assessment evidence-based?

Comments Regarding Etiologic Questions

Notwithstanding a considerable number of animal, genetic, clinical, and other studies the cause of AS is—more than 30 years after the association of AS and the HLA allele B27 was first described in 1973—still largely unknown (11). This association was even stronger than the one between this human leukocyte antigen and reactive arthritis or Reiter's disease. Bacteria that might trigger this condition such as *Shigella*, *Salmonella*, *Yersinia* or *Campylobacter* species were already known by that time. Therefore, it was widely suspected that the microorganism that supposedly triggered

AS would soon be known. A number of studies, mostly by Ahmadi et al. (12), have suggested that *Klebsiella* species might act as the causative agent. By the year 2015 more definite answers regarding the etiology and in particular the microbial agents that may cause AS are to be expected. However, one should not be too optimistic in this respect. The decline in the incidence of rheumatic fever in Western countries or the successful treatment of gout with uric acid-lowering drugs—enabling the prevention of joint damage due to tophi—has clearly turned attention away from studying etiologic issues. The same might happen in the field of AS. Anti-TNF treatment of AS patients might inhibit funding of studies that address unraveling the etiology and pathogenesis of this potentially disabling disease. In other words, if modern treatment with biologicals turns out to be largely curative then this may have negative effects on the search for the etiology of AS.

Other studies assessed whether all subtypes of HLA-B27 convey the same degree of susceptibility of developing AS. The number of reported subtypes increased steadily from year to year. The risk for a few subtypes, in particular HLA-B2706 or HLA-B2709, does not seem to be increased (13–16). However, it should be noted that HLA-B27-positive first-degree relatives of HLA-B27-positive AS patients have a considerably increased risk of developing the disease as compared to their HLA-B27-positive counterparts in the general population (17). This might be due to the admixture of other HLA-associated or non-HLA-associated susceptibility genes in the families of these AS patients (18–20). Clearly these relatives show the same B27 subtypes as B27-positive persons in the general population. The next decade will provide insight into the genetics of AS. This will expectedly enable us to delineate susceptibility genes and genes associated with severity of the disease in terms of progression and final damage.

Another yet unresolved etiologic question is what exactly explains the association between chronic inflammatory bowel disease and AS? Further, what are the implications of this association for successfully treating both conditions?

Comments Related to Diagnostic and Classification Issues

Clearly, early diagnosis is of paramount importance if treatment at an early stage provides better outcome. Currently, contrary to the Rome criteria, the (modified) New York criteria do not allow to classify a patient officially as having AS as long as radiographs of the sacroiliac joints do not yet show clear-cut evidence of sacroiliitis (grade 2 bilaterally, or grade 3 or 4 unilaterally) (5). However, patients may already be symptomatic for a considerable period of time. The time interval between the first complaints of AS and the moment of establishing a definite diagnosis often exceeds a period of four years (17). Such a state of disease could currently be labeled as pre-AS. Clearly, criteria allowing patients to be classified as AS at an earlier stages of their disease are badly needed. This includes a better definition of what we now call AS or what would possibly better be named as spondylitic disease. One might expect that the international Assessment in Ankylosing Spondylitis (ASAS) group (http://www.asas-group.org) will have accomplished this target within the next decade. However, new and more sensitive criteria will not do the job by their own. Awareness of AS among the general public and among symptomatic individuals, but of course also among health providers needs to be improved to effectively shorten the delay between onset of symptoms and establishing the diagnosis (21). The question, however, is who should be most aware of AS? The answer probably is a combination of the medical community as a whole, especially at the level of the primary health care and those people in the population who experience persisting low back pain of insidious onset. In particular, however, this applies to the relatives of AS patients. What type of educational intervention is needed to effectively raise the awareness of AS at the appropriate time among these target groups? Educational research in this field is badly needed. Hopefully answers to these important issues will already be available before the year 2015.

Comments on Prognostic and Preventive Issues

We do not yet understand how limitation of spinal mobility, bad posture, and functional limitations arise in the absence of syndesmophytes (see case scenario). What exactly is the anatomical substrate underlying these phenomena? Within the next decade we will definitely know much more about these aspects by applying modern imaging techniques such as MRI and positron emission tomography (PET) scanning. This will hopefully enable us to better predict prognosis and to guide treatment.

Genetic studies will also help in predicting not only susceptibility for the disease, but also the outcome of AS by natural history for individual patients, and in predicting patient's response to treatment (22). Moreover, we expect to see more data on (change in) life expectancy of AS patients (23,24).

Comments on Questions Dealing with Pharmacological Therapy

Until recently pharmacological interventions in AS primarily aimed at modifying symptoms such as pain and stiffness. NSAIDs therapy was usually not considered to have disease-modifying properties. A recent report supports an older case–control study suggesting that this notion is possibly incorrect. Daily use of these drugs might supposedly retard the development of syndesmophytes in contrast to intermittent use of NSAIDs (25,26). However, the cause and effect relationship of these findings has to be clarified. The effect of co-interventions such as performing daily exercises should be taken into consideration as both use of NSAIDs and performing physiotherapeutic exercises might be associated with patients' habits. Regular daily use of NSAIDs by AS patients and daily physical exercises at home might be strongly correlated as a trait of patients' compliance. Clearly, further research in this field is needed.

Current evidence for the use of TNFα blockade treatment in AS relates only to symptomatic benefit, but this will definitely change in the years to come (27–30). Clearly, reduced inflammation and lower pain levels, with substantial improvement in general well-being do not necessarily reflect changes in mobility or prevention of radiological damage (osteoporosis with the risk of spinal fractures, or syndesmophytes) (31–33).

Another currently not yet fully clarified issue is the following. Does the erythrocyte sedimentation rate (ESR) or C-reactive protein (CRP) level, or the HLA-27 status, after correction for sustained activity of disease influence the likelihood of response to TNF alpha blockade treatment (34)? Some data seem to suggest that this might be the case, but more and disease-activity adjusted data are needed.

What are the most appropriate dosages and intervals for treatment with these biologicals? Can treatment be stopped in the course of time? Clearly, there is an urgent need to re-evaluate doses and interdose intervals in individual AS patients once stable benefit is achieved. How effective are the new biological drugs not only in the prevention, but also in the treatment of otherwise unresponsive acute anterior uveitis? Do the several biologicals have different potential in this respect?

Does the response to treatment with TNFα blockade depend on the presence of symptomatic or asymptomatic inflammatory bowel disease? Should a thorough search for bowel disease be done before starting TNFα blockade? Therefore, to what degree do the several biologicals have different potential in the case of associated bowel disease and how can this be explained? Is monotherapy with TNFα blockade sufficient or can its efficacy be further improved by combinations with, for example, methotrexate?

Will we—within the next decade—have reliable estimates of treatment effects, and also of the risk to incur important adverse effects and complications of treatment through international registers? What will we know about the long-term safety of these drugs by then? Hopefully, the answer will be confirmative and reassuring.

Early diagnosis and treatment is of utmost importance if there exists a window of opportunity, for example, if treatment with biologicals should be provided at an early and active phase of the disease to better prevent radiological damage (syndesmophytes and osteoporosis). However, at this stage (the year 2005) we do not yet definitely know whether treatment with anti-TNFα has disease-modifying properties beyond potent symptomatic relief. Can physical disability be prevented and patient's outcome be improved (35–41)?

Also cost-effectiveness issues of treatment will need to be addressed (42–45). To what degree can modern treatment increase the proportion of patients that are able to maintain full employment and thus reduce sick leave or work disability and thereby at the same time reduce indirect medical costs of illness? Will modern treatment with biologicals translate into a reduced need for orthopedic surgery and also in reduced mortality of AS patients?

Further, will the incidence of spinal fractures that now occur in up to 14% of AS patients decrease (31)? Is society still able to provide the financial resources needed for treatment of AS (and other "expensive" and chronically ill) patients? How will patients' preferences influence therapeutic decisions and to what degree will the patient's role in this respect be different by the year 2015 from the current situation?

Comments on Questions Dealing with Nonpharmacological Therapy

To what degree can physiotherapy, including spa exercise, prevent decline of functional capacity (45–48)? In addition, we like to know how these interventions work, in particular we may want to study what kind of biological effects regular exercises and spa therapy have. For example, do these interventions influence the level of anti-inflammatory cytokines? Further, is it possible to increase the clinical effectiveness of such treatment modalities?

Generally speaking considerations of costs will increasingly get attention in the next decade. Therefore, one should also address the question to what degree will not only evidence-based pharmaceutical but also nonpharmaceutical interventions affect the cost-effectiveness of treatment of AS? The result of such economical analyses will be important for patients, payers, and providers of health care as the outcome will influence whether or not AS patients have access to these facilities.

Comments on Outcome Assessment

What is the best way to assess activity of disease, response to treatment, and remission in terms of which instruments to use for assessment (34,49–52)? What are the best evidence-based methods to assess function, mobility, or quality of life (53,54)?

How will physician-assessed findings and patient-reported data be integrated into final judgments about the state and activity of the disease (55)? Can current instruments be improved upon any further? Clearly, the ASAS International Working Group (http://www.asas-group.org) has something to accomplish before the year 2015. Finally, which instruments will we use routinely in daily practice in the year 2015?

In summary, by the year 2015 we hope to know exactly which AS patients to treat (including issues such as when to treat and how treatment should be applied), and which patients not to treat pharmaceutically or nonpharmaceutically (or to treat differently). Given the research agenda and the progress already made in recent years and given also ongoing studies we probably will see a lot of progress in achieving these purposes by or even before the year 2015.

REFERENCES

1. Wright V. Aspects of ankylosing spondylitis. Br J Rheumatol 1991; 30:1–4.
2. Copeman WSC. Introductory note on the nomenclature and classification of the rheumatic diseases. In: Copeman WSC, ed. Textbook of the Rheumatic Diseases. 4th ed. Edinburgh: Livingstone, 1969:12–18.
3. Wright V, Moll JMH. Seronegative Polyarthritis. Amsterdam: North Holland Publishing Company, 1976.
4. Dougados M, van der Linden S, Juhlin R, et al. The European Spondylarthropathy Study Group preliminary criteria for the classification of spondylarthropathy. Arthritis Rheum 1991; 34:1218–1227.
5. van der Linden S, Valkenburg HA, Cats A. Evaluation of diagnostic criteria for ankylosing spondylitis. A proposal for modification of the New York criteria. Arthritis Rheum 1984; 27:361–368.
6. Khan MA, van der Linden SM, Kushner I, Valkenburg HA, Cats A. Spondylitic disease without radiologic evidence of sacroiliitis in relatives of HLA-B27 positive ankylosing spondylitis patients. Arthritis Rheum 1985; 28:40–43.
7. Braun J, Bollow M, Eggens U, Konig H, Distler A, Sieper J. Use of dynamic magnetic resonance imaging with fast imaging in the detection of early and advanced sacroiliitis in spondylarthropathy patients. Arthritis Rheum 1994; 37:1039–1045.
8. Wittram C, Whitehouse GH, Williams JW, Bucknall RC. A comparison of MR and CT in suspected sacroiliitis. J Comput Assist Tomogr 1996; 20:68–72.
9. Geijer M, Sihlbom H, Gothlin JH, Nordborg E. The role of CT in the diagnosis of sacroiliitis. Acta Radiol 1998; 39:265–268.
10. van Tubergen A, Heuft-Dorenbosch L, Schulpen G, et al. Radiographic assessment of sacroiliitis by radiologists and rheumatologists: does training improve quality? Ann Rheum Dis 2003; 62:519–525.
11. Taurog JD, Maika SD, Satumtira N, et al. Inflammatory disease in HLA-B27 transgenic rats. Immunol Rev 1999; 169:209–223.
12. Ahmadi K, Wilson C, Tiwana H, Binder A, Ebringer A. Antibodies to *Klebsiella pneumoniae* lipopolysaccharide in patients with ankylosing spondylitis. Br J Rheumatol 1998; 37:1330–1333.
13. Nasution AR, Mardjuadi A, Kunmartini S, et al. HLA-B27 subtypes positively and negatively associated with spondyloarthropathy. J Rheumatol 1997; 24:1111–1114.
14. Ball EJ, Khan MA. HLA-B27 polymorphism. Joint Bone Spine 2001; 68:378–382.

15. Lopez-Larrea C, Sujirachato K, Mehra NK, et al. HLA-B27 subtypes in Asian patients with ankylosing spondylitis. Evidence for new associations. Tissue Antigens 1995; 45:169–176.

16. Garcia-Fernandez S, Gonzalez S, Mina Blanco A, et al. New insights regarding HLA-B27 diversity in the Asian population. Tissue Antigens 2001; 58:259–262.

17. van der Linden SM, Valkenburg HA, de Jongh BM, Cats A. The risk of developing ankylosing spondylitis in HLA-B27 positive individuals. A comparison of relatives of spondylitis patients with the general population. Arthritis Rheum 1984; 27:241–249.

18. Brown MA, Kennedy LG, MacGregor AJ, et al. Susceptibility to ankylosing spondylitis in twins: the role of genes, HLA, and the environment. Arthritis Rheum 1997; 40:1823–1828.

19. Robinson WP, van der Linden SM, Khan MA, et al. HLA-Bw60 increases susceptibility to ankylosing spondylitis in HLA-B27+ patients. Arthritis Rheum 1989; 32:1135–1141.

20. Lopez-Larrea C, Mijiyawa M, Gonzalez S, et al. Association of ankylosing spondylitis with HLA-B*1403 in a West African population. Arthritis Rheum 2002; 46:2968–2971.

21. Khan MA, Khan MK. Diagnostic value of HLA-B27 testing ankylosing spondylitis and Reiter's syndrome. Ann Intern Med 1982; 96:70–76.

22. Zhang G, Luo J, Buckel J, et al. Genetic studies in familial ankylosing spondylitis susceptibility. Arthritis Rheum 2004; 50:2246–2254.

23. Lehtinen K. Mortality and causes of death in 398 patients admitted to hospital with ankylosing spondylitis. Ann Rheum Dis 1993; 52:174–176.

24. Khan MA, Khan MK, Kushner I. Survival among patients with ankylosing spondylitis: a life-table analysis. J Rheumatol 1981; 8:86–90.

25. Boersma JW. Retardation of ossification of the lumbar vertebral column in ankylosing spondylitis by means of phenylbutazone. Scand J Rheumatol 1976; 5:60–64.

26. Wanders A, Heijde D, Landewe R, Behier JM, Calin A, Olivieri I, Zeidler H, Dougados M. Nonsteroidal antiinflammatory drugs reduce radiographic progression in patients with ankylosing spondylitis: a randomized clinical trial. Arthritis Rheum 2005; 52:1756–1765.

27. Braun J, Sieper J. Therapy of ankylosing spondylitis and other spondyloarthritides: established medical treatment, anti-TNF-alpha therapy and other novel approaches. Arthritis Res 2002; 4:307–321.

28. Gorman JD, Sack KE, Davis JC Jr. Treatment of ankylosing spondylitis by inhibition of tumor necrosis factor alpha. N Engl J Med 2002; 346:1349–1356.

29. Maksymowych WP, Inman RD, Gladman D, et al. Spondyloarthritis Research Consortium of Canada (SPARCC). Canadian Rheumatology Association Consensus on the use of anti-tumor necrosis factor-alpha directed therapies in the treatment of spondyloarthritis. J Rheumatol 2003; 30:1356–1363.

30. Braun J, Pham T, Sieper J, et al. ASAS Working Group. International ASAS consensus statement for the use of anti-tumour necrosis factor agents in patients with ankylosing spondylitis. Ann Rheum Dis 2003; 62:817–824.

31. Geusens P, Vosse D, van der Heijde D, et al. High prevalence of thoracic vertebral deformities and discal wedging in ankylosing spondylitis patients with hyperkyphosis. J Rheumatol 2001; 28:1856–1861.

32. Cooper C, Carbone L, Michet CJ, Atkinson EJ, O'Fallon WM, Melton LJ III. Fracture risk in patients with ankylosing spondylitis: a population based study. J Rheumatol 1994; 21:1877–1882.

33. Graham B, Van Peteghem PK. Fractures of the spine in ankylosing spondylitis. Diagnosis, treatment, and complications. Spine 1989; 14:803–807.

34. Garrett S, Jenkinson T, Kennedy LG, Whitelock H, Gaisford P, Calin A. A new approach to defining disease status in ankylosing spondylitis: the bath ankylosing spondylitis disease activity index. J Rheumatol 1994; 21:2286–2291.

35. Guillemin F, Briancon S, Pourel J, Gaucher A. Long-term disability and prolonged sick leaves as outcome measurements in ankylosing spondylitis. Possible predictive factors. Arthritis Rheum 1990; 33:1001–1006.

36. Ward MM, Kuzis S. Risk factors for work disability in patients with ankylosing spondylitis. J Rheumatol 2001; 28:315–321.
37. Boonen A, Chorus A, Miedema H, et al. Withdrawal from labour force due to work disability in patients with ankylosing spondylitis. Ann Rheum Dis 2001; 60:1033–1039.
38. Chorus AM, Boonen A, Miedema HS, van der Linden S. Employment perspectives of patients with ankylosing spondylitis. Ann Rheum Dis 2002; 61:693–699.
39. Boonen A, Chorus A, Miedema H, van der Heijde D, van der Tempel H, van der Linden S. Employment, work disability, and work days lost in patients with ankylosing spondylitis: a cross sectional study of Dutch patients. Ann Rheum Dis 2001; 60:353–358.
40. Gran JT, Skomsvoll JF. The outcome of ankylosing spondylitis: a study of 100 patients. Br J Rheumatol 1997; 36:766–771.
41. Amor B, Santos RS, Nahal R, Listrat V, Dougados M. Predictive factors for the long term outcome of spondyloarthropathies. J Rheumatol 1994; 21:1883–1887.
42. Boonen A, van der Heijde D, Landewe R, et al. Work status and productivity costs due to ankylosing spondylitis: comparison of three European countries. Ann Rheum Dis 2002; 61:429–437.
43. Boonen A, van der Heijde D, Landewe R, et al. Direct costs of ankylosing spondylitis and its determinants: an analysis among three European countries. Ann Rheum Dis 2003; 62:732–740.
44. Ward MM. Functional disability predicts total costs in patients with ankylosing spondylitis. Arthritis Rheum 2002; 46:223–231.
45. Van Tubergen A, Boonen A, Landewe R, et al. Cost effectiveness of combined spa-exercise therapy in ankylosing spondylitis: a randomized controlled trial. Arthritis Rheum 2002; 47:459–467.
46. Hidding A, van der Linden S, Boers M, et al. Is group physical therapy superior to individualized therapy in ankylosing spondylitis? A randomized controlled trial. Arthritis Care Res 1993; 6:117–125.
47. Dagfinder H, Hagen K. Physiotherapy interventions for ankylosing spondylitis (Cochrane review). In: The Cochrane Library. Oxford: Oxford Update Software, 2001.
48. van Tubergen A, Landewe R, van der Heijde D, et al. Combined spa-exercise therapy is effective in patients with ankylosing spondylitis: a randomized controlled trial. Arthritis Rheum 2001; 45:430–438.
49. Calin A, Garrett S, Whitelock H, et al. A new approach to defining functional ability in ankylosing spondylitis: the development of the bath ankylosing spondylitis functional index. J Rheumatol 1994; 21:2281–2285.
50. van der Heijde D, Calin A, Dougados M, Khan MA, van der Linden S, Bellamy N. Selection of instruments in the core set for DC-ART, SMARD, physical therapy, and clinical record keeping in ankylosing spondylitis. Progress report of the ASAS working Group. Assessments in ankylosing spondylitis. J Rheumatol 1999; 26:951–954.
51. Anderson JJ, Baron G, van der Heijde D, Felson DT, Dougados M. Ankylosing spondylitis assessment group preliminary definition of short-term improvement in ankylosing spondylitis. Arthritis Rheum 2001; 44:1876–1886.
52. Doward LC, Spoorenberg A, Cook SA, et al. Development of the ASQoL: a quality of life instrument specific to ankylosing spondylitis. Ann Rheum Dis 2003; 62:20–26.
53. Spoorenberg A, van der Heijde D, de Klerk E, et al. Relative value of erythrocyte sedimentation rate and C-reactive protein in assessment of disease activity in ankylosing spondylitis. J Rheumatol 1999; 26:980–984.
54. Haywood KL, Garratt AM, Jordan K, Dziedzic K, Dawes PT. Spinal mobility in ankylosing spondylitis: reliability, validity and responsiveness. Rheumatology 2004; 43:750–757.
55. Cohen SB, Strand V, Aguillar D, Olman JJ. Patient-versus physician-reported outcomes in rheumatoid arthritis patients treated with recombinant interleukin-1 receptor antagonist (anakinra) therapy. Rheumatology 2004; 43:704–711.

Index

About the Editors

BAREND J. VAN ROYEN is Associate Professor and Consultant Orthopaedic Surgeon at the Department of Orthopaedic Surgery of the VU University Medical Center, Amsterdam, The Netherlands, with a special interest in spinal surgery. Dr. van Royen received the M.D. degree (1988) from Leiden University, The Netherlands. He became a specialist in orthopaedic surgery at the Sint Radboud University Hospital and Sint Maartenskliniek, Nijmegen, The Netherlands (1994). He received the Ph.D. degree (1999) from the Vrije Universiteit, Amsterdam, The Netherlands, with the thesis: "Lumbar Osteotomy in Ankylosing Spondylitis, Biomechanical and Clinical Aspects."

BEN A. C. DIJKMANS is Professor of Rheumatology, VU University Medical Center, Amsterdam, The Netherlands. He received the M.D. degree (1973) from the Vrije Universiteit, Amsterdam, The Netherlands. He received the Ph.D. degree from the University of Leiden, The Netherlands (1984). Professor Dijkmans became a specialist in internal medicine (1980) and rheumatology (1986) at the University Hospital Leiden, The Netherlands. In 1996 he was appointed as Professor and Head of the Department of Rheumatology, VU University Medical Center, Amsterdam, The Netherlands.

Printed and bound by CPI Group (UK) Ltd, Croydon, CR0 4YY

23/10/2024

01778250-0012